Health, Equity and Human Rights:
Perspectives and Issues

Health, Equity and Human Rights:

Perspectives and Issues

Editors

C.P. Prakasam
K.E. Vaidyanathan
U.V. Somayajulu
N. Audinarayana

INDIAN ASSOCIATION FOR SOCIAL SCIENCES AND HEALTH (IASSH)

SERIALS PUBLICATIONS
NEW DELHI (INDIA)

First Published – 2010

ISBN: 978-81-8387-396-3

Published by

SERIALS PUBLICATIONS
4830/24, 1st Floor, Ansari Road
Darya Ganj, New Delhi-110002 (India)
Phone : 23245225. Fax : 91-11-23272135
E-mail: serials@satyam.net.in

Contents

Preface

Indian Association for Social Sciences and Health (IASSH) is an Indian Chapter of Asia-Pacific Network (APNET) of the International Forum for Social Sciences and Health (IFSSH). The major objectives of IASSH are to bring together scientists, researchers, policy makers from various disciplines to one forum to explore and work in the areas of social and cultural dimensions of illness, health and health care in the country; to strengthen networking with similar organizations in India and abroad, linking social scientists, health activist and policy makers; and to initiate steps to evolve an equitable health care system in the country through appropriate and affordable health sector reforms.

IASSH had its first conference in Tirupati in November, 2003, the second in Mumbai in February 2005, the third conference was held in Delhi in March 2006, the fourth conference was held in Surat in February 2007 and fifth conference was held in Bhubaneswar during April 2008. Sixth was at School of Social Sciences & International Studies, Pondicherry University, Puducherry in March 2009. Our membership has grown to 510 from 23 during these six years.

This volume is an outcome of the research papers submitted to the Sixth National Conference of Indian Association for Social Sciences and Health (IASSH) on the topic "Health, Equity and Human Rights" held at Pondicherry University, Puducherry during 7th and 8th March, 2009, consists of twenty eight research papers, classified into seven sections. These sections deal with the research work focusing on: Ethics and Human Rights Issues, Inequalities in Health Care Utilization, Maternal Health, Gender Dimensions of Health, Policies and Health Programs to reduce Vulnerability, Nutrition and Health, Social aspects of Health.

The Alma Ata declaration in 1978 had propounded the goal of "Health for All" by the end of the century (i.e. by year 2000) with a view that every person is entitled to have healthy life, and that resources essential for satisfying health needs should be available within reach of every one . Yet this goal has remained a distant dream in most developing countries including India. There are wide disparities between Indian states in majority of development indicators which measure Health. The risk of dying within one year of age in 1980 was 114 declines to 70 but the gap between the male, female and between the states remains in the same level. The issues are well-known viz: non availability of health facilities, lack of reproductive and child care, high maternal mortality, low socio economic status, poverty at the household, lack of implementation of health programs to the vulnerable and deprived population etc. These are often discussed in the research forums and have raised the consciousness of the Programmers and Policy makers in the country but lot more to be done in this direction. Less well-known are the *disparities within states, with in social status and Gender* in health status. There is a wide gap in Equity and Equality in Social dimension, Economic dimension, Gender dimension in the society. At the house hold level gender disparities are more visible interns of giving education, food, and clothing to the girl child. More so when it is known her parents are vulnerable to disease and poverty. There is a need to *empower* housewife to enhance the status of the family which leads to healthy family and health community to achieve the goal of "Health for All" in the coming decades.

These twenty eight research papers under seven sections deals with health, equity and brings out the issues with suggestions and may be useful for drawing appropriate strategies to reduce disparities.

It has to be noted that the arguments made in this volume focuses the research issues and not related to organizations they belong nor intended to any particular person. We are sure this volume on "HEALTH, EQUITY AND HUMAN RIGHTS: PERSPECTIVES AND ISSUES" will throw light on the emerging issues of health equity and will be useful for the researchers.

C.P. Prakasam, K.E. Vaidyanathan,
U.V. Somayajulu, N. Audinarayana

Acknowledgements

Our sincere thanks are due to Mr. Nesim Tumkaya, Country Representative, UNFPA, New Delhi and Dr. Pavitra Mohan, Health Specialist, UNICEF, New Delhi for their financial and academic support in organising the conference at Pondicherry. Sincere thanks are also due to Prof. J.A.K.Tareen, Vice Chancellor, and Prof. T. Subramanyam Naidu, conference Director and Director of School of Social Sciences & International Studies, Pondicherry University, Puducherry for organising the Sixth IASSH conference and extended their full co-operation in enhancing IASSH activities. Bringing out this volume is possible because of their co-operation and support.

Our thanks are due to contributors who have followed editorial suggestions and revised the research papers for incorporation in to this volume in bringing out the issues related to Health and Equity.

Our special thanks are due to M/s SERIALS PUBLICATIONS, New Delhi who has accepted in publishing this volume, which enlightens the emerging issues on "HEALTH, EQUITY AND HUMAN RIGHTS".

C.P. Prakasam, K. E. Vaidyanathan
U.V. Somayajulu, N. Audinarayana

List of Contributors

Ms. Anindita Chowdhury, 24/G, Jyotish Roy Road, Newalipore, Kolkata-700053, aninditachwdhry@gmail.com

Dr. Aradhana Srivastava, Consultant, D-15 Green Park, New Delhi 110016, ara.sriv@gmail.com

Dr. Arun Kumar Sharma, Professor, Humanities and Social Sciences Department, IIT Kanpur Kanpur, 208 016, arunk @iitk.ac.in

Dr. Ashish Kumar Mishra, Senior Monitoring and Evaluation Officer, Pathfinder International - India Representative Office, B-5/5, Safdarjung Enclave, New Delhi, Pin-110 029, amishra@ pathfind.org

Dr. N. Audinarayana, Professor and Head, Department of Sociology and Population Studies, Director, School of Social Sciences, Bharathiar University, Coimbatore–641 046. audi narayana.bu@gmail.com

Ms. Deepshikha Tarai, M. Phil in Population Studies, Center for the study of Regional Development, School of Social Sciences, Jawaharlal Nehru University, New Delhi, deepshikha.tarai @gmail.com

Dr. N. Dhanabagyam, Chief-in charge, Population Research Centre, Gandhigram Institute for Rural Health & Family Welfare Trust, Ambaturai (RS) Gandhigram Post , Dindigul District- 624302 drdhan@rediffmail.com

Ms. Disha Tewari, 2/116-A, Sector-2, Rajender Nagar, Sahibabad, Ghaziabad, tewaridisha@gmail.com

Dr. M. Ganesan, Senior Project Officer ,IITM's Rural Technology and Business Incubator, ESB # 331, Indian Institute of Technology Madras (IITM), Chennai - 600 036, ganesan@ tenet.res.in

Dr. Girish Chandra Tripathi, Professor, Department of Economics, University of Allahabad, Allahabad

Prof. T.R. Gopalan , Course Chairman ,Department of Clinical Nutrition ,Sri Ramachandra University & Hospital ,Porur, Chennai - 600116, drtrg@yahoo.co.in

Dr. A.J. Hemamalini , Assistant Professor ,Department of Clinical Nutrition ,Sri Ramachandra University & Hospital ,Porur, Chennai- 600116, hemajanardh@rediffmail.com

Mr. Jagannath Behera, Research Scholar, Center for Study of Regional Development, JNU, New Delhi-67, jagannathjnu08 @gmail.com

Dr. Kalpagam Polasa, Scientist 'F' & Head, Food and Drug Toxicology Research Centre, National Institute of Nutrition, Jamai-Osmania (PO), Hyderabad- 500007, kpolasa@yahoo.com

Mr. A. Krishnamurthy, 14, West Chetty Street, Aduthurai (Post), Thanjavur (Dt), Tamil Nadu-612101, krishna_200872@ yahoo.com

Dr. Meenakshi Gautham, Team Leader (First Care Health) , IITM's Rural Technology and Business Incubator , ESB # 331, Indian Institute of Technology Madras (IITM), Chennai - 600 036, meenakshi@firstcarehealth.in

Ms Monisha Vaid, Consultant, 31, Arjun Marg, DLF Phase-I, Gurgaon - 122002, Haryana, monisha.vaid@gmail.com

Mr. P. Muniappan, State Demographer of Tamil Nadu, Directorate of Family Welfare, 359 Annaisalai, Teynampet, Chennai-600006, muniappandemo@yahoo.co.in

G. Muthulakshmi, Dietician, Department of Clinical Nutrition, Sri Ramachandra University & Hospital, Porur, Chennai – 600116, gmuthul@yahoo.com

Dr. Pradeep Kumar Parida, Assistant Professor, Department of Sociology, Pondicherry University, Puducherry–605014 pradeepparida2003@yahoo.com

Dr. C.P.Prakasam, Retired Professor, C2-5/2:3, Sector-4, Vashi-400703, New Bombay, Maharashtra, prakasam60@ gmail.com

Prof. Prasanta Pathak, Faculty Member, Population Studies Unit, Indian Statistical Institute, Kolkata, India, prasanta.pathak @gmail.com

Prof. S. Ramachandran, Professor, Dept. of Population Studies, Annamalai University, Annamalai nagar–208 002, srampondy@gmail.com

Dr. A.K. Ravishankar, Lecturer, Dept. of Population Studies, Annamalai University, Annamalai nagar – 208 002 akravishankar @sify.com

Ms. Rekha Gupta, C/O- Dharamshila Bhavan, Kachari Gali, Bhikhana Pahari, Saidpur, Patna-800004, rekhaeco@gmail.com

Mr. Sangram Kumar Rout, Research Scholar, Department of Politics & International Studies, Pondicherry University, Puducherry-605014,sangramkumarrout@gmail.com

Mr. Sanjeev Bakshi, Senior Research Fellow, Population Studies Unit, Indian Statistical Institute, Kolkata, India, bakshisanjeev@gmail.com

Ms. Shilpi Tiwari, Research Scholar, Department of Economics, University of Allahabad, Allahabad, shilpi.tiwari31@ gmail.com

Dr Siddharth Agarwal, Executive Director, 89/4, Krishna Nagar, Safdarjang Enclave, New Delhi-110029, siddharth@uhrc.in; sids62@yahoo.com

Dr. U.V. Somayajulu, Director, Sigma Research and Consulting Pvt Ltd, C 23, South Extension I, New Delhi 110 049, ulimiri_vs@yahoo.com

Prof. H.C. Srivastava,B-202, Neel Sidhi Ornate, Krishna CHS Ltd., Plot no. 4 & 4A, Sector-8, Kharghar, Navi Mumbai-410210, harish_srivastava@hotmail.com

G.M. Subba Rao, Scientist 'C' (Communication & Journalism), Extension & Training Division, National Institute of Nutrition (ICMR), Jamai-Osmania (PO), Hyderabad-500007,AP, gmsubb arao@yahoo.com

Prof. A. Subbiah, Professor Head, Dept. of Population Studies, Annamalai University, Annamalai nagar – 208 002, subbiahpop@ gmail.com

Dr. R.V Sudershan, Scientist 'C', Food and Drug Toxicology Research Centre, National Institute of Nutrition, Jamai-Osmania (PO), Hyderabad. 500007. AP. vemulasr@yahoo.com

Ms. Suma Prashant, Project Manager (Rural Health Initiatives), IITM's Rural Technology and Business Incubator, ESB# 331, Indian Institute of Technology Madras (IITM), Chennai - 600 036, suma@tenet.res.in

Ms. R. Swapna, Dietician ,Department of Clinical Nutrition,Sri Ramachandra University & Hospital, Porur , Chennai – 600116,

Mr. Tilak Mukherji, Chief Mentor, Sigma Research and Consulting, C23, South Extension I, New Delhi-110 049, tilak.mukherji@gmail.com

Dr. Tushar Joshi, Director, Occupational and Environmental Medicine Programme, Centre for Occupational and Environmental Health (COEH), Ground Floor, B. L. Taneja Block, Maulana Azad Medical College, New Delhi-110 002 e-mail: kantjoshi@ gmail.com

Dr. K.E. Vaidyanathan, 3028, 13th Main Road, Anna Nagar, Chennai-600040, vaidyake@hotmail.com

Dr. M.V. Vaithilingam, Department of Fertility Studies, International Institute for Population Sciences (IIPS), Govandi Station Road, Deonar, Mumbai 400 088. vaidhya_iips @rediffmail.com

Dr. Vighnesh N. Bhat, 'Suvidha', N.R. Pura Road, Vidyanagar, Shimoga-577203, Karnataka, India, vighnubhat@ rediffmail.com

Dr. Vijay M. Sarode, Associate Professor of Statistics, Ashar Estate, Flat B2-501, Shree Nagar, Wagale Estate, THANE (W), 400 604, INDIA, vijaymsarode@yahoo.com

SECTION – 1

Ethics and Human Rights Issues

1

Equity, Health and Environment: The Indian Scenario

K.E. Vaidyanathan

Introduction

The Alma Ata declaration in 1978 had propounded the goal of "Health for All" by the end of the century, i.e., by the year 2000. This implies that every person is entitled to a healthy life, and that resources essential for satisfying health needs should be available within reach of every one (WHO, 1986). Yet this goal has remained a distant dream in most developing countries. There are wide disparities between nations and within nations. The risk of dying within one year of age in the least developed countries is 20 times that of the developed countries. The gap between the developed and developing nations is too wide and well-known. These are often discussed in international forums and have raised the consciousness of the international community. Less well-known are the *disparities within countries* in health status. Analysis of these disparities is important for discovering the factors and conditions producing these disparities and for drawing appropriate strategies to reduce the disparities (World Bank, 2000).

India's National Health Policy, 2002 devotes an entire section on equity and concludes "It is a principal objective of NHP-2002 to evolve a policy structure which reduces these inequities and allows the disadvantaged sections of society a fairer access to public health services" (GOI, 2002). Interestingly the NHP does not define the term "inequity", but it is commonly understood that inequity is synonymous with inequality which is unacceptable and unfair. The measures proposed include raising public health investment with focus on primary health care and increased investment in programmes to improve the reproductive and child health care. It also envisages the implementation of the National Rural Health Mission (NRHM) with special focus on 18 States with weak public health indicators and/or weak infra-structure.

This paper attempts to show the inequalities that persist in India, and how these inequalities affect the health status of the population. Environment is also a factor that affects the health status of the population. Environment is too broad an area, and it is necessary to limit this analysis to one or two areas-such as urban and rural residence, water and sanitation, type of housing, nature of fuel used etc. The main source of data for this study is from the National Family Health Surveys (NFHS) carried out by the International Institute for Population Sciences (IIPS), Mumbai in association with Macro International. There were three such surveys -NFHS1 (1992-93), NFHS2 (1998-99) and NFHS3 (2005-06). The main focus of the surveys was demography, reproductive health and family planning, but the surveys also provide some data on health and environmental aspects. All three surveys covered large samples of households from the entire country and were designed to provide key indicators at national and state levels. For example, NFHS3 included a sample of 109041 households, 124385 women in the age group 15-49 years and 74369 men of age 15-54 years. The surveys provide comparable data for most indicators and are therefore a preferred source for this analysis.

Socio-economic Inequalities in India: An Overview

India is a vast country of a billion people (as of 2001 census) distributed over 29 states and six union territories. The Indian population is highly heterogeneous divided into six major religions, 20 languages and hundreds of dialects and thousands of castes and sub-castes. According to 2001 Census, the Hindus constitute about 80.5% of the population. The minorities, who constitute 19.5 per cent, include Muslims (about 13.4%), Christians (2.3%), Sikhs (1.8%), Buddhists (0.8%) and Jains (0.4%) and others (0.7%). The Hindus are

Table 1
Socio-Economic Inequalities in India, 2005-06

(Percentages with Specified Characteristic)

Background Characteristics	*Persons 15-49 with 12+ Education*		*Persons 15-49 Exposed To Media*		*U5 Children Birth Reg.*		*Child Labor 5-14*
	F	*M*	*F*	*M*	*Total*	*With Certi.*	
Residence							
Urban	24.4	30.5	87.4	93.8	59.3	46.0	8.6
Rural	5.9	13.5	54.6	74.7	34.8	20.2	12.9
Religion							
Hindu	12.2	20.7	65.6	82.0	40.4	25.6	12.1
Muslim	6.6	11.7	59.8	76.3	39.3	28.6	10.8
Christian	23.5	22.7	69.7	86.7	56.8	41.7	7.4
Sikh	19.8	20.3	73.5	89.3	78.4	56.1	9.5
Jain	9.7	19.3	96.9	99.9	86.7	59.5	7.1
Caste							
SC	6.3	13.4	61.1	78.9	36.7	23.8	11.6
ST	3.9	8.7	42.6	62.2	39.0	17.6	16.5
OBC	9.8	18.6	63.2	82.6	34.1	21.6	12.2
OC	19.9	27.6	75.9	87.0	55.0	39.5	9.7
Wealth Index							
Lowest	0.4	2.4	26.3	50.7	23.9	11.2	13.2
Second	1.1	6.2	44.9	70.6	31.0	17.3	12
Third	3.9	11.0	65.1	84.0	39.4	25.0	12.2
Fourth	10.9	21.7	83.8	93.3	53.8	37.6	9.3
Highest	38.4	47.7	96.1	98.3	72.4	57.3	6.4

Source: National Family Health Survey - 3, Vol. 1, 2005-2006.

further divided into different caste groups broadly termed as the Scheduled Castes, (SCs), the Scheduled Tribes (STs), the Other Backward Classes (OBCs) and others. The SCs account for 16.2 per cent and the STs accounts for 8.2 per cent of the country's total population. In the absence of specific Census data, it is not possible to give an exact figure for the OBCs, but according to NFHS and NSS estimates they constitute about 32-37 per cent. The constitution of India guarantees equal rights to every-one and safeguards for protection and promotion of interest of the SCs/STs, the OBCs and the minorities are enshrined in the constitution. Nevertheless, in such a complex society disparities are inevitable, and these are examined in this section.

Table 1 presents evidences of inequalities among the above mentioned groups in India in some key indicators - of education, exposure to media, registration of births, and prevalence of child labour. These indicators are the ones available in NFHS-3 for the different social classes that are under examination. There is a substantial rural and urban and gender differential in the indicators presented. Among females, the proportion of those having 12 years of education in urban is four times that of females in rural, whereas among males the urban proportion is only twice that of rural. The proportion of males and females having exposure to media is close to 90 percent in urban, where as only one half of females and three-fourth of males is exposed to media in rural areas. While only a fifth of the births are registered in rural, the extent of registration in urban is close to 50 percent. The extent of child labour in the age group 5-14 years is far greater in rural in comparison to urban.

Among the religious groups, Muslims have the lowest levels in all the indicators presented except for child labour, and Christians have fared better than other religious groups. The Scheduled Tribes have the lowest levels in terms of education; media exposure, birth registration and child labour, and they are closely followed by Scheduled Castes. The lower segment of Table 1 presents the changes in these indicators as we move from the lowest quintile in wealth index to the

Table 2

Inequalities in Housing Characteristics in India by States, 2005-06

(Percentages with Specified Characteristic)

State	*With Electricity Water*	*With Drinking Water*	*With Toilet Facility*	*Cooking With Solid Fuel*	*Living in a Pucca House*	*Persons Sleeping in Room*
India	67.9	87.9	44.6	70.8	45.9	3.3
North						
Delhi	99.3	92.1	92.4	9.3	94.9	3.1
Haryana	91.5	95.6	52.4	69.1	61.1	3.3
Himachal Pradesh	98.4	88.4	46.4	68.9	52.7	2.5
Jammu Kashmir	93.2	80.8	61.7	59.5	50.3	2.9
Punjab	96.3	99.5	70.8	54.9	68.9	3.1
Rajasthan	66.1	81.8	30.8	77.2	50.1	3.6
Uttaranchal	80.0	87.4	56.8	61.7	49.8	3.0
Central						
Chattishgarh	71.4	77.9	18.7	86.7	21.7	3.0
Madhya Pradesh	71.4	74.2	27.0	80.3	26.2	3.6
Uttar Pradesh	42.8	93.7	33.1	81.7	28.8	3.8
East						
Bihar	27.7	96.1	25.2	89.7	20.4	3.3
Jharkhand	40.2	57.0	22.6	89.1	28.3	3.2
Orissa	45.4	78.4	19.3	88.6	31.9	3.1
West Bengal	52.5	93.7	59.6	79.2	39.5	3.1
North East						
Arunachal Pradesh	76.9	85.0	80.6	67.7	20.8	2.7
Assam	38.1	72.4	76.4	75.8	19.8	2.7
Manipur	87.0	52.1	95.6	64.7	10.7	2.6
Meghalaya	70.4	63.1	71.3	72.2	35.1	2.9
Mizoram	92.3	85.0	98.0	34.1	22.9	3.5
Nagaland	82.9	62.8	85.6	76.0	20.7	2.6
Sikkim	92.1	77.6	89.0	52.4	51.0	2.3
Tripura	68.8	76.1	96.7	80.4	12.1	2.9
West						
Goa	96.4	80.1	76.0	33.3	73.6	2.7
Gujarat	89.3	89.8	54.6	52.3	67.3	3.6
Maharashtra	83.5	92.7	52.9	48.1	59.0	3.5
South						
Andhra Pradesh	88.4	94.0	42.4	66.3	56.3	3.2
Karnataka	89.3	86.2	46.5	63.8	55.1	3.4
Kerala	91.0	69.1	96.1	71.4	85.1	2.2
Tamil Nadu	88.6	93.5	42.9	60.5	69.9	2.9

Source: National Family Health Survey-3, Vol. 1, 2005-2006.

highest quintile, and this indicates that the economic status has a bearing in their performance in the other indicators; the direction of causation could be in either direction.

Table 2 presents the indicators of housing characteristics across the states of India. It is evident that there are great disparities between states in the indicators presented. 95 per cent of households have electricity in four states-Delhi, Himachal Pradesh, Goa and Punjab. At the other extreme less than fifty percent of the households have electricity in five states-Orissa, Uttar Pradesh, Jharkhand, Assam and Bihar. Over 95 per cent of households have access to improved drinking water in three states-Punjab, Haryana and Bihar. Over one third of the households do not have access to improved drinking water in four states- Manipur, Jharkhand, Meghalaya and Nagaland. Over 95 per cent of households in four states - Manipur, Kerala, Tripura and Mizoram have improved toilet facility, less than 25 per cent of households have a toilet facility in four states-Chhattisgarh, Orissa, Jharkhand and Bihar. The use of solid fuels for cooking (a major health hazard) ranges from 9 per cent in Delhi to over 85 per cent in four states Chhattisgarh, Orissa, Jharkhand and Bihar. Two thirds or more of the households live in a Pucca (properly built) house in five states–Delhi, Kerala, Goa, Tamil Nadu, Punjab and Gujarat, there are two states - Tripura and Manipur where less than 15 per cent of households live in Pucca houses. In terms of overall performance Kerala, Tamil Nadu, Goa, Himachal Pradesh and Maharashtra are the most advanced states in terms of these indicators, while Bihar, Madhya Pradesh, Uttar Pradesh, Rajasthan (the so called BIMARU states) and Orissa have performed poorly in these indicators.

Impact of Residence and Social Inequalities on Health

Table 3 presents the health indicators by socio-economic classes for rural and urban. There are two sets of health indicators given, one set reflecting the health status, and the second set relating to access to health care. The indicators of health status included are the proportion of births with weight

Table 3
Health Indicators by Residence/ Social Classes India, 2005-06

		Residence		*Education*		*Wealth Index*		*Caste*	
Category	*Indicator*	*Rural*	*Urban*	*None*	*12+*	*Low*	*High*	*SC*	*OC*
Health Status									
Infant	Births with wt<2.5Kg	23.3	19.3	26.2	15.7	25.4	17.4	23.7	20.7
	Mortality Rate	62.2	41.5	69.7	25.9	70.4	29.2	66.3	48.0
U5 Children	Mortality Rate	82.0	51.7	94.7	29.7	100.5	33.8	88.1	59.2
	Wt for Ht <-2SD	20.7	16.9	22.7	12.8	25.0	12.7	21.0	16.3
	Wt for Age <-2SD	45.6	32.7	52.0	17.9	56.6	19.7	47.9	33.7
Adult Females	Diabetes PR	641.0	1371.0	690.0	878.0	371.0	1503.0	798.0	1189.0
	Asthma PR	1719.0	1648.0	1914.0	1217.0	1723.0	1639.0	1494.0	2035.0
	Goitre +others PR	758.0	1339.0	646.0	1856.0	529.0	1739.0	754.0	1240.0
	Anemia PR	57.4	50.9	60.1	44.6	64.3	46.1	58.3	51.3
	% with BMI <18.5	40.6	25.0	41.7	21.8	51.5	18.2	41.1	21.4
Adult Males	Diabetes PR	860.0	1383.0	1172.0	1454.0	705.0	1957.0	991.0	1336.0
	Asthma PR	1799.0	1329.0	2440.0	984.0	2416.0	1248.0	1688.0	1919.0
	Goitre +others PR	392.0	369.0	390.0	378.0	384.0	454.0	348.0	424.0
	Anemia PR	27.7	17.7	33.7	14.8	37.9	14.2	26.6	20.9
	% with BMI <18.5	38.4	26.5	40.3	19.3	48.3	19.1	39.1	28.9
Access to Health Care									
Children <6	% Covered by ICDS	34.8	23.4	31.6	22.1	36.7	15.6	36.1	28.3
Children 12-24 yrs	% fully immunized	38.6	57.6	26.1	75.2	24.4	71.0	39.7	53.8
	% with Vacci. Card	34.5	46.2	25.1	56.8	25.5	55.9	34.8	46.0

Contd.

		Residence		Education		Wealth Index		Caste	
Category	*Indicator*	*Rural*	*Urban*	*None*	*12+*	*Low*	*High*	*SC*	*OC*
	% not immunized	5.7	3.3	7.4	2.0	9.1	0.9	5.4	4.3
Women	% Pregnant, covered by ICDS	23.6	16.8	20.7	15.1	26.4	9.6	27.5	15.0
	% Lactating, covered by ICDS	18.3	12.9	16.1	10.8	21.5	6.8	21.5	11.2
	% Receiving ANC	59.7	82.1	44.4	83.5	42.6	91.9	61.8	76.3
	% Delivery by doctor	26.1	61.8	16.3	80.6	11.7	76.1	29.4	47.4
	% Delivery in Hosp.	28.9	67.4	18.5	86.3	12.8	83.6	33.0	51.1
	% Receiving PNC	33.9	65.7	23.6	82.8	19.3	79.3	37.1	52.6
Households	% with Health Insur.	2.2	10.4	–	–	0.1	16.4	3.3	7.8
	% HF Visit/3Mths(F)	33.6	41.5	31.1	43.1	28.8	42.2	26.7	39.2
	% HF Visit/3Mths(M)	29.9	30.2	25.7	31.5	26.5	41.3	30.6	30.4
	% HW contact/3Mths (F)	20.8	10.0	18.3	12.2	21.7	10.0	19.9	15.2

Source: National Family Health Survey-3, Vol. 1, 2005-06.

Notes:

R = Rural; U = Urban; SC = Scheduled Castes; OC = Other Castes not regarded as backward.

PR = Prevalence Rate expressed as rate per 100000 population.

ANC = Antenatal check up; PNC = Post-natal check up; HF = Health Facility; HW = Health workers.Children Immunized refers to the children 12-24 months who had received basic immunization, namely,

BCG, measles and three doses each of DPT and polio vaccine excluding polio vaccine given at the time of birth.

ICDS stands for Integrated Chid Development Services programme, which provides health care services and supplementary food to children under-6 years of age and to pregnant and lactating women.

less than 2.5 kg, infant mortality rate, Under five mortality rate, proportion of children under 5 with weight for age and height for age less than 2 SD, the prevalence rate for common diseases, the proportion of males and females with body mass index (BMI) less than 18.5. All the indicators except prevalence of diabetes shows that rural areas have poorer health status compared to urban, and females have poorer health status compared to males. The indicators show that persons with no education have poorer health status compared to persons with 12 plus years of education and scheduled castes (SC) have lower health status compared to other castes (OC).

The differentials by religion are not shown in the table, but nevertheless, they are significant. The infant mortality rate for Hindus 44.3 per thousand is much higher than for Christians (16.3 per 1000) and Muslims (35.5 per 1000), and the average for India as a whole (41.5 per thousand). Similarly, child mortality and under-five mortality rates are again higher for the Hindus followed by Muslims and Christians. The probability of dying between 1 and 5 years of age is 10.6 per thousand Hindu children, while this is 9.6 per thousand for Muslims and 9.4 per thousand for Christians. In case of under-five mortality rate, again the level is much higher for the Hindus (54.7 per thousand live births). The level was much lower for the Christians 25.5 and 44.8 for Muslims which are well below the national average of 51.7 per thousand live births. The anthropometric measurements in the NFHS-3 survey show that 42.5 per cent of the children have weights for their age low compared to international standards and are classified as undernourished. Further the survey reveals that undernourished prevails generally among all religious groups except among Christians (29.7%) and Sikhs (22.0%). It is high among children belonging to SCs and STs as about 47.9 per cent and 55.5 per cent, respectively.

The indicators of access to health care include vaccination of children; vitamin A supplementation; antenatal check-up; TT injection and Iron and Folic acid supplements; institutional delivery; and medical assistance at birth. The coverage is far from being universal, only about 43.5 percent of children received all the recommended doses in India. There is difference between three major religious groups, Christians and Hindus have, over 56.3 per cent and 44.4 per cent, whereas and Muslims with (36.3%) that less than national average of 43.5 per cent full immunisation. Among caste groups the rate of immunisation (full vaccination) was higher for OCs about 53.8 per cent and lower for STs about 31.3 per cent of children and 39.7 per cent for SCs. Antenatal care refers to pregnancy related health care and included adequate doses to tetanus taxoid (TT) vaccine and other health check-up. The NFHS-3 estimates that during 2005-06 the ante-natal check-up by qualified professionals covered 74.2 per cent of births. The proportions who received antenatal check-up were Christians (80.8%) as compared to Hindus (74.5%), Muslims (71.7%) and other religious groups (46.6%). Among the caste groups the proportions who received antenatal care are: SCs (70.8%), STs (61.1%), and OCs (82.9%).

Majority of deliveries (61%) and especially in rural areas (71%) take place at home irrespective of caste and religion. But this is relatively low among Christians. The percentage of deliveries at home is about 46.5 per cent for Christians and about 60.6 per cent for Hindus and 66.8 per cent for Muslims. Among caste groups, the percentage is very high for SCs/STs about 66.8 per cent for SCs and 81.9 per cent for STs and relatively low for others (48.8%). About 46.6 per cent of deliveries were assisted by a professional, i.e. a doctor or trained midwife/health workers 38.7 per cent among the Muslims, 47.4 per cent among the Hindus, and 60.4 per cent among the Christians. The proportion of SC/ ST mothers receiving medical assistance during delivery is only 40.7 per cent among SCs, 25.3 per cent among STs and 57.8 per cent for others. The above analysis shows that, there is inequality among social groups in health status and access to health care.

Health Status and Use of Health Care according to Wealth Quintiles

Table 4 presents some indicators of health according to wealth quintiles from the NFHS-3 (2005-06).

Table 4
Indicators of Health Status and Use of Health Care by Wealth Quintiles

(Figures are Percentage to total)

	Wealth Index					
Health Status Indicators	*Lowest*	*Second*	*Third*	*Fourth*	*Highest*	*Total*
Babies with <2.5 Kg	25.4	25.4	23.7	21.8	17.4	21.5
IMR	70.4	68.5	58.3	44.0	29.2	57.0
U5 MR	100.5	89.6	71.9	51.2	33.8	74.3
Weight for age <2SD	56.6	49.2	41.4	33.6	19.7	42.5
Weight for Height <2 SD	25.0	22.0	18.8	16.6	12.7	19.8
U5 children with anaemia	76.4	73.6	69.3	64.8	56.2	69.5
Women with BMI <18.5	51.5	46.3	38.3	28.9	18.2	35.6
Men with BMI<18.5	48.3	42.4	37.4	29.6	19.1	34.2
Women with any anaemia	64.3	60.3	56.0	52.2	46.1	55.3
Men with any anaemia	37.9	30.2	24.8	18.8	14.2	24.7
ANC by Professionals	54.0	65.9	77.3	88.1	96.5	74.2
Recd. 2+ TT	59.7	70.2	79.3	87.2	92.9	76.3
Hospital Delivery	12.8	23.5	39.2	57.9	83.6	38.6
Recd. PNC	19.3	27.7	42.9	56.8	79.3	42.4
U5 Children with Basic vaccinations	25.4	33.2	46.9	55.3	71.0	43.5
CMW currently using modern FP	43.5	49.8	55.2	58.0	48.5	34.6

Source: National Family Health Survey-3, Vol. 1, 2005-06.

The first ten indicators are health status indicators and the last six indicators are indicators of health care utilization. This table shows an improvement in health status as we move from the lowest wealth quintile to the highest wealth quintile. There is a decline in the proportion of babies with low birth weight, underweight (according to weight for age), wasting (according to weight for height) among children and men and women with low body mass index (BMI). Equally significant, the infant mortality rate and child mortality rate and the prevalence of anaemia decline first lowest to the highest quintile. Among the indicators of health care utilization such as mothers receiving ANC by professionals, PNC, hospital delivery, use of family planning there is an improvement as we move form lowest quintile to the highest quintile.

Socioeconomic inequalities in health outcomes are large within India overall, but more pronounced in Uttar Pradesh (UP), Madhya Pradesh, Bihar and Rajasthan. This suggests that the poor have benefited less from publicly provided health services (Peters et al., 2002; Gwatkin et al., 2000). Associated with these inequities in health outcomes are inequities in health care utilization across India, and in UP in particular (Peters et al., 2002; Mahal et al., 2001). According to their analyses, poorer Indians use health services much less than the rich. The distribution of inpatient days, outpatient treatments, and obstetric care at public facilities favors the higher expenditure quintiles, although immunizations and ante/post natal care at public facilities and outreach programs are much more evenly distributed. Financial barriers and user dissatisfaction are suggested as important reasons the poor not benefiting from the public health services.

Health Status of the Poor and Non-poor

Table 5 presents some indicators of health for the non-poor and the ratio of poor to non-poor for these indicators.

Table 5
Health Status Indicators for Poor / Non-poor

Category	*Probability of dying between ages 15 & 59 per 1000*	*Probability of dying between birth and age five per 1000.*
Males Non-poor	16	33
Poor Non-poor Ratio	2.1	4.5
Females Non-poor	8	40
Poor Non-poor Ratio	3.7	4.3

Source: World Health Report, 1999, (Annex Table 7), WHO.

Although we do not have information on incidence of infectious diseases among the poor and non-poor, we do have enough evidence to show that poor are exposed to greater mortality and morbidity than the non-poor. The probability of dying between ages 1 and 5 (child mortality) is more than four times higher for the poor as for the non-poor, while the probability of dying between 15 and 59 (adult mortality) is two to four times greater for the poor than for the non-poor. The tuberculosis prevalence rates for the poor are 2.5 times the rate observed for the non-poor, which indicates greater vulnerability of the poor to tuberculosis (WHO, 1999). It will be wrong to conclude that poverty alone is a factor contributing to this situation. The poor are also likely to be less educated and live in slums and shanty towns with poor quality housing and polluted environment. Consequently, the lack of education, unhealthy housing conditions and lack of access to health care etc are also contributing to the higher prevalence of infectious diseases among the poor. The direction of causation can be both ways. The poor are more vulnerable to infectious diseases. At the same time infectious diseases are contributing to the poverty of the households through lower productivity, loss of wages due to illness, and wastage of household resources to treatment rather than improving the quality of life. Reducing the incidence of infections can greatly contribute to the achievement of reducing poverty (MDG 1) by breaking the vicious circle of poverty and disease (Montgomery and Smith, 2004).

Environmental Factors and Infectious Diseases

One of the millennium development goals (MDG 7) adopted in the millennium declaration of September 2000 is environmental sustainability and another one (MDG 6) relates to the reduction of infectious diseases. Achievements of these goals are related (UNDP, 2003). Figure 1 provides a schematic view of the influence of environmental factors on the incidence of various infectious diseases In the absence of cause of death statistics and morbidity data classified according to environmental factors an attempt has been to gather some limited evidences for India ailments during the two weeks prior to the survey tabulated according to some environmental characteristics. Rural populations have higher morbidity than urban population in most cases; likewise those having low standard of living have higher morbidity than that of others. Lower rates of infections have been recorded for those using piped water and boiled or filtered water (IIPS and ORC Macro, 2000: 217-218).

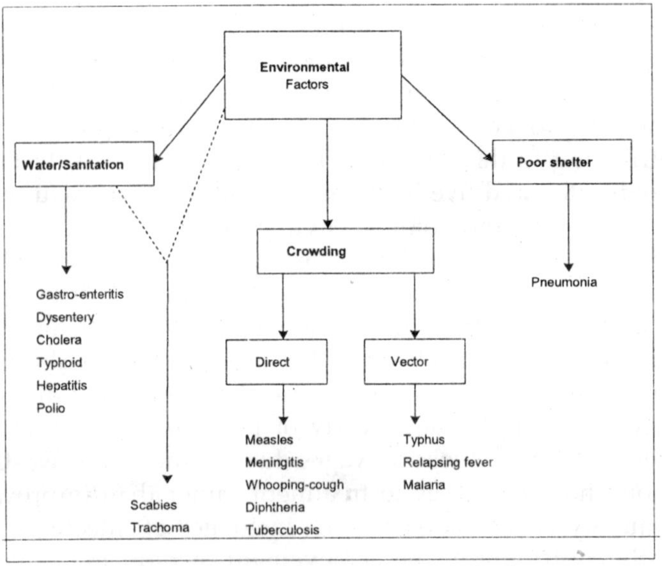

Fig. 1: Environmental Factors and Infections

Environmental Problems

India has very low levels of hygiene and environmental sanitation, which are further accentuated by water logging and flooding during the monsoons and water shortages at other times. Lack of latrines is a major problem in rural areas. Arsenic in the ground water in some states and high iron content and pesticide residues in most areas is another serious problem. In addition, the over-crowding, poor housing and an increase in the number of vehicles and waste matter like sewerage and plastic bags have resulted in the pollution in urban areas. These environmental factors cause frequent illnesses, especially among children (Northridge et al., 2003).

The target of environmental sustainability set for MDG 7 is to reduce by one-half the proportion of people without access to safe drinking water and sanitation. In the absence of more reliable indicator of "safe water" and "sanitation" the measures derived from the NFHS are examined here. Table 6 presents two environment-related indicators, namely, the

Table 6
Indicators of Household Environment

(Percent of total households)

Indicator		*1992-93*	*1998-99*	*2005-06*
Household having piped water or hand pump	Total	68.2	77.9	87.9
	Urban	87.6	92.6	95.0
	Rural	60.9	72.3	83.5
Household having flush toilet or pit latrine	Total	30.2	35.9	43.9
	Urban	75.6	80.7	82.3
	Rural	12.8	18.8	25.3
Households using Solid Fuels	Total	81.4	74.6	73.2
	Urban	43.1	30.1	31.7
	Rural	96.0	91.5	90.5
Households living in Kutcha (poor) house	Total	48.5	32.5	13.7
	Urban	17.2	9.4	2.5
	Rural	60.4	41.4	19.1
Households with 7 plus Members sleeping in a room	Total	5.0	4..2	5.6
	Urban	4.7	3.5	4.0
	Rural	5.0	4.5	6.4

Source: NFHS-1 (1992-93), NFHS-2 (1998-99), and NFHS-3 (2005-06).

percentage of population with access to improved water source and the percentage of population with access to improved sanitation, proportion of households using solid fuel, households living in kutcha houses (a measure of quality of housing) and the number of persons sleeping in a room (a measure of crowding).

There have been some impressive improvements in the availability of piped water and sanitation. The proportion of population with access to improved water sources in India increased from 68.2 per cent in 1992-93 to 87.9 per cent in 2005-06; the recorded improvement being 19 percentage points. According to NFHS-3 in 2005-06 the percentage of population having improved water supply is 95 per cent in urban and 83.5 per cent in rural areas. These figures are extremely doubtful, since the definition of "safe" or "improved" water source is highly subjective. In India, protected water supply is unheard of in most villages and metropolitan water supply systems are often contaminated with sewerage. In cities like Madras (India), bottled water has become a flourishing business. Unless samples of water are taken and rested, it is difficult to conclude that the drinking water is an improved one.

The proportion of population having improved sanitation in 2005-06 is 43.9 per cent of population as against 35.9 per cent in 1998-99 and 30.2 per cent in 1992-93. In 2005-06 the proportion of households having improved sanitation are 82.3 per cent in urban and 25.3 in rural, an increase from 18.7 per cent in urban and 18.8 per cent in rural in 1998-99. The caveat about the reliability of the data on improved sanitation applies because of the possibility of exaggeration of the improved sanitation facility by the respondents.

In 2005-06, nearly three fourth of the households are using solid fuels, 31.7 per cent in urban and 90.5 percent in rural. Overall there is very little change in the proportion of households using solid fuels, with a slight decline in rural areas and a slight increase in urban areas. The slight increase in the use of solid fuels urban areas is surprising in view of the expansion of LPG outlets in urban areas.

The NFHS-3 also shows an improvement in quality of housing in the country, the percentage of households living in kutcha (poor quality) housing had declined to 13.7 per cent in 2005-06 from 48.5 per cent in 1992-93. The improvement in quality of housing is noticeable in both urban and rural. As in the case of other indicators rural area lags behind urban in housing quality. The percentages of households living in Kutcha houses in 2005-06 is 19.1 per cent in rural against only 2.5 per cent in urban.

The indicator of crowding, namely the percentage of households having 7+ persons sleeping in a room shows an increasing trend in both rural and urban areas. This is not surprising in view of the increasing cost of accommodation and shortage of affordable housing.

Impact of Environment on Health: The Case of Infectious Diseases

Infectious diseases constitute a disproportionate share of the burden of disease as measured by DALYs. Out of the estimated 287.9 million DALYs for India in 1990, communicable diseases accounted for 117.4 million DALYs or 41 per cent. Out of these 83.1 million DALYs (or 29% of the total DALYs) is contributed by infectious and parasitic diseases and 34.3 million DALYs (8%) by respiratory infections. The largest contribution for DALYs comes from Acute Respiratory Infections (ARI), diarrhoea, tuberculosis, childhood diseases, measles and tetanus. Children under five years of age account for two-thirds of the deaths due to infectious diseases. Nutritional deficiencies are the major risk factors for death due to infectious diseases (Zaidi et al., 2004). Interventions such as the Integrated Management of Childhood Diseases (IMCI) have resulted in substantial decline in mortality due to ARI and diarrhoea. However, a large proportion of children do not receive timely and appropriate care due to reasons such as lack of recognition of the seriousness of the illness by the parents, low income, and poor access to referral health facilities etc. Neonatal infections are major causes of death among children, and these are preventable by proper nutrition of the mothers during pregnancy, tetanus toxoid immunization, skilled birth attendance at the time of delivery, clean delivery practices, and exclusive breast-feeding of the babies at least for one year.

The impact of environment on health in India can be illustrated with data on the incidence of Tuberculosis in India. Tuberculosis has emerged as a major public health problem in India, as in many other developing countries. TB is also the leading cause of death among HIV positive persons. The National Tuberculosis Control Programme in India is one of the largest health programmes in the country with an outlay of Rs. 680 crores (US$130 million) in the Tenth Five Year Plan (2002-07). The National Family Health Survey of 2005-06 included a question whether any of the household members were suffering from TB and whether he/she received any treatment. The Prevalence Rate for number of persons suffering from tuberculosis and the number treated for tuberculosis were worked out expressing these as a ratio of 100000 of the population of the households covered. These rates could be underestimates because of the stigma attached to TB. At the same time certain amount of over reporting is also possible due to mistaken reporting of other respiratory ailments like asthma as tuberculosis. The figures of medically treated TB cases may be more accurate than all cases recorded in the survey. Table 7 presents the data on Tuberculosis Prevalence Rate by gender, residence and broad age groups:

Looking at the medically treated TB cases, there are differences in the prevalence rate by residence, sex and age, the rates being higher for men than for women, higher for rural residents than for urban residents, The prevalence rate also increases with age, the rate for the elderly (60+) being twice as high as that for 15-59 and about nine times as high as that for children under 15 years of age. Both age and sex differentials are greater for rural population than for urban population (NFHS-3, 2005-06). The higher prevalence of

Table 7
Tuberculosis Prevalence Rate by Gender, Residence and Broad Age Groups, India, 2005-06

(Number per 100000 Resident Population)

Age Group/ Gender	*URBAN*		*RURAL*		*TOTAL*	
	All Cases	*Treated Cases*	*All Cases*	*Treated Cases*	*All Cases*	*Treated Cases*
Age Group						
< 15	98	98	115	114	110	110
15 - 59	367	354	853	605	555	519
60 +	768	727	1180	1102	1066	998
Gender						
Women	247	246	371	337	334	309
Men	385	364	634	602	554	526
All	319	307	502	469	445	418

Source: National Family Health Survey-3, 2005-06 (Table 13.1.1).

tuberculosis among males in India has been observed for many years in the general population and also among medically treated cases. This is probably due to the greater prevalence of smoking habit among males or due to work in a polluted environment (IIPS, 1995; IIPS and ORC Macro, 2000). South Asian countries are implementing the WHO's "Directly Observed Therapy Short Course" (DOTS) strategy. Although some progress has been made in implementing DOTS strategy, major constrains have been the weak public health infrastructure, shortage of staff especially in the primary health centres, inadequate funding, lack of awareness about DOTS among private practitioners, resistance to multi-drug therapy etc. Moreover, occurrence of tuberculosis in conjunction with HIV infections further complicates treatment of both (Zaidi et al., 2004).

Table 8 presents evidences of environmental factors associated with tuberculosis prevalence revealed by the NFHS-3. The data show that the prevalence of TB was higher among household cooking inside the house without a separate kitchen, compared to the households that cook in a separate kitchen. The prevalence of TB among those cooking indoors is lower than among those cooking outdoors, or elsewhere. The probable explanation for this is that those cooking outdoors are more likely to use sold fuels like firewood or charcoal, since it was found that TB prevalence rate was higher among those who used solid fuels. It was also found that the TB prevalence rate was lower among those who had chimney, which is probably because the chimney allows the smoke to escape. Households using an open fire under a chimney reported the lowest TB prevalence rate while those using solid fuels without a chimney reported he highest TB prevalence rate. A breakdown of the data according to rural and urban would have been more revealing, but regrettably such data are not available. Some studies indicate that indoor smoke can cause respiratory infections among children and chronic obstructive pulmonary disease (COPD) among women (Mishra et al., 2004).

Table 8
Prevalence of Tuberculosis by Type of Housing and Fuel /Cooking Arrangements

(Prevalence Rate per 100000 usual household residents

Housing and Cooking/ Fuel Arrangements	*All Cases of TB*	*Medically Treated TB*	*No of Household Members*
Persons per Room Used for Sleeping			
< 3	484	456	423196
3 – 4	282	259	84196
5 – 6	218	218	11394
7 +	388	388	3141
Cooking Fuel			
Electricity of Gas	220	217	124028
Kerosene	564	550	13511
Coal/lignite/charcoal	472	436	12001
Wood	463	430	257123
Straw/shrubs/grass	1012	924	38038
Agricultural crop residues	703	703	20972
Dung cakes	440	416	65681
Other	755	755	640
Place for Cooking			
In the house, separate room	303	294	223520
In the house, no separate room	562	518	160729
In a separate building	567	423	44393
Outdoors	573	543	91479
Others	1223	1223	533
Type of Fire/Stove for Using Solid Fuels			
Stove with a chimney	0	0	118
Open fire (chullah) under a Chimney	295	278	32641
Stove without a chimney	426	426	617
Open fire (chullah) not under a Chimney	533	497	350132
Other	1516	1516	175
Total	445	418	522027

Source: National Family Health Survey-3, 2005-06 (Table 13.1.2).

Environmental Factors and Other Common Ailments

Malaria is another major cause of morbidity in India. Estimates are provided by the NFHS of 1992-93 and 1998-99 based on a question on the incidence of malaria in the households during the three months preceding the survey. According to these surveys the malaria incidence rate per 1, 00,000 populations was 3324 and 3697 persons in 1992-93 and 1998-99, respectively. Malaria incidence is known to vary according to seasons and in a vast country like India bouts of malaria occur in different parts of the country at different times. It cannot be concluded that malaria incidence has increased in India during the intervening period. The surveys show that the malaria incidence rate in the rural population (4254 per 1, 00,000 population in 1998-99) is twice the rate in the urban population (2156 in 1998-99). There is no significant difference between the incidence of malaria among males and females in the two surveys, the reported incidence of malaria being only 2 to 3 per cent greater among males than among females. Even though malaria accounts for less than 5 per cent of deaths among children in South Asia, it remains a major contributor to morbidity and chronic anaemia among children (WHO-SEARO, 2002).

Hepatitis B and C infections are reaching epidemic proportions in India with prevalence rates ranging from 2 per cent to 8 percent in different population groups. Hepatitis C infections are also rising and the prevalence rates are estimated to be between one and four percent. The high incidence of Hepatitis B and C is attributable to unsafe blood supply, use of contaminated syringes, lack of maternal screening, and lack of immunisation by Hepatitis B vaccine. There have been outbreaks of typhoid, dengue fever and dengue haemorrhage disease, but reliable data on the number of cases are not available since this would require laboratory tests for confirmation. High incidence rate of typhoid fever (980 per 1,00,000 population) are reported for the slums of Delhi, and the infection rates for children under five years of age are even higher (Zaidi et al., 2004).

A description of the infectious diseases scenario in India will not be complete without a mention about the growing resistance to the commonly used anti-microbial drugs. The increasing drug resistance is due to misuse of drugs arising from empirical use of antibiotics for a wide range of illnesses, prescription by unskilled medical practitioners, or because of

Table 9
Prevalence of Acute Respiratory Infection (ARI), Fever and Diarrhoea

(Percentages of children suffering from the ailments in the two weeks preceding the survey)

	Fever		Diarrhoea		ARI	
Environmental Characteristic	*Cough with fast breathing (ARI)*	*Fever*	*Any Diarrhoea*	*Diarrhoea with Blood*	*Number of Children*	*% with ARI taken to a health facility or provider*
Source of Drinking Water						
Piped water	15.1	28.4	19.3	1.8	9,697	75.7
Hand Pump	21.7	29.6	19.2	3.2	13,343	60.1
Well Water	21.1	30.9	18.5	2.5	5,834	61.1
Surface Water	19.3	30.0	22.1	3.8	783	47.3
Other	17.6	34.6	16.8	1.4	200	(66.3)
Purification of Water						
Straining by cloth	18.6	29.0	22.0	2.3	5,151	71.2
Alum	20.3	29.0	18.8	1.6	323	76.1
Water filter	12.2	25.4	15.2	0.9	1,159	78.9
Boiling	16.9	31.2	16.5	1.8	2,059	75.7
Other	23.3	30.3	25.2	3.3	216	80.0
Nothing	19.9	29.6	19.0	2.8	21673	61.1
Residence						
Urban	16.2	28.8	19.6	1.6	6,768	75.1
Rural	20.3	29.7	19.0	2.9	23,096	61.4
Standard of Living Index						
Low	21.0	29.8	19.9	3.2	10,710	55.1
Medium	19.4	30.1	19.7	2.6	13,906	67.4
High	15.7	26.7	16.1	1.3	4,889	76.9
Total	19.3	29.5	19.2	2.6	29,864	64.0

Source: National Family Health Survey-2, 1998-1999, (Table 6.16).

self-medication by patients. Such resistance to drugs has made the treatment of common infections (tuberculosis, malaria, and pneumonia. dysentery, typhoid, neonatal sepsis and urinary track infections) a challenge to the medical profession (Zaidi et al., 2004).

Table 9 presents data from the National Family Health Survey of India, 1998-99 relating environmental factors to the percentage of children suffering from various diseases. Regrettably NFHS-3 does not provide cross tabulation of environmental factors such as type of house, kind of fuel used and the kind of toilet facility etc with the prevalence o common ailments and this has limited our analysis. It appears that the use of pipe water greatly reduces the prevalence of the common ailments – fever, malaria and ARI. Likewise, using a water filter or boiling water contributes to a reduction in the incidence of these ailments. The prevalence rate is substantially lower in urban than in rural areas, presumably because of better sanitation in urban areas.

Conclusions

The paper presents evidences of inequalities in India in various socio economic indicators by residence (rural/urban), by gender (male/female), religion, caste and wealth quintiles. The socio-economic indicators used include education, exposure to media, and registration of births and extent of child labour. This shows that urban areas are better off than rural, males fare better than female and SCs and Muslims are faring badly in comparison to other communities. These inequalities persist when the health status of the population is examined by rural and urban, by gender and by caste and religious groups. While the direction of causation could be either way, it is more likely that the social and economic inequalities are affecting the health status of the different communities. An examination of the poor /non poor differentials in health status by gender shows that even the non-poor females fare badly compared to non-poor males in the probability of dying between ages 15 & 59 (per 1000) and probability of dying between birth and age five per 1000.

There are substantial differentials between the poor and the not so poor in respect of survival prospects as well as prevalence of infectious diseases. The poor have three to four times the probability of dying as the non-poor, among males as well as females.

Environmental factors account for a substantial proportion of infections; consequently there is a close relationship between environmental sustainability and control of infectious diseases. The available indicators show that India is not achieving the Millennium Development Goals relating to environmental sustainability and the control of infectious diseases (Vaidyanathan, 2004). Environmental factors such as type of drinking water, method of purifying the water, standard of living, urban and rural residence have an influence on the incidence of fever, diarrhoea and acute respiratory infections. The age-old method of controlling infections is vaccination, unfortunately this is not effectively implemented, and less than one-half of the children were able to show their vaccination cards, and the proportion who had complete vaccination is even less. Providing clean drinking water and improves sanitation could bring about a drastic reduction in mortality and morbidity especially among children.

It must be pointed that the paper has raised more research questions than it has found answers. If the Hindi-speaking states are performing poorly in health outcomes and health utilization, is it due to problems of governance, or is there a fundamental behavioural and cultural problem in these states. By the same token if the SCs and STs are having a poor health outcome or utilization, is it due to discrimination by the authorities or due to problem of attitudes and behaviour. It would be interesting to assess the extent to which project interventions enable Muslims, lower caste Hindus and the poor to make use of health services and gain satisfaction and to assess how they fared relative to better-off groups in similar circumstances.

References

Government of India (GOI), (2002), *India's National Health Policy*. New Delhi: Ministry of Health and Family Welfare.

Gwatkin, D., Rutstein, S., Johnson, K., Pande, R., and Wagstaff, A., (2000), *Socio-Economic Differences in Health, Nutrition and Population in 44 countries*. Washington, D. C.: The World Bank, Health, Nutrition and Population Department.

International Institute for Population Science (IIPS), (1995), *National Family Health Survey (NFHS-1), 1992-93, India*. Mumbai: IIPS.

International Institute for Population Science (IIPS) and ORC Macro, (2000), *National Family Health Survey (NFHS-2), 1998-99, India*. Mumbai: IIPS.

International Institute for Population Science (IIPS) and Macro International, (2007), *National Family Health Survey (NFHS-3), 2005-06, India*. Mumbai: IIPS.

Mahal, A., Singh, J., Afridi, F., Lamba, V., Gumber, A., and Selvaraju, V., (2001), *Who Benefits from Public Spending in India?* New Delhi: National Council of Applied Economic Research.

Mishra, V.,R.D. Retherford and Smith K.R. (1999), "Biomass Cooking Fuels and Prevalence of Tuberculosis in India", *International Journal of Infectious Diseases* 3(3): 119-129.

Montgomery, Mark, and Paul Hewett (2004), *Urban Poverty and Health in Developing Countries*. New York: Population Council.

Northridge, Mary E., Gabriel No. Stover, Joyce E. Rosenthanl, and Donna Sherard, (2003), "Environmental Equity and Health: Understanding Complexity and Moving Forward", *American Journal of Public Health* 93(2): 209-214.

Peters, D. H., Yazbeck, A. S., Sharma, R., Ramana, G. N. V., Pritchett, L., and Wagstaff, A., (2002), *Better Health Systems for India's Poor: Findings, Analysis, and Options*. Washington, D. C.: World Bank.

UNDP (2003), *Population and Environment Nexus*. New Delhi: UNDP.

Vaidyanathan, K.E. (2004), "Infectious Diseases and Achievement of Millennium Development Goals: The South Asian Perspective", Paper presented at a *Workshop on Infectious Diseases*, Asian Meta Centre for Population and Sustainable Development, Singapore.

WHO (1986), *Inter-sectoral Action for Health: The Role of Inter-sectoral Co-operation in National Strategies for Health*. Geneva: WHO.

WHO (1999), *World Health Report, 1999: Making a Difference*. Geneva: WHO.

WHO-SEARO (2002), "India's Health System Profile", In: *Regional Health Situation for SEA Region*. New Delhi: WHO-SEARO.

World Bank (2000), *Socio-economic Differences in Health, Nutrition and Population*. Washington D. C.: HNP/Poverty Thematic Group.

World Bank (2001), *Environmental Health in India: Priorities in Andhra Pradesh*. Washington: Environmental and Social Development Unit.

Zaidi Anita, Shally Awasthi, and Janaka Da Silva (2004), "Burden of Infectious Diseases in South Asia", *British Medical Journal* 328(7443): 811-815.

2

Some Conceptual Issues Concerning Health and Human Rights

Vighnesh N. Bhat

Introduction

There is an ongoing and extensive debate today on the nature, dynamics and significance of health in individual and societal development and the vice versa in sociological literature for quite sometime now. Perspectives on health in these current debates reflect the rapidly changing realities and opportunities in today's globalised world with the firm belief that responding to health needs is ultimately determined by how we address the issue of rights and access to power and resources. In this sense, human rights, health and development represent interdependent sets of values, aspirations and disciplines. Promoting and protecting health, and respecting, defending and fulfilling human rights are seen as inextricably linked. The domains of health and human rights as development partners are currently on the forefront of political and policy debates. This is reflected in civil society movements around the world as well as in political statements heralding greater global equality, poverty reduction, improved democratic governance and protection of public health and security, all in the context of geopolitical shifts, economic globalization and environmental changes. These sentiments are echoed unequivocally in the rights movements in India as well.

Every country in the world is now party to at least one human rights treaty that addresses health-related rights, including the right to health and a number of rights related to conditions necessary for health and the global attempt now is to strengthen all possibilities in providing technical, intellectual and political leadership in the field of health and human rights. Drawing on these domains, this paper offers a theoretical and practical framework for the analysis, application and assessment of health, justice and progress. It attempts to explore the links between human rights concerns, improving the health of individuals and communities, and the goals and processes of development that are central to improving people's living standards and life chances.

Health is an imperative precondition for, and desirable end product of, human development and societal progress. Health is '...directly constitutive of the person's well being and it enables a person to function as an agent, that is, to pursue the various goals and projects in life that she has reason to value'. Health is also the most widely considered constituent of individual well-being and community's advancement. It is often judged as a necessary condition for the fulfillment of all other personal and public aspirations. In the words of Marmot (2004), it is "a marker, a way of keeping score of how well the society is doing in delivering well-being".

A brief look at the significance of this stance may not be out of place here. Myrdal (1969/1974) told us in no uncertain terms that "people are poor because they are sick, they are sick because they are poorer, poorer because sicker... the vicious cycle continues" thus. On the same line, the World Bank, almost two decades ago, acknowledged the reciprocal dependency between progress in health and economic development[1]. This acknowledgment was not an earth-shaking revelation, particularly to those who worked in the field of health and development in Asia and Africa where the bubonic plague of HIV had already begun a heavy toll. Yet this revelation brought in a turning point in the World Bank's lending guidelines along with the emerging global movement towards poverty alleviation, consistently emphasizing the vitality of community's health status in the reduction of poverty. It was not until 2001 that the international community, through the *World Health Organisation Commission on Macroeconomics and Health*, documented that poverty leads to ill-health, but also that ill-health leads to poverty (WHO 2002 & World Bank)[2]. This is no secret now that ill health is one of the prime culprits of underdevelopment - both at the individual and the collective level.

By now it is well known that the World Health Organization defined health as "a state of complete physical, mental and social well-being and not merely the absence of disease or infirmity". The definition has been modified later to include the ability to lead a 'socially and economically productive life'. Researchers have identified health as a key determinant of the ability of an individual or group to benefit from a broader set of rights and entitlements. Public health, defined as 'the art and science of preventing disease, promoting health, and prolonging life through the organised efforts of society' and challenges facing in the field. It also reinforces widespread recognition that promoting health requires multi-sector and 'upstream' efforts to address the determinants of health, much more than simply improving access to health care. Subsequently, health has been understood in more comprehensive terms incorporating human rights elements. It has been thus proposed that health is 'created by caring for oneself and others, by being able to take decisions and have control over one's life circumstances, and by ensuring that the society one lives in creates conditions that allow the attainment of health by all its members'[3].

The eight Millennium Development Goals (MDGs) - which set targets for 2015, amongst other things, to halve abject and absolute poverty, halt the spread of HIV/AIDS and improve health and education - have been agreed to by all the nations as well as leading development institutions (UNDP 2005). It is important to note that all these stated 'Goals' are coupled with health status either by their direct bearing on health outcome and the needed services (e.g. through efforts to reduce child and maternal mortality, HIV, malaria and other diseases), or by emphasizing the principles central to public health policy (for instance, gender equality), or else by calling for the creation of policies addressing the underlying conditions for progress in health (e.g. education, environmental sustainability, global partnerships). The Millennium Development Goals, as we all know, highlight a number of important health indicators that deserve research attention. Public health is a critical component in each of these goals. None of these goals could be achieved unless and until the human community achieves a desirable level of health status across countries.

The term 'human rights', at times, is used so vaguely and generically that there is also a sense of skepticism among law interpreters that has led to the question of 'what exactly are human rights and why do citizens need them'? Human rights, in their most common and agreed upon practice, are best seen as articulations of a commitment in social ethics because their ethical status is socially more relevant and functionally more useful than their legal position[1]

It may be appropriate to make a distinction between human rights and legal rights. While human rights often motivate law, they are not by themselves legal rights. In fact, human rights exist on their own merit whether or not the lawmakers and legal interpreters have had the opportunity and wisdom to turn them into actual legislations.

Human rights constitute a set of normative principles and standards, which can be traced back to ancient times in the cradles of human civilization. Although these concerns for and commitment to social ethics of community development without discrimination have a long history, they received their fastidious modern indentation greatly through the works of political philosophers and leaders of 17th century Europe. Later, the activists, through networks of activities and movements, have developed and expanded upon their ideas often bringing in radical and distinct flavors to them. Today, in its modern and measurable adaptation, the concept of 'human rights' is no longer a mere academic subject but a tool to challenge any prejudiced practices in terms of class, caste, gender, age, ethnicity, language or such other inequalities. Enriched by new perspectives, human rights today play an important role in shaping public policies, programs and practice aimed at improving actual and potential individual and social welfare.

Health and Human Rights

Viewed as a globally desired human aspiration, the notion of 'good' health as the attainment of physical, mental, social and spiritual well being, the right of the individual to live and lead a life to exploit his/her total potential becomes the fundamental prerequisite. In this sense, health of the individual obviously leads to the realisation of all human rights. From the same perspective, the gratification by everyone of the highest achievable standard of physical and mental health is widely regards as a human right (UN CESCR General Comment 14). From a global normative perspective then, the health status and the satisfaction of enjoying his/her human rights remain closely intertwined and interdependent. This position is echoed in many international treaties and declarations and supported by mechanisms of monitoring and accountability[2]. Further, in the globalised social context, development is measured individually and collectively in various ways with indicators such as *status* (for example, measured as income or health status), *capacity* (for example, as human capital in the form of knowledge and skills), *participation* (for example, as individuals' access to employment and capacity to engage with institutions) and *possibilities* (for example, as the presence of pathways to future development). Each one of these indicators clearly demonstrates the positive and juxtaposing relationship between individual rights and his/her health. Each one is intertwined with human rights and health. While there are differences between societies in terms of the intensity of the relationship between these two factors due to variance in terms of history, culture, technology and institutions and how these differences both can and should translate into varied "local" responses to regional or global processes, and varied strategies for development, their intricate and in-depth relationship cannot be denied.

Health and human rights individually occupy advantaged places in public discourse, political debates, civic policy and the media. Both topics are at the top of human development deliberations that do not conclude without references to justice, security, health, housing, education and employment opportunities as essential prerequisites to development. Important it is to note that while the above said goals are not necessarily framed as 'human rights' but the fact that they are nevertheless contained in human rights treaties and often translated into national constitutions and legislations. Hence they provide policy and legal support for efforts in these areas. Incorporating the relationship of health and human rights into public health policy therefore amounts to responding to the demands of people, policy makers and political leaders for outcomes that meet public aspirations. Such a public debate also creates an opportunity for helping decipher how all human rights and other determinants of well being and social progress interact, by allowing progress to be measured towards these goals, as well as shaping policy directions and agendas for action.

The right to health does not mean the right of the individual to remain healthy as such, but embodies an obligation on the part of the government to create the conditions necessary for individuals to achieve their optimal health status. In 2000 the United Nations Committee on Economic, Social and Cultural Rights adopted a General Comment explicating the substance of government obligations relating to the right to health (UN CESCR General Comment No 14). In addition to clarifying governmental responsibility for policies, programs and practices influencing the conditions necessary for health, it sets out requirements for the delivery of health services, including their *availability, acceptability, accessibility* and *quality*. It lays out directions for the practical application of Article 12 and proposes a monitoring framework indicating the ways in which the State's responsibility can be implemented through national law. Currently, over 100 national Constitutions have recognized a right to health and this number continues to increase as Constitutions are rewritten or updated.

As suggested by Gruskin and others (2001, 2007), affixing public human rights strategies in community health agendas certainly supplements the concepts and methods used to attain health objectives, by drawing attention to the legal and policy context within which health interventions occur, as well as bringing in rights principles such as non-discrimination and the participation of affected communities in the design, implementation, monitoring and evaluation of health programs and interventions[3]. It is now generally agreed that the introduction of human rights into public health work is about constructing approaches and processes and their application towards maximising public health gains in achieving comprehensive development. It does not only preordain how the work is done, but also what its ultimate outcome will be. For example, using human rights standards with a focus on health systems requires attention to their availability, accessibility, acceptability, quality and outcomes among different population groups. Furthermore, it needs to be realized that the application of human rights principles of health require that benchmarks and targets be set and ensure transparency and accountability apply to decisions made and their ultimate outcomes.

Achieving development implies a qualitative change in environmental, social, economic or political conditions of the society that improve the welfare of individuals, communities and nation States in the ultimate analysis. Realisation has dawned that vulnerability to ill health can be reduced by taking steps to respect, protect and fulfill human rights. Thus nations have shown serious commitments in enacting legislations resulting in freedom from discrimination on account of ethnicity, sex and social status and the rights to food and nutrition, water, education and adequate housing. In India, there has been a gradual awareness at the public level that violations or lack of attention to human rights, such as harmful traditional practices, slavery, torture and inhuman and degrading treatment, violence against women, etc. can have serious health consequences. Thus health has come to be treated as a fundamental human right.

The interrelatedness of human rights and improved health status as a measure of development can be seen clearly in the context of the right to health. Rights relating to autonomy, information, education, food and nutrition, freedom of association, reproduction, equality, sexuality, participation and non-discrimination are integral and indivisible elements of the achievement of the highest attainable standard of health. So too is the enjoyment of the right to health, inseparable from the enjoyment of most other rights guaranteed by the Constitution or society. Such rights may be classified as civil, political, economic, social or cultural rights depending on the definition of that particular societal context. The literature on women's rights in general-and gender, reproductive and sexual rights in particular-highlights the interdependency of human rights and health. A woman's right to health cuts across the economic, social and cultural as well as civil and political rights, affecting the individual, as well as the entire family unit as researchers have demonstrated. This recognition is based on empirical observation and on a growing body of evidence which establishes the serious impact that lack of fulfillment of these rights has on people's health status–education, non-discrimination, food and nutrition epitomize this relationship. Ill health may constrain the fulfillment of all rights, as the capacity of individuals to claim and enjoy all their human rights may depend on their physical, mental and social well-being[4].

Health-Human Rights Incongruity: The Indian Scenario

While there has been considerable improvement in human living during the last few centuries thanks to the rapid pace of science and technology application, the benefits have not been shared equally between countries, communities and categories. True, that better education, improved nutrition and environmental advances, including better water and sanitation, safer working conditions and improved housing, have enhanced health outcomes in general, and life expectancy has greatly increased in many medium and high-income countries. It is also equally true that major causes of mortality in early childhood, in particular, have been, or have the potential to be, addressed in most nations and technical expertise to tackle infectious diseases, injuries and non-communicable diseases, as well as to treat and manage ill-health have been greatly enhanced. However, in spite of these significant achievements, the benefits of economic advances, human security and access to health care, have not been shared equitably. Vital statistics at the global level provide ample evidence to this fact.

Like in many other countries, India is also facing a paradoxical situation in the case of health and human rights nexus. Following the globalization, liberalization and privatization waves that have swept the trends across the world, the role of the Indian State in health services provision and in securing the basic needs required for health and development has been challenged and in many cases undermined. Increasingly, the private sector and other non-State actors have been brought into the process of providing care, often within an economic and ideological framework which positions health care as yet another commodity, without recognizing the existence of significant market failures. Powerful private actors are increasingly involved in shaping the agenda around public health. Large networks of private hospitals, multilateral organisations, private foundations and the like have in many cases become more influential than the Government in shaping public health policies and health care service resulting in increased inequalities and human rights violation. This is a matter of grave concern for everyone today. True, that health is increasingly understood as a human rights issue, related to a wide range of non-health determinants, and there is recognition that health is far more than health care, but strategies to secure the commitment and resources required to overcome inequities in access to these determinants of health seems to be greatly is lacking. Therefore, what is important today for the researchers in health to debate is not the health services proper, but the ability to shape and frame how inequalities and inequities are seen, the way in which they are defined and tackled, and from where the resources to address them should come. Rights, politics and power have become prominent actors on the health scenario in India, moving to centre stage.

The pragmatic discussion centering on public health and human rights in India needs to emphasise the importance of outcome and impact, measured in public health terms by the reduction of mortality, morbidity and disability, but that is not enough. In development terms, it needs to contemplate on the improvement of quality of life, along with the development of the human potential. The extent tc which the outcomes measured include the fulfillment of human rights is a moot question to be tackled. For example, there is an on-going debate over the functional significance of sex education in the Indian schools today. In this context, it is appropriate to see the value of policies which promote sex education in school measured not only in terms of reduction of unwanted teenage pregnancy or the incidence of sexually-transmitted diseases, but how the right of the child to information is fulfilled in this way, how it affects further demands for health-related, life-saving information, and how access to this information prepares young people to benefit fully from psycho-social and cultural development. Likewise, when assessing the effects of policies that prioritize childhood immunisation, one would want to know not only how immunizations make future population healthier both early and later in their childhood, but also how the right of the child to growth and development, and the right to education by improving attendance and performances at school, are factored in.

Bringing health and human rights together in the socioeconomic developmental context means examining the circumstances in which they function and seeking to identify opportunities for the elaboration of sound policy and programs. It requires ensuring that the processes of policy and program development, implementation and monitoring are informed by best knowledge and practice relevant to both domains with a comprehensive and deep understanding of Indian realities. World Health Organization's (2005) rights-based approach to health is consequential here. His approach makes explicit reference to human rights from the outset, does not invent the content of rights and does not name the relevance of rights only in retrospect. Rather than being mere referential, it emphasizes building capacity and does not use human rights norms as a way of naming violations after they have occurred. In other words, it promotes a way of preventing violations from occurring in the first place and is based on implementation of one or several core rights concepts including nondiscrimination, participation, accountability and transparency.

Following are a few important areas where health and human rights merge into integral parts of comprehensive development: (a) health status and reduction in human rights power (b) Vulnerability to ill health due to weakening of human rights (c) human rights violation and promotion of ill health (d) violation of human rights through skewed health development (e) right to water, information, sanitation, food and nutrition, and education (f) right to freedom of movement, right to participation, right to work and health promotion (g) harmful social and cultural practices (h) violence against women, children, disabled and the destitute (i) Freedom from discrimination and right to privacy. Each of these areas needs specialized attention and study before action programmes are initiated to promote better health and exercise of human rights. There is much important legislation in this direction but an effective way of implementing them for public welfare is yet to see the light of the day[5]

Thus far we have argued the need for human rights based health system to achieve individual and societal development. Given the systemic constraints in India today, the issues are truly complex and complicated making such an attempt easier said than done. However, a broad conceptual scheme is presented here for critical debate in pragmatic terms. Health institutions, health policy makers and health-related movements can deal with poverty and health within a framework encompassing equity and human rights concerns in five broad-spectrum ways:

Institutionalizing the Methodical and Regular Application of Equity and Human Rights Perspectives to Actions concerning Public Health

While most public health efforts in India are intended to benefit the weaker sections of the population, experience over the last six decades has shown that a strategic approach is necessary to overcome the tendency for the poor or marginalised to benefit too little from even the best intentioned government efforts. Countering this, at the minimum, requires a continuous and built-in monitoring of social inequalities in health, delivery of health care, health care financing, and allocation of health care resources. Further, this also calls for an ongoing mechanism of translating findings into action programmes that fill the gaps. Equity and human rights perspectives systematically call attention to factors that are not within the purview of the traditional health sector, and includes a check on gender-based, racial/ethnic and other forms of discrimination, as well as perceived poor quality of available health services, and lack of infrastructure or adequately trained and compensated medical personnel in areas where the poor and disadvantaged live.

Strapping and Expanding the Public Health Functions beyond Health Care that Creates a Positive Environment for Effective Health

The health sector could conceive itself in a comprehensive way beyond traditional patient care services. It can make a major contribution through other socially relevant functions such as setting and enforcing standards for major health determinants. They may include areas like clean water and sanitation, food and drug safety, tobacco control, access to health-related education and information. Other spots such as standards for safe working, housing, transport, and environmental conditions also can be monitored by health agencies in association with other related departments. These actions benefit society as a whole but particularly the poor and disadvantaged; like police and fire services, they represent essential public goods that should not be determined by market forces.

Approaches focusing on poverty, equity, or human rights in relation to health have sometimes been viewed as conflicting or competing, and champions of the poverty-health relationship have sometimes viewed equity and human rights concerns as too abstract or insufficiently relevant. In addition, links between health, equity and human rights have not previously been examined rigorously. We explore the concepts of poverty, equity, and human rights in relation to health and to each other, suggesting operational implications and opportunities for effective action by health institutions.

Executing Just and Unbiased Health Care Financing, which helps Diminish Poverty while Increasing Access for the Poor

The impact of economic globalization on health and human rights, as well as how current global health issues are being addressed under such paradigms as social justice, bioethics, humanitarianism, utilitarianism, or the concept of 'Global Public Goods' should be further explored towards ensuring greater equity in the limitations they face require further research. Meeting the above research needs will be best served by a combination of methods normally used in an array of disciplines, including those applied to policy, legal, strategic and economic analyses as well as epidemiological, behavioural, anthropological and social research.

Ensuring that health services respond effectively to the major causes of preventable ill-health among the deprived and underprivileged:

Health institutions will need to make systematic and sustained efforts to build infrastructure, to overcome the complex barriers to receiving health care that often accompany poverty and social disadvantage, and to achieve comprehensive and high-quality universal services. Access and quality must be considered together; perceived low quality is a widespread barrier to use of available health services by the poor and disadvantaged. To assess whether services are received by those who need them and are effective, systems must be in place for the routine monitoring of poor and disadvantaged groups (in relation to those that are more advantaged) with respect to health status, receipt of care, and health care financing and resource allocation.

Monitoring, promoting and taking action to address the potential health equity and human rights implications of policies in all sectors affecting health, not only the health sector:

Health professionals have a vital responsibility on their shoulders. They are to become more active in countering discrimination by, for example, providing simple, accurate information to users of health services, using technology to reduce information and knowledge gaps, and prioritizing research and development in areas where the poorest are left unprotected, such as neglected tropical diseases. Protection of patient privacy, confidentiality, and dignity, and ensuring informed consent prior to any intervention, are also paramount.

Conclusions

There is an acute need to advance the research field of health and human rights to further build the evidence base that a human rights approach to health and development is both effective and necessary. Potential research topics may include documenting how and to what extent compliance with human rights principles enhances health, and documenting and analysing the ways and extent to which the neglect or violations of human rights impact on health and development. Further, there is an absolute need for good governance in regard to health, human rights and community development.

This calls for the public institutions providing equal distribution of services, ensuring privacy and confidentiality, permitting the right to information, promoting dignity, and creating effective mechanisms of accountability. Research in this area may focus on promoting improved governance of public institutions in relation to health, human rights and development principles. In addition, addressing discrimination, inequalities and inequity in access to services and systems is an important element of a human rights-based approach to health and development.

It is humbly but firmly proposed that an indispensable trait needed by those working in both public health and human rights is sanguinity. Such optimism is conceived as a basic need in large part because of the appalling situations in India as well as in the world in terms of community health. While addressing the challenges posed by the country and global public health and human rights crises, sanguinity must be joined with a critical view of the structural causes of the challenges. There is an absolute need to stand against social structural inequities that exist at different levels as the result of inequitable power structures.

The solution is complex but certainly achievable with professional commitment, intellectual honesty, critical comprehension and societal dedication. Through the use of leadership skills, creativity, and optimism, coupled with an eye towards correcting unjust power structures and eliminating inequities through rights-based approaches, a clear pathway can be paved through the intersection of health and human rights in order to move further towards the realization of the right to health and other human rights envisioned by many leaders in this area.

Endnotes

1. See WHO 2002 & The Annual Report of the World Bank, *World Development Report 1993*, Introduction, page 7 for this position. Also refer to WHO statement that 'The role of health in economic growth has been greatly undervalued. Evidence presented by the Commission suggests that each 10 per cent improvement in life expectancy is associated with an increase in economic

growth of about 0.3 per cent to 0.4 per cent per year, other growth factors being equal' (WHO 2002).

2. This definition is taken from Article 3, of the Ottawa Charter 1986.
3. Under international human rights law (IHRL), the right to health includes freedoms (e.g., the right to be free from nonconsensual and uninformed medical treatment, medical experimentation, forced HIV testing, and degrading treatment) and entitlements (e.g., the right to a system of prevention, treatment, and control of disease, access to essential medicines, reproductive healthcare, and education to prevent unhealthy or risky behavior). IHRL does not prescribe how health care should be delivered; rather it calls for a public heath system that guarantees services are available to all, especially the poor, vulnerable, and marginalized. According to the UN Committee on Economic, Cultural, and Social Rights, public health facilities, goods, services, and programs must be: (a) available; (b) accessible, both physically and financially; (c) acceptable, i.e., gender sensitive, confidential, culturally appropriate; and (d) of good scientific medical quality.
4. An interesting PhD research work on *Health and Social Status of the Aged in Karnataka'* has empirically established the fact that without the freedom to exercise one's individual rights regarding various social issues, the general health status of the individual and that particular groups suffers considerably.
5. Following are the major Acts and Rules promulgated by Government of India in terms of health and human rights:
   - Health Facilities & Services
   - Disease Control & Medical Care
   - Human Resource
   - Ethics & Patients Rights
   - Pharmaceuticals & Medical Devices
   - Radiation Protection
   - Hazardous Substances
   - Occupational Health & Accident Prevention
   - Elderly, Disabled, Rehabilitation & Mental Health
   - Family, Women & Children
   - Smoking Alcoholism & Drug Abuse
   - Social Security & Health Insurance
   - Environmental Protection
   - Nutrition & Food Safety
   - Health Information & Statistics
   - Intellectual Property Rights
   - Custody, Civil & Human Rights

References

Gruskin S, Tarantola D., (2001), "HIV/AIDS, Health and Human Rights" In: Lamptey P, Gayle H, Mane, P. (eds.) *HIV/AIDS Prevention and Care Programs in Resource-Constrained Settings: A Handbook for the Design and Management of Programs*. Arlington, Va: Family Health International, pp. 661–678.

Gruskin S, Tarantola D., (2007), "Health and Human Rights", In: Detels R, Beaglehole, R. (eds.), *Oxford Textbook on Public Health*. Oxford, England: Oxford University Press.

Marmot, M., (2004), *Status Syndrome: How Your Social Standing Directly Affects Your Health and Life Expectancy*. London: Bloomsbury, p. 312.

Myrdal, G. (1968/1974), *Asian Drama: An Inquiry into the Poverty of Nations: A Twentieth Century Fund Study*. London: Penguin Books, p. xxx 2284.

Sen, Amartya (2007), "Children and Human Rights", *Indian Journal of Human Development* 1(2): 235-45.

Shetty, V. (2007), Health and Social Status of an Aging Population: A Comparative Study of Urban and Rural Bangalore. Unpublished Ph.D. Thesis, Kuvempu University.

3

Ethics in Social Research on Health: Review of Guidelines

U. V. Somayajulu, Tilak Mukherji

Introduction

What do we mean by Ethics?

Ethics is concerned with the conduct of human beings and the scientific activities, including those by the social scientists, are conducted with the participation of human beings or have an impact on human beings or on the wider society and environment. In view of this, it is highly essential that scientists/researchers understand ethical issues as well as the implications of their scientific work and act in accordance with these.

For making ethical judgement, the scientists/researchers rely upon various standards of ethics, which could be universal or specific to the culture(s) or localities. Indeed, it is essential that researchers share and discuss the ethical issues in their work and evolve collective standards of their own.

Need for Ethics

Of late, ethical considerations have come to the forefront across the research community. This is due to the legislative change in human rights and data protection and increased public concern about the limits of inquiry. There has also been enhanced concern for responsible action within the workplace with many large organisations expressing a desire for higher ethical standards in customer relations and in investment related decisions.

Growing corporate responsibility entails a clear recognition that business and public service activities are not value-free and cannot set standards merely by the meeting of measurable performance indicators. Responsibility entails thinking about the consequences of one's actions upon others and the establishment of clear lines of accountability for the redress of grievances.

There has been a steady growth of research in the social sciences and in social science research in health in India. A wide range of research topics and issues including the ones that have the potential to seriously invade the privacy and security of individuals are being studied. Methodologies employed for such research studies have also expanded in range and depth. There is a considerable increase in the types and numbers of individuals and institutions undertaking such research and those sponsoring and funding it.

It is encouraging to note that social science research in health is getting the attention it deserves. But growth of research without social and ethical commitment could adversely affect credibility of research, autonomy of researchers, quality of research and rights of the participants. In fact, there is a growing concern about indifference to ethics in some the social science research in the field of health in India.

Social and ethical commitment and self-regulation are, thus imperative for all parties in research, namely, institutions undertaking research, researchers, funders/ sponsors and those who publish material generated from research. Their individual and joint efforts are needed in order to achieve consensus on a common framework for research, and to improve and strengthen the system and environment in which research is conducted. Thus enunciation of ethical principles and formulation of necessary guidelines for research are a part of such process, and also a necessary and desirable step.

Objectives

The role of ethics in health related social research perhaps has not been given adequate attention in India due to various reasons. There is also a need to provide review of the current status in terms of existing guidelines. This paper is an attempt to review the ethical guidelines that are in place at national as well as international level through review of the relevant documents that are available.

International Efforts

Self-regulation and ethics have been issues for debate in medical research more often than in social sciences. The Second World War and the Nuremberg trials of doctor-researchers exposed the horrors of the fascist politics as well as unethical biomedical research. In the post World War period, the scientists paid increased attention to ethics in biomedical research. In the process, the quality and validity of unethical research was questioned, the human rights of participants were recognised and ethical codes were formulated. The Nuremberg Code (1947) was followed by the Declaration of Helsinki in 1964, which was amended subsequently (WMA, 1989). The Council for International Organisations of Medical Sciences (CIOMS) and the World Health Organisation (CIOMS & WHO, 1993) also proposed guidelines in 1983 and adopted them in 1992.

In the post World War period, there has been growing pressure on social science professionals to self regulate and evolve their own code of conduct. There has been a continuing debate between the view of making the social sciences "value free" and "objective" and the view that social scientists could not remain value free simply because they deal with contemporary society and because there is an explicit connection between research and social action or political viewpoint. The former tries to make social scientists attain a status of professionals and often puts them in ivory tower situations, while the latter tries to make them aware of the impact of their activities on the society. In both the cases, ethics of social inquiry and application of expertise of social science to current social problem need adequate attention.

Internationally, the associations of Applied Anthropology and the Psychologists formulated their codes 1940s and 1950s. The controversy regarding the Project Camelot and its cancellation in 1965 led to increased discussion on ethics among the social scientists and eventually paved the way for formulation of guidelines by major social science associations (Barnes, 1979).

The universities have also tried to establish formal guidelines to protect student research and their exploitation by the teachers. Most associations of sociologists, anthropologists, political scientists, psychologists etc. have formulated and refined their ethical guidelines in the last three decades. In the past one and half decades, these associations of science and social science disciplines combined their efforts to evolve joint guidelines.

Medical Research Council of Canada, Natural Sciences and Engineering Research Council of Canada and Social Sciences and Humanities Research Council of Canada appointed a joint committee (Tri-Council Working Group) to formulate "The Code of Ethical Conduct for Research Involving Humans". In 1997, these three councils adopted the Tri-Council report as a common code of ethics. One can notice some similar processes in USA as well. These developments emphasise that the principles governing all research on humans by all disciplines of sciences have many things in common and the researchers must respect and protect human rights of the participants of research.

The core principles adopted at international level include: Obligations to Society, Obligations to Funders and Employer, Obligations to Colleagues, Obligations to Subjects, Widening the scope of social research, Considering conflicting interests, Pursuing objectivity, Assessing alternatives impartially, Guarding privileged information, Maintaining confidence in research, Ensuring safety and minimising risk of harm to field researchers, Avoiding undue intrusion, Obtaining informed consent, Protecting the interests of subjects, Enabling participation, Maintaining confidentiality of records, Preventing disclosure of identities and Confidentiality and Anonymity

The Professional Associations involved actively in ensuring ethics in research include: British Sociological Association, British Psychological Society, MRS Code of Conduct, European Code developed by ESOMAR, The Association for Practical and Professional Ethics, Office for Human Research Protections (OHRP), The US Centre for Disease Control et al.

National Efforts

The international developments inspired several such initiatives at the national level and in various specific fields of biomedical research. In 1980, the Indian Council of Medical Research (ICMR) formulated "Policy statement on ethical considerations involved in research on human subjects" and in 1997, it brought out the draft of "Consultative Document on Ethical Guidelines on Biomedical Research Involving Human Subjects".

The issue of ethics in social sciences, unlike in medical research, has been given less importance in India. Though many social scientists did pay serious attention to the appropriate conduct of research and set personal examples, they are often not discussed as ethics and no efforts are made to formalise guidelines based on such experiences. The national councils for social science research and their institutions have many guidelines either as administrative orders or for improving the quality of research. But enough efforts have not been made to bring them together as comprehensive ethical guidelines. In the absence of such comprehensive guidelines, ethics are hardly there in the social science education curriculum.

The efforts to formulate ethical guidelines for research in social sciences and health in India began in 1998. After a rigorous documentation of the guidelines for medical as well as social science research in India and outside, a multidisciplinary national committee was constituted in 1999. The committee brought out the final guidelines including the ethical framework based on four moral or normative principles and ten principles that are relevant for ethics in research in India. Though these guidelines are not administrative rules, they are approximate standards informing the choice of action in a concrete situation. Concern for and protection of the human rights of the participants is fundamental to understanding and applying the ethical principles and guidelines. The guidelines formulate rights and responsibilities of the four major players in research; namely, the researchers, the institutions, the sponsors and funders and the gatekeepers.

Lastly, the development of organisational mechanism for ethics in social science research in health has been kept as an open process to be evolved by the community researcher and institutions. The national meeting of researchers in May 2000 felt that such a mechanism could be different for different types of institutions and projects; and that only by practising ethics within institutions; one can arrive at appropriate models for the organisational mechanism. Such a process would also create a critical mass of individuals and institutions having experience in integrating ethics and guidelines in their institutional environment and the research process. This should be essentially a collective endeavour of networking, sharing, discussing and providing assistance to each other.

Principles of Ethics

Moral Principles

The four moral principles that constitute the basis for ethics in research include:

(i) *The Principle of Non-malfeasance:* Research must not cause harm to the participants in particular and to people in general

(ii) *The Principle of Beneficence:* Research should make a positive contribution towards the welfare of people

(iii) *The Principle of Autonomy:* Research must respect and protect the rights and dignitv of participants

(iv) *The Principle of Justice:* The benefits and risks of research should be fairly distributed among people

General Ethical Principles

The Ten general ethical principles, relevant for social science research in health, include:

(i) *Essentiality:* It is necessary to make all possible efforts to get and give adequate consideration to existing literature/knowledge and its relevance, and the alternatives available on the subject/issue under the study

(ii) *Maximisation of Public Interest and of Social Justice:* Research, a social activity, carried out for the benefit of society, should be undertaken with the motive of maximisation of public interest and social justice

(iii) *Knowledge, Ability and Commitment to do Research:* sincere commitment to research in general and to the relevant subject in particular and readiness to acquire adequate knowledge, ability and skill for undertaking particular research are essential prerequisites for good and ethical research

(iv) *Respect and Protection of Autonomy, Rights and Dignity of Participants:* Research involving participation of individual(s) must not only respect, but also protect autonomy, rights and dignity of participants. The participation of individual(s) must be voluntary and based on informed consent

(v) *Privacy, Anonymity and Confidentiality:* All information and records provided by participants or obtained directly or indirectly on/about the participants are confidential. Permission of the participants is essential for revealing or sharing any information that may identify them

(vi) *Precaution and Risk Minimisation:* As all types of research studies carry some risk to the participants and society, taking adequate precautions and minimising and mitigating risks is essential

(vii) *Non-exploitation:* Research must not unnecessarily consume the time of participants or make them incur undue loss of resources and income. It should not expose them to risks due to participation in the research. The relationship within the research team should be based on the principle of non-exploitation. Contribution of each member of the research team should be properly acknowledged and recognised

(viii) *Public Domain:* All persons and organisations connected to research should make adequate efforts to make public in appropriate manner and form, and at appropriate time, information on the research undertaken and the relevant results and implications of the completed research

(ix) *Accountability and Transparency:* The conduct of research must be fair, honest and transparent. It is desirable that the institutions and researchers are amenable to social and financial review of their research by an appropriate and responsible social body. They should also make appropriate arrangements for the preservation of research records for a reasonable period of time.

(x) *Totality of Responsibility:* The responsibility for due observance of all principles of ethics and guidelines devolves on all those directly or indirectly connected with the research. They include institution(s) where the research is conducted, researcher(s), sponsors/ funders and those who publish material generated from research.

Rights and Responsibilities of Researchers/Institutions

Responsibilities of Research Institutions

The responsibilities of research institutions include:

- Respecting the autonomy of researchers and the ethical guidelines for research
- Creating and maintaining an environment with adequate support systems to enable researchers to follow the ethical guidelines
- Taking appropriate and adequate steps for protection against pressures inimical to the observance of ethical guidelines for research.

Protection and Promotion of Integrity in Research

Researchers have a right, as well as a responsibility, to refrain from undertaking or continue undertaking any research that contravenes ethical guidelines, violates the integrity of research and/or compromises their autonomy in research, including study design/ methodology, analysis and interpretation of findings and publication. If they feel that their rights are being violated, or that the study is unethical, the researchers should make all possible efforts towards making corrections. In the event of failure of remedial measures, the researchers should exercise their right to terminate the study or to opt out of it.

Other Responsibilities of Researchers are as follows :

- Should undertake only such research that according to their understanding will be useful to the society or for the furtherance of knowledge on the subject.
- Should not undertake secret or classified research, any secret assignment under the garb of research or research whose findings are to be kept confidential.
- Should make all necessary efforts to bring the research and its findings to the public domain in an appropriate manner.
- Should make reasonable efforts to anticipate and guard against possible misuse and undesirable or harmful consequences of research. Researchers should take reasonable corrective steps when they come across misuse or misrepresentation of their work.

- Should ensure honesty and transparency at every stage of research as these are indispensable for good and ethical research.
- Should ensure that there is no fabrication, falsification, plagiarism or other unethical practices at any stage of the research; and that the findings of research are reported accurately and truthfully. They should also ensure protection of historical records and preservation of study material.
- Should inculcate and practice sensitivity and respect for culture and other aspects of the group or community studied.
- Must ensure respect, protection and promotion of rights of participants. Criteria for the selection of participants of research should be fair, besides being scientific.
- Should make peer review an essential part of every research endeavour or initiative, and should be sought at various stages of research.

Relationship among Researchers

Principal researchers are responsible for the ethical conduct of research by all juniors, assistants, students and trainees. Juniors, assistants, students and trainees also have an equal responsibility for ethical conduct and observance of ethical guidelines.

Juniors, assistants, students and trainees have a right to receive, while principal researchers have a responsibility to provide/impart proper training and guidance regarding all aspects of research, including ethical conduct. The principal researchers should delegate to the juniors, assistants, students and trainees only those responsibilities that they are reasonably capable of performing on the basis of their education, training or experience, either independently or under supervision.

Researchers should not engage, personally or professionally, in discriminatory, harmful or exploitative practices, or any perceived form of harassment. Researchers should not impose views/beliefs on or try to seek personal, sexual or economic gain from anybody, including other researchers, juniors, assistants, trainees and students.

Researchers should not deceive or coerce other researchers, including juniors, assistants, trainees and students into serving as research subjects/participants, and not use them as cheap labour.

Researchers should be cooperative, responsive and respectful about the interest opinion/view, capability and work of other researchers, including juniors, assistants, trainees and students.

All team members working on a research project, have a right to know and document all aspects of research including ownership of the data. This applies to the participation of students doing their own research in a project team. Thus the students have the right to opt out of a research project without having to face adverse consequences.

Other individuals such as administrative staff of the organisation conducting research or that of the research setting, associated with the research should be briefed on ethical issues and the guidelines, including the need to protect the rights of participants and the confidentiality of identifiable data.

Data Sharing

Sharing of data should be done in consonance with the interests and rights of the participants. Full responsibility of ensuring protection and promotion of interest and rates of participants while sharing or making the data available to public lies with researchers and the Institute where the study is conducted.

The researchers involved in the research and the institution where the research is conducted, have a joint right over and ownership of all raw data, including those identifying the participants. They should take full responsibility for ensuring that when such data, including those that identify participants, are shared with other researchers, all necessary measures are taken and followed to maintain confidentiality, by those researchers with whom data are shared.

Data that do not identify participants and their whereabouts, in the form of anonymous or abstracted facts, may be commonly shared, if necessary even before the publication of the study, among researchers, peer reviewers, or may even be made available to the public.

Researchers and institutions should ensure to the extent possible that relevant summary findings of the research are taken back to the research participants in a form and manner that they can understand and also take necessary steps to prevent possible social harm that such information might cause to the research problem.

Reporting and Publication of Research

Reporting of research and its results is the right as well as duty of every researcher and institution that conducted the study. When they agree to delegate this responsibility to funder(s)/sponsor(s) or any other individual(s)/organisation(s), they should do it only if they received mutually agreed and expressed commitment to publish/disseminate the results/report within a stipulated period.

The results should be reported irrespective of whether they support or contradict the expected outcome(s). Researchers should also disclose in their publications, the source(s) of funding and sponsors, if any, unless there is a compelling reason not to do so. The findings should also explain the methodology used, as well as how, in actual practice the ethical guidelines were followed, ethical dilemmas encountered and resolved, etc.

Authorship Credit

The guidelines to be followed with respect to giving authorship credit while reporting the research in any form are listed below:

Authorship, and its sequence in case of more than one author, should be based on the quantum of contribution made in terms of ideas, conceptualisation, and actual performance of the research, analysis and writing of the report or any publication based on the research. Authorship and its sequence should not be based on the status of the individual in the institution or elsewhere.

All other individuals not satisfying the criteria for authorship but whose contribution made the conduct and completion of research or publication possible should be properly acknowledged.

A student should be listed as principal or first author on any multiple authored publications that substantially derives from the student's dissertation or thesis. Appropriate credits should be given where data or information from other studies or publications is quoted or included.

Researchers should avoid dissemination of the research results before they are peer-reviewed or published in appropriate journals. When such results are disseminated through the popular media, extra care should be taken to ensure that even those media persons not specifically trained in social science and health issues and research, are able to comprehend the limitations and implications of research results. Journalists and the media that publish these research results have a responsibility to do so truthfully and honestly.

The institutions and/or researchers publishing a report or any other documents based on research should make adequate efforts to ensure their easy availability and accessibility.

Rights of Participants

Relationship with the Participants

Participants should be seen as indispensable and worthy partners in research. Researchers should recognise and ensure that respect, protection and promotion of the rights of participants are made intrinsic to every stage and level of research undertaken by them.

Research undertaken should not adversely affect the physical, social and/or psychological well being of the participants. The risks and benefits of the research to the prospective participants must be fully considered. Research that could lead to unnecessary physical harm or mental distress should not be undertaken. Researchers should make adequate provision for the comfort of the participants as well as for protection against all possible and potential risks.

The criteria for selecting research participants should be fair. Easy accessibility of the participants alone does not constitute a fair criterion for their inclusion in research as that will make them bear an unfair share of the direct burden of participation. No particular group or groups should be unfairly excluded from research, as that could exclude them from the social understanding of their situation, and can also unfairly exclude them from direct, indirect or potential benefits of research.

Unless consent on mutually beneficial arrangement is obtained, institution and student should not use community or research setting as a constant and long-term resource for data collection for curricular research or training in an institution.

The relevant social, cultural and historical background of the participants should be taken into consideration and given appropriate importance in the planning and conduct of research.

Researchers should not impede the autonomy of participants by resorting to coercion, promise of unrealistic benefits or inducement. Participants and communities should not be exploited and the time taken for data collection from these sources should not be inordinately long.

Participants should be considered as autonomous agents and must have the right to choose whether or not to be part of the research. They also have the right to change their decision or withdraw the informed consent given earlier, at any stage of the research without assigning any reason.

Informed Consent

Voluntary and informed participation of individuals or communities is necessary for research. Their participation should be based on informed consent. Greater the risk to participants, the greater is the need for it. Informed consent is essential to protect the participants, not the researchers and institutions.

Consent for participation in research is voluntary and informed only if it is given without any direct/indirect coercion and inducement, and is based on adequate briefing given to the participants about the details of the project. The briefing should be given both verbally and in writing in a manner and language that the participants know and understand. In India, often, it may not be possible to obtain signed informed consent of the participants in social science research in health. It is essential that the participants are provided written information with adequate details of the research. Researchers have a duty to ensure that the participants comprehend the information given.

The verbal and written briefing of the participants, in the manner and language they understand, should include the following details:

(a) *Purpose of Research*: The goal and objective of research should be presented in simple local language.

(b) *Identity of the Researchers*: Name and address of researcher(s), the institution(s) and the main person of the ethics committee/ethical review board or any such ethics group of the institution.

(c) *Identity of Others Associated with the Research*: Name(s) and address of chief consultant(s), funder(s) or sponsor(s), etc., if any.

(d) *Why Selected*: Reasons or method for selecting the particular locality, community and/or any other setting and individual(s) or group(s) within that, for participation in the study.

(e) *Harms and Benefits*: The possible, anticipated and potential benefits and/or harms (direct/indirect, immediate/long term) of research and their participation.

(f) *Privacy, Anonymity and Confidentiality*: Information on the extent of privacy, anonymity and confidentiality that will be provided to participant(s). This at least must include the firm commitment that privacy, anonymity and confidentiality of data identifying participants will be strictly maintained. In case the data identifying participants is to be shared with or made available to individuals/organisations not in the research team, information about them (their names, addresses etc.) should be provided.

(g) *Future Use of Information*: The future possible use of the information and data obtained, including use as a database, archival research or recordings for educational purposes, as well as possible use in unanticipated circumstances, like its use as secondary data should be made known to participants. Such use should be only of anonymous or abstracted information and data, and should in no way conflict with or violate the maintenance of privacy, anonymity and confidentiality of information identifying participants.

(h) *Right not to Participate and Withdraw*: Participants should also be informed about their right to decline participation outright, or to withdraw consent given at any stage of the research, without undesirable consequences, penalty and so on. The participants should be informed that they are free to object to and refuse to allow the use of data gathering devices, such as camera, tape recorder etc.

(i) *Right to get Help*: The researcher should try and get all the possible help that the participants might require. The researcher also has a responsibility to help the participant(s) in cases of adverse consequence or retaliation against the participant(s) by any agency due to their participation in the research. Information, which may contribute to the improvement of quality of life of the participants, should be passed on to concerned person(s), official(s) or the agencies.

If the data collection from the participant(s) is done in more than one sitting or contact and there is a long time period between the sittings/contacts, informed consent should be sought each time.

Revealing the identity of the group of participants, groups, village(s), neighborhood(s), etc, in the report could have an adverse effect on members/residents in other cases. Researchers should take care that the study communities and/or localities are not identified or made identifiable in the report unless there are strong reasons for doing so. If the researcher(s) and institution intend to identify them participants in the report, participants' informed consent allowing such disclosure should be obtained.

(j) *Non-disclosure of All Information*: In case of some specific situations and research issues, it is not practically possible to carry out research if all the details of the study are revealed to the participants. This may be due to genuine difficulties in accessing participants, possibility of affecting change in behaviour or responses, etc., when the details are revealed. It may not be possible to obtain informed consent in the same way as described and in such cases, the following should be done:

(i) A detailed justification for not revealing all necessary information must be provided in the research proposal and methodology and should be subject to peer and ethical review. Only on approval in peer review, should such research be undertaken.

(ii) The participants' right to privacy, anonymity and confidentiality gains additional importance in such cases as they do not know fully the real purpose or objective for which they provide information.

(iii) Even if it is accepted through a peer review process that some of the information about the study need not be revealed, participants must be provided the rest of the information. Under no circumstance should the researchers withhold the information regarding physical risks, discomfort, unpleasant emotional experiences, or any such aspect that would be a major factor in taking the decision to participate.

(iv) As far as possible, debriefing should be done with the participants after completion of the research, giving reasons for not providing full information. As a part of the debriefing process, it might be necessary to provide services such as counselling and referral.

(k) *Consent where Gatekeepers are Involved*: In a few cases there may be a need to obtain permission of the 'gatekeeper' to access the participants for research. The following steps must be taken in such cases:

(i)) *Permission Obtained from the Gatekeeper* must not be substituted for the need to take separate and full informed consent of the participants. The rights of participants in such cases are the same as in all other cases and need determined protection.

(ii) For obtaining permission of the gatekeeper, no pre-condition demanding sharing of information or data obtained should be accepted.

(iii) In the process of research or data collection, adequate care should be taken to ensure that the relationship between the gatekeeper and the participants is not jeopardised.

(iv) Greater care should also be exercised in protecting participants and their interest while publishing and disseminating results of research.

(l) *Informed Consent in the Case of Research with Children* (below 14 years) should be sought from the parents/ guardians as well as the children themselves. Where the parents/guardians consent to participate, and the children have declined, the rights of the children should be respected. The consent from parents/ guardians should be waived only in special cases such as child abuse. Peer review is indispensable and the protection of children especially from the immediate consequences of research gains prime importance.

(m) *Privacy, Anonymity and Confidentiality*

(i) Anonymity and confidentiality are the inherent of all participants. The right whether to remain anonymous or to be identified lies with the participant. It becomes important in research projects dealing with stigmatised, sensitive or personal issues and information.

(ii) Possibility of the breach of confidentiality and anonymity should be anticipated, addressed and explained to the participants.

(iii) Appropriate methods should be devised to ensure privacy at the time of data collection. These methods are also essential to ensure the validity of data.

(iv) The obligation to maintain privacy, anonymity and confidentiality extend to the entire research team, other researchers in the institution, the administrative staff, and all those (from or outside the institution) not directly associated with the research that may possibly have access to the information.

(v) As regards what information should be regarded as private or confidential, the perspective of the participant(s) on the matter should be given adequate importance.

(vi) Researchers should maintain appropriate anonymity and confidentiality of information in creating, storing, accessing, transferring and disposing of records under their control, whether these are written, automated or in any other medium.

NACO Guidelines

Ethics Committee

NACO Ethics Committee for Research is responsible to ensure that the ethical implications of any research undertaken are afforded serious consideration prior to the commencement of a project and that such research is consistent with legislative and statutory requirements.

The ethical approval is required to ensure that the process of research is conducted 'ethically' and responsibly and ensures protection of privacy and not exploitative of participants. This involves establishing procedures for the informed consent of those subjects involved in research, as well as appropriate handling of the research findings (e.g. secure storage of data) and material. The highest ethical standards must be upheld when collecting behavioural or biological data on HIV/AIDS the study participants may experience psychological, social, physical or economic harm due to stigma and human rights issues around HIV/AIDS,

All the research activities involving human participants should be conducted in accordance with the four basic ethical principles viz: autonomy (respect for person/participant) beneficence, non-malfeasance (do no harm) and justice. The guidelines laid down are directed at application of these basic principles to research involving human participants.

The basic responsibilities of NACO Ethics Committee are:

(a) To protect the dignity, rights and well being of the potential research participants.

(b) To ensure that universal ethical values and international scientific standards are expressed in terms of local community values and customs.

(c) To assist in the development and the education of a research community responsive to local health care requirements.

The NACO Ethics Committee for Research consists of the experts in epidemiological, behavioural and social disciplines, legal expert and a representative from the community. The

Chairman of the Committee should not be appointed from the NACO so that independence of the committee can be maintained. The Member Secretary should be the officer in-charge for Operational Research in NACO who should organise the functioning of the Committee. The number of members in the Ethics Committee should range between 8 and 12.

Principles for Ethical issues in Research with human beings

Any research using the human beings as participants shall follow the general and specific principles given below. There are twelve *general principles* that are common to all areas of research include:

Principles of essentiality, Principles of voluntariness, Principles of non-exploitation, Principles of privacy and confidentiality, Principles of precaution and risk minimisation, Principles of professional competence , Principles of accountability and transparency, Principles of the maximisation of the public interest and of distributive justice, Principles of institutional arrangements, Principles of public domain, Principles of totality of responsibility, and Principles of compliance

The Specific Principles include

Informed Consent of Participants, Essential information for prospective research participants, Confidentiality for Prospective research participants, Conflict of Interest, International collaboration/assistance in Evaluation and Operational Research, Researcher's relations with the media and publication practices.

Ethical Issues in Epidemiological Research

The welfare of the individual has to be balanced against the welfare of the community and society at large. The C.I.O.M.S/ W.H.O Guidelines for Epidemiological Research assume that the individuals or population groups being studied are capable of giving informed consent understanding the implications of the study. For with low large segments of our population with low level of education, the full understanding may not be achievable. How the principle of "do no harm" is ensured under such circumstances without being paternalistic is a major issue that has to be taken into consideration in ethical guidelines.

In cohort or survey techniques for incidence and prevalence of various diseases, a major issue that has to be considered pertains to how much of intervention is justified and whether one is justified in withholding interventions. Health education or other interventions including non-health interventions can be quite expensive. An alternate strategy that may be followed involves making curative therapy available to the population at their own request. This usually involves running a clinic, which is readily accessible to the population without any other intervention. However, it is generally considered unethical to withhold intervention or services. Surveillance studies to obtain true HIV burden rates most likely lead to ethical dilemmas regarding maintenance of confidentiality and prevention of stigmatization, wherever applicable *anonymous* could solve these problems when the information is required to be placed in public domain.

Research and Programme Evaluation

Whenever a programme evaluation and surveillance is launched, the monitoring and evaluating mechanisms should clearly be planned and cleared by NEC (NACO Ethics Committee) before initiation

Community Participation

A community can be defined as a group of people sharing the same location, beliefs, culture, ideals, goals, age, gender, profession, lifestyle, common interests, geographical locations or settings or disease. When research participants are drawn from a specific community, members of that community can be involved to discuss any concerns it may have regarding the research. If an ethics committee does not have a member from the community, it may ask a local community representative to be the voice for all participants. On the other had, community representatives can formally join together to form a group termed as Community Working Group, or Community Advisory Group, which takes part in the research at all stages of the study.

In international studies, particularly on issues involving communities, representation from this body ensures that the community's health needs and expectations are addressed, informed consent is appropriate, and access to research benefits is provided through research that is designed and implemented in the best interests of science and community. Community representation should be ensured before, during and after the study. Before the study is initiated the community is informed to see if it agrees that the research addresses a need or problem relevant to that community and to confirm that the design is culture specific and brings some benefits to research participants or the community. The community representation is needed to assist in developing appropriate ways to protect the participants. During the study, the association with community representatives continues to educate others about the research and to alert the researcher to ethical issues related to the research. Post completion of the study, community representatives can help in making the results known to the entire community. The community representatives should be made to understand the results. Person for intervention responsible and conditions under which this would be done, duration of availability of intervention, methods of improving the quality of health care in the community and any expected desirable behavioural change in the community.

Ethical Issues for Studies through Questionnaire Based Research

A questionnaire is a common research methods used in the field of epidemiology, social sciences, psychology, etc. Success of research studies depends on the trust and cooperation the researcher gains from the participants. It is essential to establish ethical standard.

Ethical Issues in Focus Group Discussion

Ethical considerations for focus group discussions are the same as for most other methods of social research. When selecting and involving participants, researchers must ensure that full information about the purpose and use of participant's contributions is given. Being honest and keeping participants informed about the expectations of the group and topic, and not pressuring participants to speak is good practice. A particular ethical issue to consider in case of focus groups is the handling of sensitive material and confidentiality given that there will always be more than one participant in the group. Participants need to be encouraged to keep confidential what they hear during the meeting and researchers have the responsibility to anonymise data from the group.

Internet Based Research

The fundamental tenets governing the protection of human subjects in research studies apply to internet based research also. The complexity of internet research through, for example, e-mail surveys, web based surveys or on-line discussion groups present different challenges that need to be addressed in accordance with the Ethics Committee. The general principles are applicable as well as the specific guidelines/issues should be followed while conducting internet based research. These include:

- Identification of who will have access to the data, how long the data will be protected (secure protection of information during the study, removal and storage of records following completion of the study minimum primary investigator, faculty advisor, or department and accessible if review of the data is necessary).
- Statement affirming that web surveys are password protected using a secure server without inclusion of identifying information.
- Contact persons for questions about the research.

- Statement that the participant has read the informed consent statement, all questions has been answered, and his/her willingness to complete the questionnaire or participate in the research implies consent.
- Access to results (posting a summary or abstract or sent via e-mail).

These procedures may not apply to research involving children or other vulnerable groups who are not, according to federal regulations, empowered to authorise consent for themselves. While the child may assent, the parents or guardians must provide consent. With internet use, the identity/age of the participant is not easily determined. In general, as risk level increases for participants, the use of the internet may not be advisable.

The use of the Web for recruitment of subjects, data collection, and data analysis may be advantageous in securing larger or more specific samples more efficiently and at a lower cost. Careful attention must be given to the treatment and protection of research participants and, specific to student research, research advisors must be vigilant about use of on-line data analysis.

References

Amar Jesani, Tejal Barai: "*Ethical guidelines for Social Science Research in Health*", http://www.hsph.harvard.edu/bioethics/guidelines/ethical.html

Barnes J. A. (1979), *Who Should Know What? Social Science, Privacy and Ethics*. Cambridge: Cambridge University Press.

CIOMS and WHO (1993), *International Ethical Guidelines for Biomedical Research Involving Human Subjects*. Proposed Guidelines, 1983, Revised and adopted 1992, Geneva: CIOMS/WHO

ICMR (1980), *Policy Statement on Ethical Considerations Involved in Research on Human Subjects*. New Delhi: Indian Council of Medical Research.

ICMR (1997), *Consultative Document on Ethical Guidelines on Biomedical Research Involving Human Subjects*. New Delhi: Indian Council of Medical Research

International Tribunal of Nuremberg (1947), *"The Nuremberg Code"*, In: Scholl Connor Suzan, Fuenzalida-Puelma Herman L. (ed.), *Bioethics: Issues and Perspectives*. Washington DC: Pan American Health Organisation, pp. 217-218.

NACO (2008), *Ethical Guidelines for Operational Research on HIV/ AIDS*. New Delhi: National AIDS Control Organisation.

4

Inequities in Occupational Health: A Human Rights Perspective

Tushar Joshi

Introduction

The World Health Organization believes that 100 million workers are injured and 200,000 die each year in occupational accidents and 68-157 million new cases of occupational disease are attributed to hazardous exposures or workloads. These high numbers of severe health outcomes contribute to one of the most important impacts on the health of the world's population.

Occupational injuries and diseases play an even more important role in developing countries where 70% of the working population of the world lives. By affecting the health of the working population, occupational injuries and diseases have profound effects on work productivity and on the economic and social well-being of workers, their families and dependents.

According to recent estimates, the cost of work-related health loss and associated productivity loss may amount to significant per cent of the total gross national product of countries of the world.[1] These are telling observations from an organization that has been pursuing the goal of health for all for more than 60 years. Despite such high costs of work related illness and injures, much more needs to be done in India to secure safe and healthful workplaces, in particular in unorganized sectors like agriculture and construction where a large workforce is employed.

This paper provides a review of the status and inequities in occupational health in India on the basis of the official data and reports.

Occupational Diseases and Injuries in India

One of the main stumbling blocks in formulating a sound policy and action plan for labour protection in India is inadequacy of data. The official government of India site of Director General of Factory Advise Service and Labour Institutes (DGFASLI) at Central Labour Institute, Mumbai does not furnish statistics on occupational diseases affecting workers in India.[2]

Under The Factories Act, 1948, amended in 1987, a number of obligations were stipulated which employers were obliged to meet to raise the standards of occupational health care for workers, [3] these were as under:

Every occupier of a factory involving any hazardous process shall:

(a) Maintain accurate up-to-date health records or, as the case may be, medical records, of the workers in the factory who are exposed to any chemical, toxic or any other harmful substances which are manufactured stored, handled or transported and such records shall be accessible to the workers subject to such conditions as may be prescribed;

(b) Appoint persons who posses qualifications and experience in handling hazardous substances and are competent to supervise such handling within the factory and to provide at the working place all the necessary facilities for protecting the workers in the manner prescribed :

Provided that where any question arises as to the qualifications and experience of a person so appointed, the decision of the Chief Inspector shall be final;

(c) Provide for medical examination of every worker -

(i) before such worker is assigned to a job, involving the handling of, or working with, a hazardous substance, and

(ii) While continuing in such job, and after he has ceased to work in such job, at intervals not exceeding twelve months, in such manner as may be prescribed.

Protecting the Health of the workers

It requires special training for physicians to be able to meaningfully assess the factories or workplaces for inadequacies in working conditions and working environment. They also have to undergo training in specific disciplines like industrial medicine, toxicology, industrial hygiene, ergonomics, work physiology, safety sciences and others to be able to identify occupational illness. Quoting the correspondence with the Chief Inspector of Factories in various states and union territories, the DGFASLI says that a total of 133703 factories were inspected by a mere 37 certifying surgeons between 1999-2003. It is not known how many of them were actually qualified in the discipline of industrial medicine and occupational health. There is no mention if they identified any occupational illness, and if so, where and when, and what was the nature of such illness. There is however reporting of injuries as shown in Table 1.

A cursory look at the data indicates that many states do not even record and report injuries. This shows the interest respective states are taking in promoting occupational safety and health. Further analysis of data provided on injuries in ports and docks and in mines confirms that the numbers do not reflect the reality. Such an apathy and lack of interest in providing occupational health and safety to vast majority of

Table 1
Total Number of Industrial Injuries in Factories by State (1999 - 2003)

State/Union Territory	*1999*	*2000*	*2001*	*2002 (P)*	*2003 (P)*	
Andaman & Nicobar	NA	NA	NA	37 (-)	53 (-)	
Andhra Pradesh	3325 (115)	3241 (121)	3010 (118)	2316 (99)	1976 (100)	
Arunachal Pradesh	NA	NA	NA	NA	NA	
Assam		133 (7)	139(6)	149 (15)	62 (11)	65 (6)
Bihar		606 (21)	NA	NA	NA	NA
Chandigarh	NA	24 (1)	4 (-)	5 (-)	81 (11)	
Chattisgarh	NA	NA	NA	NA	NA	
Dadra Nagar Haveli	3 (1)	NA	NA	NA	NA	
Delhi		74 (11)	43 (9)	28 (6)	NA	NA
Goa		190 (5)	NA	142 (4)	185 (13)	145 (3)
Gujarat		10724 (211)	NA	6417 (175)	NA	NA
Haryana		428 (48)	NA	NA	245 (34)	181(25)
Himachal Pradesh	234(48)	NA	NA	NA	NA	
Jammu & Kashmir	NA	NA	NA	NA	NA	
Jharkhand	NA	NA	NA	NA	NA	
Karnataka	1107(50)	1044 (NA)	NA	2132(44)	2013(50)	
Kerala		3849(25)	NA(!5)	NA	NA	NA
Lakshadweep	NA	NA	NA	NA	NA	
Madhya Pradesh	5115 (66)	3321(51)	2232(32)	1947(49)	2065(48)	
Maharashtra	14477(155)	11873(168)	9679(178)	7616(150)	6416(159)	
Manipur		NA	NA	NA	NA	NA
Meghalaya	NA	47(2)	NA	NA	NA	
Mizoram		NA	NA	NA	NA	NA
Nagaland		NA	NA	NA	NA	NA
Orissa		1049(22)	1031(30)	812(20)	709(34)	700(49)
Pondicherry	862(2)	856(2)	592(4)	559(5)	581(8)	
Punjab		262 (23)	1049 (35)	492(5)	466(8)	NA
Rajasthan		2245 (59)	1300(44)	2555(33)	1997(57)	1748 (58)
Sikkim		NA	NA	NA	NA	NA
Tamil Nadu	2702 (41)	NA	2245 (37)	2172 (36)	NA	
Tripura		4(1)	8(2)	7(NA)	5(-)	4(1)
Uttar Pradesh	NA	NA	NA	NA	NA	
Uttaranchal	NA	NA	NA	NA	NA	
West Bengal	NA	NA	NA	NA	NA	

Note: Number in parenthesis indicates number of factories,
NA: Not available, P: Provisional

workers, leads to inequities in health status and their earning capacity. Also, of the total workforce, only those working in factories, mines, ports and docks, and in construction have a statutory protection. Further, there are loop holes in the system which provides a vast majority of employers to escape the legal net.

Since the health and safety legislation does not extend to the vast majority of workers in unorganized sector, majority of the workforce is not entitled to benefits such as preventive and protective measures, on site emergency response, health check up and record keeping as well as compensation should they suffer a serious bodily injury and impairment. The total employment in both organized and unorganized sector in the country was of the order of 450.9 million as per the last survey. Out of this, about 20.6 million were in the organized sector and the balance 430.3 million were in the unorganized sector. Out of 430.3 million workers in the unorganized sector, 260.9 million workers were employed in agricultural sector; 20.6 million in construction, and remaining were in manufacturing activities, trade and transport, communication & services. The workers in unorganized sector fall in various categories but a large number of them are home based workers engaged in occupations like *beedi* rolling, *agarbatti* making, papad making, tailoring, *jary* and embroidery work.[4]

The Silicosis Conundrum

Nothing illustrates better than the plight of silicosis affected workers who worked without any occupational health care provided to them. In case of Silicosis victims, the matters were placed before the National Human Rights Commission which took a serious view of the neglect of occupational safety and health by employers as well as the state government officials.

According to a Times of India report, hundreds of Bhil and Bhilala tribals in Jhabua and Dhar districts of Madhya Pradesh are waiting to die. In a survey conducted in 2007 by a group of doctors in 21 villages of Jhabua, 158 people were found dead of silicosis. "266 others, who have been exposed to silica dust and are sick, will also eventually die," the doctors noted. All of them had gone to Gujarat to work in the quartz crushing units there as unregistered daily wagers. In these factories, quartz stones are first broken by hammer into smaller ones, then crushed and powdered to be used to make glass. Large quantities of dust are generated in the process that the laborers inhale as they breathe deep due to the physically heavy workload involved.[5]

Those who develop impairment due to work related injuries and illness can not earn the same wages. Most do not get compensated and still others lose their job and are added to the poverty pool. The National Human Rights Commission asked the Chief Secretaries of Gujarat and Madhya Pradesh to submit their comments on a news report which highlighted the plight of the laborers employed in quartz units in Gujarat... Taking cognizance of this news report which appeared in the "The Times of India" on May 19, 2005 captioned "Silicosis Silently Killing Hundreds in MP Villages" the Commission said the news report raised a serious issue of violation of human rights of the laborers employed in quartz units in Gujarat.[6]

The International Labour Organization (ILO) and International Labour Standards

The ILO was founded during the Versailles peace negotiations at the close of World War I. It became part of the UN's predecessor, the League of Nations, along with the International Institute of Commerce. While the league eventually died, the ILO continued to function and found a new home as the UN's new specialized agency in 1946. India is one of the founding members and played a significant role in the strengthening of ILO. The organization has a tripartite structure with governments, employers and unions being the three pillars. The ILO has created instruments known as International Labour Standards based on a number of conventions and recommendations, of which nearly 40 per cent are on occupational safety and health. The ILO looks forward to the member governments to ratify these in order to ensure labour protection and creating a safe and healthful workplace, which in countries like India is important. Occupational injuries and diseases are preventable provided a set of measures are put in workplace for creating safe and healthful working conditions and environment. It is surprising that many countries including India have been slow in responding to these valid demands of the organization for ratifying key ILO conventions.

The statistics put forth by ILO recently is quite alarming. Some 2.2 million women and men around the world perish in work-related accidents or diseases every year. It is estimated that globally some 270 million occupational accidents and 160 million work-related illnesses occur annually. The

International Labour Office prepared a special ILO report, titled "Prevention: A global strategy".

According to the ILO, deaths due to work-related accidents and illnesses represent 3.9 per cent of all deaths and 15 per cent of the world's population suffers a minor or major occupational accident or work-related disease in any one year. A large number of the unemployed–up to 30 per cent - report that they suffer from an injury or disease dating from the time at which they were employed. The unemployed often cite impairment of their health as a hindrance to finding new employment.

Also the deaths and injuries due to occupational factors are unevenly distributed, with working population in Asian countries bearing the major burden. The ILO's statistical division provided data on occupational accidents and diseases, and work-related deaths in 2005 in detail which are given below:

- The number of fatal occupational accidents, especially in Asia and Latin America, is increasing. For example, between 1998 and 2001, fatal accidents at work rose from 73,500 a year to 90,500 in China, while there were nearly half a million work-related deaths in 2001. In Latin America, fatal accidents moved from 29,500 per annum in 1998 to 39,500 in 2001. According to a new ILO analysis, rapid economic expansion lies behind these figures.
- Diseases related to work cause the most deaths among workers. Hazardous Substances alone are estimated to cause 438,489 deaths a year.
- The construction industry has a disproportionately high rate of recorded accidents.
- Younger and older workers are particularly vulnerable. The ageing population in developed countries means that an increasing number of older persons are working and need special consideration.[7]

Ratifying Key ILO Conventions

Though ratifying key conventions such as Convention No.

155 on Occupational safety and health, Convention No. 161 on Occupational health services, and convention No. 162 on Asbestos exposure, and others by itself does not increase the standards of occupational health care. However, it does draw attention towards the fact that the occupational health and safety is a major determinant of workers health. Table 2 gives the conventions Indian government has ratified so far.[8]

Table 2
India – OHS Conventions Ratified by India

Convention	*Ratification Date*	*Status*
C16 Medical Examination of Young Persons (Sea) Convention, 1921	20:11:1922	ratified
C18 Workmen's Compensation (Occupational Diseases) Convention, 1925	30:09:1927	ratified
C19 Equality of Treatment (Accident Compensation) Convention, 1925	30:09:1927	ratified
C32 Protection against Accidents (Dockers) Convention (Revised), 1932	10:02:1947	ratified
C42 Workmen's Compensation (Occupational Diseases) Convention (Revised), 1934	13:01:1964	ratified
C115 Radiation Protection Convention, 1960	17:11:1975	ratified
C136 Benzene Convention, 1971	11:06:1991	ratified
C141 Rural Workers' Organizations Convention, 1975	18:08:1977	ratified
C174 Prevention of Major Industrial Accidents Convention, 1993	06:06:2008	ratified

Total Ratified: 39, Conditional ratification: 0, Declared applicable: 0, Denounced: 2

Occupational Diseases Management

The occupational health and safety is under the jurisdiction of ministry of labour and employment. Though the annual

Box 1
Provisions for Occupational Safety and Health in Indian Constitution

The Constitution of India contains specific provisions on occupational safety and health of workers in Table 13.1. The Directorate General of Mines Safety (DGMS), Dhanbad and the Directorate General of Factory Advice Service and Labour Institutes (DGFASLI), Mumbai, the two field organizations of Ministry of Labour and Employment, strive to achieve the principles enshrined in the Constitution of India in the area of occupational safety and health in mines, factories and ports.

report brought out by the ministry (Box-1) emphasizes the importance given to the subject in Indian constitution, much remains to be done to change the ground realities.

Absence of a Healthy Worker Effect

The healthy worker effect was first described by William Ogle in an appendix of the Registrar General's report on mortality in England and Wales. It was based on the observation that the working population is healthier than the general population. Ogle identified two kinds of selection responsible: one working at the time of hire, and the other working at the time of employment.[9] The first selectively attracts or rejects new workers depending on physical demands of the job and health selection, by for instance occupational physicians. The second forces people to leave industry because their health is too much impaired for the job they are in. This has been repeatedly observed in a number of studies conducted in the western world. However, a lack of this effect which we observed during our survey in Delhi indicates that the working conditions and working environment even in a city like Delhi are a matter of concern.

Table 3
Comparative Study of Selected Health Characteristics of Male Factory Workers and General Population #

	Male Factory Workers		*General Population*		
Health Characteristics	*N =581*	*Percent*	*N =846*	*Percent*	*Chi-square value*
Smoking	108	18.59	336	39.71	70.75**
Alcohol(Frequent/Occasional)	277	47.70	285	33.69	27.65**
BMI					
<19	296	50.94	246	29.0	80.00**
20-24.99	229	39.42	418	49.50	
>25	56	9.64	182	21.50	
Asthma	2	0.34	20	2.36	7.97*
TB	14	2.41	4	0.47	6.41*
Allergies/Dermatitis	55	9.47	33	3.90	17.49**
Hypertension	133	22.89	101	11.94	29.35**

A Health Survey to determine the Adverse Health Impact of Pollution in Delhi, **P<.001, *P<.01

The findings presented in Table 3 indicate that the people in community are healthier. Nearly 50 per cent workers examined were underweight against 29 per cent in community. Workers also showed a prevalence of tuberculosis to the extent of 2.41 per cent against 0.47 per cent prevalence in the general population.

Conclusions

Although India is a founding member of ILO, it lags behind in providing occupational health care to its workers. The statutes promulgated by the Indian Ministry of Labour do not cover such vitally important segments of economy as agriculture, and emerging sectors of information technology. There is no national occupational health policy despite the idea being mooted almost a decade back. The identification of occupational illness and underlying causes of injuries at work have not been seriously dealt with. Moreover recording of such data does not get the seriousness it deserves. In consequence, serious policy interventions can not be made.

At the same time globalization is depriving workers of their basic human right, i.e. to be able to work in a 'safe and healthful workplace. The authorities need to address capacity building in core disciplines of occupational health such as industrial medicine, industrial hygiene, ergonomics etc. Upgrading existing ones to train workers in health and safety is required. India can also take lead in ratifying some of the key International Labour Standards such as Convention No. 155 on occupational safety, No. 161 on Occupational Health Services, and No. 162 on Asbestos until such time its use is totally prohibited.

The poor state and neglect of occupational health and safety in the country is leading to greater inequity with workers paying a heavy price of the neglect. No country can call itself a civilized state unless a serious effort is made to provide workers their due and rightful place in the society. It is hoped that the civil society in India will take greater interest in the matters of workers' health and safety.

References

WHO/OCH/94.1© (1994), World Health Organization.

http://dgfasli.nic.in/welcome.html

http://labour.delhigovt.nic.in/act/html_ifa/page14.html

The Ministry of Labour, Government of India, *Annual Report 2006-2007.*

Nitin Sethi (2008), "Silicosis Silently Killing Hundreds in MP Villages" *Times of India,* 19 May.

http://www.andhranews.net/India/2008/May/28-NHRC-asks-Gujarat-46934.asp

International Labour Organization., *World Day for Safety and Health at Work 2005: A Background Paper*

ILOLEX - 11. 2. 2009

Occup. Environ Med. 2006 February; 63(2): 83. doi: 10.1136/oem.2005.024307

5

Human Rights and Rural Health Providers' Access to Health Information

M. Ganesan, Suma Prashant, Meenakshi Gautham

Introduction

People in rural areas frequently suffer from common diseases that are easily preventable and curable. In India, it was reported that more than 6000 children below the age of five years die every day. More than half of these deaths are due to malnutrition-mainly deficiency of Vitamin A, iron, iodine, zinc and folic acid (Micronutrient Initiative, 2007). Many primary health problems could be prevented and health of rural communities could be improved if local community based health workers had essential primary health knowledge.

In India, although 72 per cent of people live in rural areas, their healthcare is attended by less than 20 per cent of qualified medical doctors (WHO, 2007). There is ample evidence that primary health care in rural areas is mainly provided by village based informally trained private practitioners (hereafter referred to as Rural Healthcare Providers or RHPs) who are not formally trained in any medical system and do not possess a statutory medical qualification (Bhat, 1999). These RHPs are usually the first point of contact at the village level in

India for delivering primary health care. The widespread presence of RHPs across the country has been documented from the early 1970s (Gautam, 2006).

Considering the lack of good health care due to acute shortages of well trained health professionals in rural areas, the National Rural Health Mission under Ministry of Health and Family Welfare, Government of India, has proposed training and licensing of these practitioners (RHPs) in rural areas (MOHFW, 2006a). Other recent government documents and policies have also made strong recommendations for mainstreaming of RHPs through training and other linkages (MOHFW, 2006b).

Access to timely and appropriate health information is essential for any health professional. For community based health workers it is even more imperative because these health workers are in direct contact with community members and have a crucial role to play in preserving and promoting community health. If health workers lack access to essential health information, communities are deprived of good health. It is small wonder that access to essential healthcare information for health workers as well as users is slowly gaining international recognition as a human right.

The belief that health information is a human right is central to the online advocacy campaign on "Health Information for All by 2015" (HIFA, 2006) global campaign launched in 2006 to improve the availability and use of healthcare information in developing countries. HIFA and its supporters argue that the right to health information is grounded in the right to health and the right to receive safe, effective healthcare. The right to health is a human right enshrined in the Universal Declaration of Human Rights 1948 (UN).

So what does it take to translate this right into practice? In spite of all the arguments that have been presented here in support of increasing access to health information for community based health workers, the task is easier said than done. Some of the key challenges include: How does one build a regular stream of health information delivery for health workers in far flung but needy rural areas who do not have the time to attend classroom training for long periods? How does one transcend the language barriers, as much of health information is in the English language that health workers are not familiar with? How does one make the information relevant, meaningful and useful and also attractive enough for health workers to want to access it with self motivation?

The Indian Institute of Technology Madras's Rural Technology and Business Incubator (IITM's RTBI) recognized these challenges in 2007 when they decided to respond to the pressing need for strengthening rural health care providers' knowledge and skills. The RTBI launched a project "First Care" to strengthen Rural Healthcare Providers (RHPs) in India. The first project intervention was to deliver relevant health information to RHPs through a distance-learning mode. In this paper we describe how E-learning through distance mode has not just been successfully established but has also contributed to enhancing the information and knowledge levels of community based RHPs.

Methods and Materials

IITM's RTBI initiated a First Care pilot project with 22 Rural Healthcare Providers in Thiruppathur taluk of Sivaganga district in Tamil Nadu. The study area comprised villages including Thiruppathur town within a distance of 35 km with a rural population of approximately 1.9 lakhs. A survey was carried out to identify the rural healthcare practitioners. In all, 35 non MBBS RHPs practicing in Thiruppathur region were contacted through a local Practitioners' Association and invited for an orientation meeting. Following the orientation programme, 22 RHPs were selected to take part in the pilot project based on a set of criteria including a minimum 5 years of independent practice, minimum class X educational background, having clinic base and village internet kiosks availability in their respective village. The remaining RHPs were informed that they would be inducted in the future training programme. The distance E-learning mode was adopted to impart essential primary health information. These 22 RHPs were linked with computers and Internet and trained in basic computer use at their respective village where the village Internet kiosks are located and sent E-learning modules fortnightly. The 11 E-learning modules included primary health aspects of infectious and non-infectious diseases; respiratory systems; cold and flu; cough; asthma; bronchitis; pneumonia; fever; headache; eating right to stay healthy and foods that help us to stay healthy. Health content in the modules was adapted from "Where There Is No Doctor", the globally renowned primer for community health workers. All modules were translated into Tamil, the local language and hosted on a password protected website for RHPs.

Five to ten questions based on the module content, with multiple choice responses were designed and the RHPs were required to select the corrects answer before and after reading each respective module. Pre and Post module study marks of every RHP in each E-learning module were obtained through the back end database. Percentage of increase in knowledge was calculated individually and collectively. The mean scores were compared using paired t-test for their statistical significance using SPSS 7.5 version and presented the same in Table 1 and 2.

Results

The data on characteristics (sex, education, etc.) of 22 RHPs and pre/posts test marks obtained by them for each E-learning module are presented in the Tables 1 and 2. Majority of the RHPs (82 percent) were males and 68 percent were 40 years old. Most of the RHPs (86percent) studied up to 12th standard and only 14 percent studied up to 10th standard. They had diversified background including diplomas in Sidha, Homeopathy, Lab technology, Auxiliary Nursing Midwife and Pharmacy etc.

Majority of the RHPs (59%) have been practicing independently for the last 16 to 20 years in their respective villages. These RHPs are well integrated within their communities. They have their own small clinics and are available almost 24 hours as they generally lived and worked in the same place. RHPs reported that they met about 10 to 20 patients per day suffering from a variety of symptoms. The common ones included cough, fever, diarrhea, injuries and pain related symptoms.

Table 1
Distribution of Rural Health Providers by Background Characteristics

Characteristics		*Number*	*Percentage*
Sex	Male	18	(82)
	Female	4	(18)
	Total	22	(100)
Educational qualification	Up to 10th Std	3	(14)
	Up to 12th Std	19	(86)
	Total	22	(100)
Years of independent practice	0 to 5 years	3	(14)
	6 to 10 years	4	(18)
	11 to 15 years	2	(9)
	16 to 20 years	13	(59)
	Total	22	(100)

In each of the E-learning modules, the pre-test scores obtained by the RHPs collectively in all the modules are lower when compared to their post test scores. The lowest pre-test scores were recorded in case of Infectious and Non-Infectious Diseases module whereas the highest pre-test scores were recorded in Respiratory systems module as compared to other modules. The average pre-test mark for all modules combined is 67 out of 100 (all the 11 modules). The average post test score is 91 percent indicating an increase of 24 percentage points, which is significant at $P < 0.01$.

Significant increase in scores was observed for the following modules: 'Pneumonia' (53 percent at $P < 0.01$) followed by 'Headache' (34 percent at $P < 0.01$), Infectious and Non Infectious Diseases (28 percent at $P < 0.01$), 'Foods that help us to stay healthy' (39 percent at $P < 0.01$), 'Eating right to stay healthy' (28 percent at $P < 0.01$), 'Cold and Flu'

(26 percent at P< 0.01), 'Fever' (25 percent at P< 0.01), 'Bronchitis' (20 percent at P< 0.01), 'Cough' (11 percent at P< 0.05) and Respiratory systems (3percent at P< 0.05).

Table 2
Module wise Pre and Post Test Marks obtained by RHPs through Distance Learning Mode (Percentage) (N=22)

E-learning Module	*Pre-Test*	*Post-Test*	*Percent Increase over pre-test*	*'t'-value*
Infectious and non-infectious diseases	44	72	28	5.792**
Respiratory systems	89	92	3	2.159*
Cold and flu	66	92	26	5.186**
Cough	75	86	11	2.806*
Asthma	87	91	4	1.073NS
Bronchitis	74	94	20	4.500**
Pneumonia	47	100	53	43.924**
Fever	54	79	25	7.423**
Headache	66	100	34	5.631**
Eating right to stay healthy	72	100	28	7.868**
Foods that help us to stay healthy	69	100	31	10.529**
Mean	67.44	91.38	23.95	5.512**

*P< 0.05; **P< 0.01; NS- Non Significant

Discussion

The results indicate that the knowledge of RHPs significantly increased in all the E-learning modules except Asthma module. It is obvious from the pre test scores that the knowledge of RHPs for the respective health conditions was inadequate. The higher marks in post test were due to acquisition of knowledge through the E-learning process.

The modules in which the RHPs gained significantly are all extremely important modules with great public health significance. Pneumonia can be a potential killer among children, Headache is one of the most frequent complaints, Infectious and Non-Infectious diseases pertain to fundamental concepts of disease transmission, Child nutrition information is critical in our country where almost half of all under fives are malnourished, Cold and Flu are common viral infections and due to this there may be mild diarrhea especially in young children, Fever is a sign of illness, Bronchitis is an infection of the bronchi that carry air to the lungs, Cough is a very frequent complaint.. With these modules we have improved RHPs' knowledge in some of the most fundamental health issues related to rural communities.

Although distance learning courses such as the Indira Gandhi National Open University are available to urban educated Indians living in cities and big towns, these are mainly in English and rely more on printed material than the Internet. Training and knowledge development programmes for community based health workers have typically relied on conventional classroom methods that require the workers to travel quite some distance away from their home base. Ours is probably a pioneering programme in India that seeks to improve community based health workers' knowledge levels 'wherever they are', at their own pace, using internet technology. Although not so common in India, web based courses have been used successfully in other developing countries. A Web-based course was very successful in respect of nutrition in public health in Brazil (Dirce et al., 2001). Similar web based course was conducted in New Zealand. There was success in knowledge enrichment after the course in respect of health. It has been reported that Internet technology was alternative for delivering educational material and advice although there was a bandwidth limitation (David et al., 2001).

The main problems observed include low Internet bandwidth, and longer time taken to download the module. Despite this limitation, the E-learning training was very successful and a constructive tool for knowledge building. The E-learning materials were constantly reviewed and updated by the health team on the back end and the RHPs also had the opportunity to give their feedback and comments directly to the team members. Based on this course outcome, we would recommend that it should play an important role in the capacity building programme of these RHPs who are delivering primary health care to the rural people.

However it is still difficult to say how the skills of these RHPs have changed as a result of improvement in knowledge levels alone. We are developing other methods and interventions to improve the overall health care delivery services provided by these RHPs. Mobile phone, Voicenet technology and a clinical guidance system called e-Guide will be introduced to other areas where there is even poorer Internet or no Internet connection.

From this study it is suggested that E-learning is an effective and feasible tool for increasing RHPs' knowledge on essential health information required to address rural health problems. This is one step closer to helping rural communities and their health providers achieve the right to access essential health information.

References

Bhat, Ramesh (1999), *Private Medical Practitioners in Rural India: Implications for Health Policy*. Ahmedabad: Indian Institute of Management.

David Parry, Alec Holt, John Gillies and FRACP (2001), "Using the Internet to Teach Health Informatics: A Case Study", *Journal of Medical Internet Research* 3: 3. Available from http://www.jmir.org/2001/3/e26/HTML

Dirce M Sigulem, Tania B Morais, Lilian Cuppari, Sylvia C.C Franceschini, Silvia E Priore, Kátia G Camargo, Reinaldo Gimenez, Viviane Bernardo and Daniel Sigulem (2001), "Web-Based Distance Education Course in Nutrition in Public Health: Case Study", *Journal of Medical Internet Research* 3: 2.

Available from http://www.jmir.org/2001/2/e16/HTML#figure1

Gautham, M. (2006), *Quality of Care for Reproductive Tract Morbidities by Rural Private Practitioners in North India*. Unpublished Ph. D. Thesis, U.K, London University: London School of Hygiene and Tropical Medicine.

HIFA (2006), "Health Information for All by 2015".

Available from http://www.hifa2015.org/hifa2015-and-human-rights/

Micronutrient Initiative (2007), *Controlling Vitamins and Mineral Deficiency in India. Meeting the Goal*, Micronutrient Initiative

MOHFW (2006a), *Report of the Working Group on Public Health Services (including water and sanitation) for the Eleventh Five Year Plan (2007–2012)*. New Delhi: Ministry of Health and Family Welfare, Government of India.

MOHFW (2006b), *Task Force on Medical Education for the National Rural Health Mission*, New Delhi: Ministry of Health and Family Welfare, Government of India.

WHO (2007), "Not Enough Here, Too Many there", In: *Health Workforce in India*. New Delhi: World Health Organization, India Country Office.

SECTION – 2

Inequalities in Health Care Utilization

6

Public Health Facilities and their Role in Utilization of MCH Services in Indian States: DLHS-RCH, 2 Data Analysis

N. Audinarayana

Introduction

Availability of facilities in public health establishments is the basic requirement for providing the programmed services in reliable manner and thereby, attracts the public to utilize such facilities in a better way. Further, such facilities, on the one side, indicate the type of infrastructure, supply and drugs available at public health centres; on the other side, they also indicate the quality of services provided at these centres. Generally, it is observed that availability and accessibility, including economic and time costs, of maternal health services, notably antenatal care and delivery care are related to service utilisation. In Uttar Pradesh, it was found that the presence of health services in the community significantly increased the use of antenatal and delivery services (Stephenson and Tsui, 2002). In Guetamala, Glie et al. (2003) observed that the effects of the availability of private and public sector providers on the use of biomedical care during pregnancy were modest. In Viet Nam, Do (2008) found that the availability of ANC services of a public sector facility within

5 km. of the community had a strong and positive impart on whether rural women received at least three ANC visits during a recent pregnancy.

With this background, in this paper, an attempt is made to have a glimpse into how adequately the different public health centre (First Referral Units, Community Health Centres and Primary Health Centre) are equipped with specific facilities across the states of India. It is also intended to examine whether such availability of facilities in various public health centres have any association with the utilisation of maternal and child health care services.

Data and Methodology

Data for the present paper has been drawn from the Facility Health Survey, 2002-2003 as well as District Level Health Surveys conducted under the Reproductive Health Survey, Round 2 (DLHS-RCH, 2) carried out during 2002-2004 by 12 research organizations including Population Research Centres (PRCs) and the International Institute for Population Sciences designated as the nodal agency (IIPS, 2005; 2006). These studies have been conducted in 29 States and 6 Union Territories using systematic, multi-stage stratified sampling designs. However, in the present paper, data for 20 major states only have been considered for analysis. The estimates of availability of different facilities available as well as the magnitudes of maternal and child health care services for state level provided/published by the IIPS have been used here as it is.

Of the facilities available at various public health centres, the following information is made use for First Referral Unites (FRUs) and Community Health Centres (CHCs):

Percent adequately equipped (at least 60%) with:

- *Infrastructure* (INF) includes building, water, electricity, labour room, toilet facility, telephone, vehicle, staff quarters, etc.
- *Medical Staff* (STA) includes obstetrician/gynecologist, pediatrician and anesthetist,

- *Paramedical Staff* (STA) includes staff nurse, ANM, pharmacist, laboratory technician, PHN, health assistant male and female.
- *Supply* (SUP) includes tubal ring, set of standard surgiscal kits, emergency obstetric care kit, new born care kit, RTI/STI kits and delivery kit, and
- *Equipment* (EUP) includes equipment in operation theatre, cold chain equipment, Boyle's apparatus, shadow less lamp, oxygen cylinder, labour room equipment, Refrigerator, BP instrument, infant and adult weighing machine, etc.

In the case of Primary Health Centres (PHCs) similar data is taken into consideration with slight modifications. *Staff* includes here both medical and paramedical staff, whereas training aspect has been included. *Training* (TRA) includes at least one MO trained in sterilization, MTP, RCH integrated training and paramedical staff trained in the aspects of IUD insertion, checking BP, CDD/ORT, UIP, CSSM, RCH and ARI. Data related to all these facilities available at public health centres is provided in Table 1.

With regard to utilisation of maternal and child health care services the following indicators at the state level have been considered for analysis.

- % of women who received full ANC (at least 3 visits for ANC + at least one TT injection + 100 or more tablets) - *Fanc*
- % of women who utilised government health facility for antenatal care - *Ancg*
- % of women who delivered in government health institutions - *Delg*
- % of women who delivered in private health institutions - *Delp*
- % of women who had safe delivery (either institutional delivery or home delivery attended by Doctor/Nurse/TBA) - *Sdel*
- % of children age 12-35 months received full immunisation - *Cfimmu*

Table 1

Facilities Available in the First Referral Units (FRUs), Community Health Centres (CHCs) and Primary Health Centres (PHCs) Across the Major States of India, Facility Survey, 2002-2003

STATE	*% FRUS Adequately Equipped. (At Least 60%)*						*% CHCS Adequately Equipped (At Least 60%)*						*% PHCS Adequately Equipped (At Least 60%)*					
	INF	*STA*	*SUP*	*EQP*	*TRA*	*TNC*	*INF*	*STA*	*SUP*	*EQP*	*TRA*	*TNC*	*INF*	*STA*	*SUP*	*EQP*	*TRA*	*TNC*
Col. 1	2	3	4	5	6	7	8	9	10	11	12	13	14	15	16	17	18	19
Andhra Pradesh	78.3	28.3	28.3	20.0	80.5	120	75.7	7.1	12.9	5.7	82.9	70	59.2	88.4	40.3	84.5	84.5	380
Assam	60.0	40.0	40.0	40.0	40.0	30	38.5	12.8	35.9	17.7	7.7	39	21.0	35.2	50.0	32.4	29.7	290
Bihar	26.3	30.3	11.8	7.9	14.5	76	7.7	19.2	3.8	3.8	11.5	26	8.9	19.6	11.4	6.2	15.5	845
Chhattisgarh	66.1	10.2	39.0	35.6	61.0	59	43.3	0.0	33.0	17.5	48.5	97	2.8	26.3	14.1	8.8	3.8	320
Gujarat	84.3	15.7	7.8	36.3	68.6	102	76.6	1.8	2.7	29.7	58.6	111	89.0	85.7	83.4	80.6	17.1	356
Haryana	80.6	19.4	34.7	36.1	58.3	72	68.3	7.9	44.4	25.4	44.4	63	54.6	51.1	46.2	41.2	50.4	262
Himachal Pradesh	82.8	12.1	31.2	29.3	46.6	58	73.5	0.0	38.8	16.3	28.6	49	39.7	29.3	44.2	42.7	20.1	199
Jammu & Kashmir	78.9	49.1	31.6	24.6	80.7	57	59.1	31.8	13.6	4.5	63.3	22	31.4	31.4	28.6	40.3	30.3	290
Jharkhand	40.0	28.0	24.0	0.0	28.0	25	–	–	–	–	–	–	9.8	38.2	50.5	21.4	42.5	285
Karnataka	92.7	42.7	50.0	71.8	65.3	124	80.8	13.7	38.4	60.3	49.3	73	58.1	58.0	88.9	61.1	23.1	540
Kerala	91.7	66.7	8.3	83.3	75.0	12	61.5	15.4	76.9	38.5	30.8	13	42.9	91.4	55.7	34.3	18.6	70
Madhya Pradesh	73.9	27.9	69.2	40.0	65.5	165	50.6	5.0	62.1	22.8	47.2	180	10.0	35.4	32.0	26.2	11.4	628
Maharashtra	95.3	20.9	2.3	26.7	29.1	86	72.0	4.8	0.5	22.5	24.1	187	76.5	95.6	67.3	91.4	31.9	677
Orissa	66.7	69.3	52.6	41.2	58.8	114	50.6	54.0	65.5	28.7	42.5	87	3.2	0.2	3.5	15.1	13.4	595
Punjab	77.4	16.1	22.6	32.3	71.0	31	93.3	6.7	46.7	60.0	80.0	15	40.8	38.0	43.7	43.7	19.7	71
Rajasthan	75.8	42.4	19.7	44.7	65.2	132	66.5	16.2	16.8	35.1	49.2	191	33.2	25.6	69.2	53.9	14.8	671
Tamil Nadu	91.8	54.5	5.5	23.6	88.2	110	50.0	50.0	50.0	0.0	0.0	02	64.7	96.8	77.8	92.2	27.7	471
Uttar Pradesh	72.7	49.4	50.3	21.0	65.1	352	66.4	34.0	66.0	18.4	57.8	256	17.2	52.8	19.5	28.6	12.4	2081
Uttaranchal	81.5	51.9	48.1	14.8	77.8	27	68.4	36.8	68.4	10.5	73.7	19	27.8	68.1	23.6	27.1	7.6	144
West Bengal	84.7	28.2	61.2	17.6	50.6	85	42.2	1.2	47.5	12.0	3.6	83	12.0	5.7	23.0	8.6	9.1	209

Note: For the description of the Indicators provided in Cols. 2-6, 8-11 and 14-18 see the Section on Data and Methodology.
TNC = Total Number of Public Health Centres;
– = Data is not Available.

- % of women who had been visited by ANM/Health worker–*Anmhwvi*
- % of women who said health worker spent enough time with them–*Entime*
- % of women who satisfied with service/advice given by health worker–*Saadhw*
- % of women who utilised government health facility for treatment of pregnancy complications–*Tr.Pgcomg*
- % of women who utilised government health facility for treatment of delivery complications–*Tr.Delcomg*

Data related to all these indicators of maternal and child health care services for each state under consideration are provided in Table 3.

For the purpose of analysis and discussion, states have been ranked based on the facilities available and magnitudes of utilizing various maternal and child health care services. In the case of facilities available at different health centres, the ranks have been assigned for each type of facility and later pooled together and again ranked based on the pooled ranks so as to know the states that have better to poor facilities in public health centres. Later the ranks of facilities at each centre level have been pooled together and again ranked to have understanding of overall health facilities available in all public health centres together at the state level (Table 2). Similarly, ranks have been assigned to the states based the magnitudes of each and every indicator of maternal and child health care services on scale of better to poor level (Table 4). Finally, in order to see the association between facilities available at public health facilities and utilisation of maternal and child health services rank order correlation analysis is adopted and the results are presented in Table 5.

Results and Discussion

Ranking States Based on Facilities Available at Public Health Centres

Basic data and the ranking of major states based on the facilities available in different health centres (as provided in

Facility Survey, 2002-2003) are provided in Table 1 and 2, respectively. Ranking of major states based on all the facilities equipped at least 60 percent in First Referral Units (FRUs - Col. 2 of Table 2) reveal that the facilities in FRUs are much better in the states of Karnataka closely followed by Kerala, Orissa, Tamil Nadu and Uttaranchal, whereas such facilities are worst in Bihar followed by Jharkhand, Chattisgarh, Maharashtra and Himachal Pradesh. In the case of overall facilities available in Community Health Centres (CHCs - Col. 3 of Table 2), it can be seen that while Punjab is ranked as top most followed by Karnataka, Uttaranchal, Uttar Pradesh and Kerala, the Bihar ranked as the lowest followed by West Bengal, Chattisgarh, Assam and Maharashtra. Based on the overall ranking of all facilities at the Primary Health Centres (PHCs) of different states under consideration (Col. 4 of Table 2), it is interesting to note that Tamil Nadu ranked as number one followed by Maharashtra, Andhra Pradesh, Gujarat and Karnataka in the next four ranks. On the other hand, Chattisgarh ranked as the lowest in this regard followed by Orissa, Bihar, West Bengal and Madhya Pradesh. The ranks of other states in the case of each type of centres positioned in between these two extremes.

Information about the overall ranking of the states based on all facilities available in all public health facilities (FRUs, CHCs and PHCs together) is provided in Col. 4 of Table 2. From this ranking, it is evident that the public health centres are well equipped with different facilities in the state of Karnataka closely followed by Kerala, Tamil Nadu, Uttaranchal and Punjab, while Bihar placed at the bottom in these regard followed by Chattisgarh, West Bengal, Assam and Himachal Pradesh. The ranks of other states located in between these two extremes.

Ranking of States Based on the Utilisation of Different Maternal and Child Health Care Services

Data on utilisation of different maternal and child health care services at state level and ranking of states based on the magnitude of such services (as provided in DLHS-RCH, 2)

Table 2
Ranks of FRUs, CHCs and PHCs and all Public Health Facilities (PHFs) based on All Type of Facilities Available in Different Centers Across the Major States of India, Facility Survey, 2002-2003

State	*Ranks of All Facilities at FRUS*	*Ranks of All Facilities at CHCS*	*Ranks of All Facilities at PHCS*	*Ranks All Facilities at All PHFS*
Col. 1	*Col. 2*	*Col. 3*	*Col. 4*	*Col. 5*
Andhra Pradesh	15	10	3	8
Assam	12	16	12	13
Bihar	20	19	18	16
Chhattisgarh	18	17	20	15
Gujarat	11	9	4	10
Haryana	13	8	6	7
Himachal Pradesh	16	13	10	12
Jammu & Kashmir	7	12	12	9
Jharkhand	19	–	12	–
Karnataka	1	3	5	1
Kerala	2	5	7	2
Madhya Pradesh	6	11	16	10
Maharashtra	17	15	2	11
Orissa	3	6	19	8
Punjab	14	1	8	5
Rajasthan	8	7	9	6
Tamil Nadu	5	14	1	3
Uttar Pradesh	9	4	15	8
Uttaranchal	5	3	14	4
West Bengal	10	18	17	14

Note: Ranks assigned based on the pooled ranks of facilities available at different centres as well as among all public health facilities.
– =As data not available ranks have not been computed.

are provided in Tables 3 and 4, respectively. With a few exceptions, utilisation of different maternal health care services viz., antenatal and delivery care services, immunization to children, ANM visit to home, enough time spent by ANM, satisfaction with ANM visit, treatment taken for pregnancy complications and delivery complications is much better in the states of Tamil Nadu, Kerala, Maharashtra, Andhra Pradesh and Karnataka, whereas such services utilisation is very low in the states like Bihar closely followed Jharkhand, Chhattisgarh, Madhya Pradesh and Assam. The

Table 3
Utilization of Selected Maternal and Child Health Care Services Across the Major States of India, DLHS-RCH, 2002-2004

STATE	*Indicators of Women's Utilization of Maternal Health Care Services*										
	Fanc	*Ancg*	*Delg*	*Delp*	*Sdel*	*Cfimmu hwvi*	*Anm-Entime*	*hw*	*Saad – pgcomg*	*Tr. delcomg*	*Tr.*
Col. 1	2	3	4	5	6	7	8	9	10	11	12
Andhra Pradesh	43.6	32.9	22.1	38.8	69.0	62.9	13.2	87.5	90.6	72.8	66.2
Assam	9.6	33.8	13.9	12.9	33.2	19.3	3.1	54.0	84.0	39.9	42.1
Bihar	5.0	6.0	5.4	17.6	29.5	24.4	3.3	66.9	64.1	36.2	42.3
Chhattisgarh	11.6	32.7	9.6	10.6	29.1	60.9	5.6	86.3	93.2	43.5	40.6
Gujarat	25.7	23.2	12.7	39.5	62.1	57.7	12.8	84.4	88.3	54.3	55.3
Haryana	11.5	46.2	10.6	24.6	43.2	62.9	3.1	80.9	91.5	48.8	54.0
Himachal Pradesh	32.5	81.9	63.9	8.2	51.4	79.4	4.6	67.7	92.3	68.8	52.5
Jammu & Kashmir	41.5	67.3	55.9	14.6	73.1	38.6	3.0	76.1	89.9	81.0	83.1
Jharkhand	9.4	14.4	5.3	17.1	27.8	29.3	1.3	75.5	80.8	37.4	39.3
Karnataka	33.3	37.2	29.0	28.9	66.6	74.1	17.7	77.8	85.8	70.8	69.0
Kerala	73.6	34.3	40.5	57.3	98.3	81.2	12.2	83.0	89.7	76.7	72.0
Madhya Pradesh	5.7	28.3	17.6	10.6	35.5	32.5	5.4	72.8	80.8	39.9	35.7
Maharashtra	22.6	40.3	24.1	33.8	62.6	74.3	14.2	86.1	87.8	73.2	64.4
Orissa	14.8	45.6	25.6	8.7	43.5	65.1	5.5	59.8	81.9	42.5	42.0
Punjab	15.9	46.0	9.5	39.4	64.3	75.3	2.5	72.4	91.4	55.3	73.1
Rajasthan	5.0	38.7	19.4	12.0	44.4	25.4	10.2	59.6	85.9	46.3	40.0
Tamil Nadu	22.7	52.7	44.5	41.7	89.2	92.1	17.9	93.0	94.0	64.4	61.9
Uttar Pradesh	4.3	27.1	8.5	13.9	28.7	28.1	11.2	71.2	86.2	40.6	55.2
Uttaranchal	10.4	38.8	10.7	13.0	32.5	47.2	11.0	79.1	91.4	35.7	43.9
West Bengal	13.4	55.0	34.3	12.0	54.1	54.4	12.5	32.3	83.0	53.3	48.8

Note: For the description of the Indicators provided in Cols. 2-12, see the Section on Data and Methodology.

utilisation of such services is at a moderate level in other states under consideration.

Associations between Facilities Available in Public Health Centres and Utilisation of Maternal and Child Health Care Services

Rank order co-relations between facilities available in different public health centres and utilisation of various maternal health care services are presented in Table 5. On the whole, it can be seen that the rank order correlations are mostly in expected direction, but differentially across the facilities available in different public health centres under consideration. When taken into consideration all facilities in public health centres (Col. 5 of Table 5), it is conspicuous to note that the deliveries took place in private sector is positively and highly significantly correlated ($p<0.001$), which shows that in spite of facilities available at public sector, women prefer to have deliveries more in private sector. On the other hand, when it comes to treatment to delivery complications, more and more women appears to be visiting public health facilities ($p<0.01$). Likewise, the positive and moderate rank correlations have also been found in the case of facilities available in all health centres and women who had safe delivery as well as immunization to children ($p<0.05$). By and large, facilities available at FRUs and CHCs did not make much dent in utilizing maternal and child health services. But it is interesting to note that the rank order correlation between facilities available at FRUs and women delivered at institutions is positive and highly significant ($p<0.01$). Also is the case with regard to safe delivery and visit of ANM / HV to home, but to a lesser extent ($p<0.10$ in each case). Facilities available CHCs is observed to be positively correlated only with treatment taking for delivery complications ($p<0.10$).

It is conspicuous to note that almost all the indicators (except two) of utilisation of maternal and child health services under consideration are positively correlated (at different levels of significance) with the facilities available at PHCs.

Table 4
Ranking of States Based on the Utilisation of Different Maternal Health Care Services, DLHS-RCH, 2002-2004

STATE	*Fanc*	*Fucg*	*Delg*	*Delp*	*Sdel*	*Cfimmu*	*Annh-wvi*	*Entime*	*Saadhw*	*Tr. pgcom*	*Tr. delcom*
	Ranks Assigned to Indicators of Women's Utilization of Maternal Health Care Services										
Andhra Pradesh	2	14	9	5	4	9	4	2	7	4	5
Assam	15	13	12	14	15	20	17	19	15	18	14
Bihar	19	20	19	9	17	19	15	16	20	14	19
Chhattisgarh	12	15	16	18	18	10	11	3	2	16	20
Gujarat	6	18	13	3	8	11	5	5	10	9	8
Haryana	13	5	15	8	13	9	17	7	4	11	10
Himachal Pradesh	5	1	4	20	10	3	14	15	3	6	11
Jammu & Kashmir	3	2	1	11	3	14	18	10	8	1	1
Jharkhand	16	19	20	10	20	16	20	11	19	19	17
Karnataka	4	11	6	7	5	6	2	9	14	5	4
Kerala	1	12	3	1	1	2	7	6	9	2	3
Madhya Pradesh	17	16	11	18	14	15	13	12	19	18	18
Maharashtra	8	8	8	6	7	5	3	4	11	3	6
Orissa	10	7	7	19	12	7	12	17	17	13	5
Punjab	9	6	17	4	6	4	19	13	6	8	2
Rajasthan	19	10	10	16	11	18	10	18	13	12	16
Tamil Nadu	7	4	2	2	2	1	1	1	1	7	7
Uttar Pradesh	20	17	18	12	19	17	8	14	12	16	9
Uttaranchal	14	9	14	13	16	13	9	8	6	20	13
West Bengal	11	3	5	16	9	12	6	20	16	10	12

Note: Ranks assigned based on the magnitude of utilisation of various maternal health care services by women at state level.

Table 5
Rank Correlation Coefficients between the Facilities Available at Different Public Health Centres and Utilisation Maternal and Child Health Care Services Across the Major States of India, DLHS-RCH, 2002-2004

Indicators of Maternal and Child Health Care Services	*Facilities at FRUS*	*Facilities at CHCS*	*Facilities at PHCS*	*Facilities at All Public Health Centres*
Fanc	0.246	0.110	0.554**	0.350
Fancg	0.269	0.024	0.203	0.126
Delg	0.554**	-0.104	0.327	0.214
Delp	0.061	0.235	0.748***	0.567**
Sdel	0.417+	0.155	0.675***	0.511*
Cfimmu	0.220	0.229	0.538**	0.450*
Anmhwvi	0.383+	0.029	0.455*	0.361
Entime	0.005	0.066	0.572**	0.367
Saadhw	0.011	0.132	0.422+	0.300
Tr.pgcomg	0.155	0.024	0.625***	0.270
Tr.delcomg	0.322	0.423+	0.685***	0.561**

Note: +, *, ** and *** = Rank order correlation co-efficients are significant at 0.10, 0.05, 0.01 and 0.001 levels, respectively.

For instance, the rank order correlations between health facilities at PHCs and women who had full ANC ($p<0.01$), safe delivery ($p<0.001$), immunization of children ($p<0.01$), enough time spent by ANM/HV during home visit ($p<0.01$), treatment for pregnancy complications ($p<0.001$) and delivery complications ($p<0.001$) are in the positive direction. Conspicuously, as noted earlier, the correlation co-efficient between facilities in PHCs and women who had deliveries in private institutions is also highly significant in positive direction ($p<0.001$). Rank order correlation coefficients also turn out to be positively significant between the facilities in PHCs and ANM visit to home as well as women satisfied with service/advice given by health worker, but to a moderate ($p<0.05$) and lesser ($p<0.01$) extent only.

Summary and Implications

Among the major states of India, facilities available at various public health centres showed differential patterns. By and large, public health centres in the states of southern region viz., Karnataka, Kerala, Tamil Nadu and Andhra Pradesh, in addition to Uttaranchal, Maharashtra and Punjab are better placed in terms of facilities and equipment available, while Bihar placed at the bottom in these regard followed by Chattisgarh, West Bengal, Assam, Madhya Pradesh and Himachal Pradesh. With a few exceptions, utilisation of different maternal health care services viz., antenatal and delivery care services, immunization to children, ANM visit to home, enough time spent by ANM, satisfaction with ANM visit, treatment taken for pregnancy complications and delivery complications is much better in the states of Tamil Nadu, Kerala, Maharashtra, Andhra Pradesh and Karnataka, whereas such services utilisation is very low in the states like Bihar closely followed Jharkhand, Chhattisgarh, Madhya Pradesh and Assam. On of the whole, majority of the indicators of utilisation of maternal and child health care services are closely associated with facilities available at primary health centres, mostly in expected positive direction. The noteworthy unexpected phenomenon noticed here is that a positive and highly significant correlation between facilities available at public health centers in general and PHCs in particular, and institutional delivery.

These findings have some policy implications. Firstly, establishment of public health centres to a large extent with better facilities is very much in need. Of course, though the NRHM is rightly aimed in this direction, efforts have to be taken to implement the same with utmost care and commitment. Efforts are also should be taken to provide uniform infrastructure, filling up all staff positions, supply and training to staff, which are likely to motivate the women to make us of such services effectively. Provision of quality delivery care services at government health care facilities appear to be very much essential, which may be fulfilled by appointing the lady doctors especially obstetric and gynecology specialization and sufficient training to the staff.

Limitations

1. Data used in this paper is based on the macro level estimates (at state level) as provided by the DLHS-RCH, 2, which has some limitation.
2. Rank correlations have been performed, which is bivariate in nature, and has a limitation in interpreting the results.
3. Utlisation of maternal health care services would not only associated with the facilities available at public health centres, but also associated with the socio-economic background of the women, which have not been analysed here.

References

Do Mai (2008), "Antenatal Care Services Availability and Utilization in Rural Viet Nam", Asia-*Pacific Population Journal* 23 (1): 29-54

Glie, N. Goldman and G. Rodriguez (2003), "Utilization of Care during Pregnancy in Rural Guatemala: Does Obstetrical Need Matter?" *Social Science and Medicine* 57 (12): 2447-2463.

International Institute for Population Sciences (IIPS), (2005), *DLHS-RCH, 2002-2004 Data CD*. Mumbai: IIPS.

International Institute for Population Sciences (IIPS), Mumbai, (2006), *District Level Household Survey (DLHS-2, 2002-2004: India)*. Mumbai: IIPS.

Stephenson, Rob and Amy O. Tsui (2002), "Contextual Influences on Reproductive Health Service Use in Uttar Pradesh, India", *Studies in Family Planning* 33 (4): 309-320.

7

Health Problems during Pregnancy and Health Seeking Behaviour among Married Women in Uttar Pradesh

Shilpi Tiwari, Girish Chandra Tripathi

Introduction

Health is multidimensional and holistic, embracing all aspects of Individual and collective existence. A healthy person is one who enjoys a harmonious existence within himself and within his social context. World health organization (WHO) constitution defines health as a state of complete physical, mental, and social wellbeing and not merely the absence of disease or infirmity (WHO 1992). Although, this definition is a fine inspiring concept and its pursuit guarantees health professionals unlimited opportunities to carry out work in future, it may not be of much practical relevanance (Doll, 1992) and it seems to work against its effective functioning (Saracci, 1997).In the Indian epic Mahabharata, a woman was always blessed as "*sau putravati bhabah*" (be the mother of hundred sons), because in those days the prime role of women was childbearing. The situation has not changed much since then as till date in many parts of India, mainly rural areas, the main role assigned to her is that of a child bearer. Thus pregnancy is one of the most important events in life of an

Indian woman. While glancing at data show that over the last two decades the fertility rate in India has considerably declined but a closer look confirms that in some of the states, for example in Uttar Pradesh, the results are not satisfactory. This implies that women in such areas experience repeated pregnancies taxing their health. In Uttar Pradesh it is a common feature in most of the households for women to bear the major chunk of the household chores. However, this work is not supplemented by proper diet due to gender bias against the situation does not change even during pregnancy thus leading to various problems during pregnancy.

In rural areas the picture is worse as owing to agricultural economy women also help in the fields apart from performing the household chores. This accompanied by malnutrition is responsible for various problems during pregnancy. Other than nutrition another important factor influencing the health of women during pregnancy is her health-seeking behaviour, especially antenatal checkups. Antenatal care (ANC) refers to pregnancy-related health care provided by a doctor or a health worker in a medical facility or at home. A review of literature shows that women who do not avail of antenatal care are more likely to suffer from problems during pregnancy. However, the health-seeking behaviour of women is again the function of the interplay between various socio-economic conditions including caste, place of residence, education level of both woman and her husband, work status of woman and standard of living. This paper therefore attempts to analyze the problems during pregnancy among married women in Uttar Pradesh and also tries to examine the health-seeking behaviour among these women against certain socio-economic backgrounds. The data used in the analysis is obtained fro m National Family Health Survey (NFHS) 2, 1998-99.

Objectives

The main objectives of the paper are as follows:

1. To analyze the pattern of problems during pregnancy among married women in Uttar Pradesh.

2. To examine the influence of antenatal care on pregnancy problems.

Data and Methodology

Data were collected from National Family Health Survey-2 (NFHS-2). For the present paper women who gave live birth during the three years preceding the survey (1996-98) have been considered and pregnancy problem during recent birth is taken into account. There were 3759 women data has been analysed for the present study. NFHS-2 has identified seven problems during pregnancy-: night blindness, blurred vision, convulsions (not from fever), swelling (of the legs, body or face), excessive fatigue, anaemia and vaginal bleeding. These problems are based on woman's self report and are not clinically tested. Hence the results are to be interpreted with care. Night blindness, i.e., difficulty seeing at dusk is the result of chronic Vitamin A deficiency and is often seen in pregnant women in areas where Vitamin A deficiency is endemic. Blurred vision is also caused by deficiency of Vitamin A. Anaemia is one of the major problems faced by most of the Indian women. It is characterized by a low level of hemoglobin in the blood and usually results from a nutritional deficiency of iron, folate, Vitamin B12 or some other nutrients. Another problem reported is convulsion, which results from toxemia and other physiological problems. If it is accompanied by signs of hypertension it can be symptomatic of eclampsia, a potentially fatal condition. However, a combined outcome of toxemia, anaemia and malnutrition is swelling of legs, body or face. Similarly if a pregnant woman suffers from malnutrition accompanied by overwork she experiences excessive fatigue. Vaginal bleeding, unlike the other above-mentioned problems, results from release of secretions from glands and also might be due to certain infections. Thus, all these problems are related to the nutritional status of the woman during pregnancy.

Results

Percentage of women expressing "excessive fatigue" during pregnancy (Fig 1) found to be high among married women in

Uttar Pradesh. Figure 1 shows the distribution of problems during pregnancy in Uttar Pradesh. Thus, it is seen that most of the problems experienced by pregnant women are the outcome of Vitamin deficiency and malnutrition. As mentioned in the patriarchal Indian society women bear the major burden of the household chores and it is not compensated with balanced diet. Even during pregnancy she is not given any concession from the household work and there is hardly any improvement in her diet. Thus in most of the cases she is malnourished and is overexerted, which worsens her condition during pregnancy.

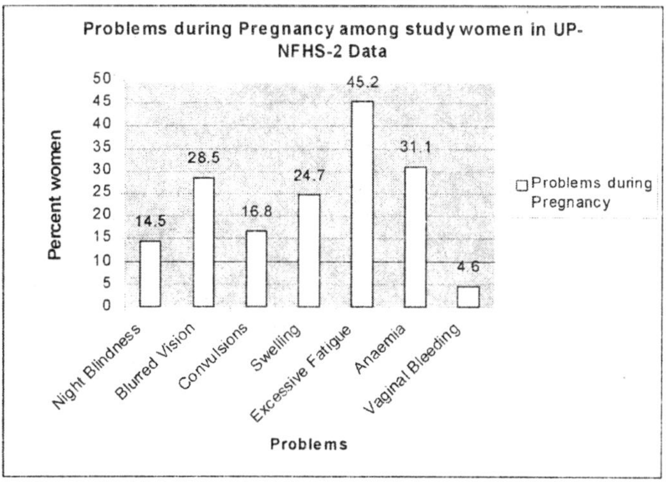

Fig. 1: Problems During Pregnancy Among Study Women in UP-NFHS-2 Data

Anaemia is another major problem during pregnancy and 31.1 per cent women in Uttar Pradesh report it. A woman should consume sufficient quantity of liver, green leafy vegetables, Vitamin B11 and folic acid to prevent anaemia. But her food basket often does not contain such items. Women in India have so much internalized the patriarchal system that even in matters related to food she does not have her own preferences. Therefore, in a household not much attention is given to the food consumption pattern of women from her childhood. As a girl child she is discriminated against her male siblings in share of food and often has to be satisfied with what she gets after the male members (father and brother(s)) have had their share. After marriage her fate does not improve as she usually gives preference to her husband's choice. When she becomes a mother and is in-charge of the household, by tradition she prioritizes her husband and male children in matters of share and liking of food and hence the trend continues. As a result it leaves a woman malnourished and anaemic. Considering the anaemic nature of Indian women Government of India recommends a dose of 100 iron and folic acid tablets is prescribed during pregnancy. But this dosage has its own shortcomings. One of the main side effects of such tablets is it causes acidity. 28.5 per cent of the women suffer from blurred vision and 14.5 per cent experience night blindness during pregnancy in Uttar Pradesh. As discussed earlier malpractice in food intake of woman prevents her from consuming sufficient Vitamin A through various food products (butter, egg yolk, liver, milk, carrots, leafy green vegetables, fish liver oil). The other problems that are significant among pregnant women in Uttar Pradesh are swelling of legs, body or face (24.7 per cent) and convulsions not from fever (16.8 per cent). However, vaginal bleeding does not seem to be a common problem among these women as it is reported by only 4.6 per cent. Birth weight of the child is often used as a proxy variable to measure the nutritional status of the mother. In the present study more than 85 per cent of the children were not weighed after birth and therefore, this variable could not be used in the analysis.

Nutritional Status of Women

A widely used indicator of nutritional status is the body mass index (BMI), which is defined as the weight in kilograms divided by the height in metres squared (Kg/m^2) this indicator is used to assess both thinness and obesity. It is helpful in detecting the risk of health and nutritional disorders. A BMI of less than 18.5 indicates chronic energy deficiency (CED). Chronic energy deficiency refers to an intake of energy less than the requirement for a period of several months or years.

At the other end of the spectrum, women with a BMI of 25.0-29.9 are considered to be overweight and those with BMI of 30.0 or above are identified as obese. Table 1 shows the percentage of ever married women in the age group 15-49 in Uttar Pradesh who has a chronic energy deficiency and the percentage that are overweight or obese.

Table 1
Percentage Ever Married 15-49 Age Group Women in Uttar Pradesh with Percentage Chronic Energy Deficiency and Over-weight by Background Characteristics

Background Characteristic	*Percentage with BMI below 18.5 Kg/m²*	*Percentage with BMI of 25.0 Kg/m² or More*	*Number of Women*
Age			
15-19	46.8	2.1	5,877
20-29	38.1	6.8	12,379
30-39	31.0	13.5	15,041
40-49	26.4	17.4	13,547
Residence			
Urban	25.0	17.4	20,330
Rural	40.6	6.2	55,940
Education			
Illiterate	41.7	5.9	43,989
Literate, < Middle school complete	37.2	8.6	15,086
Middle school complete	34.1	10.7	6,295
High school complete and above	35.0	10.9	10,891
Standard of living indexLow	51.5	1.6	24,414
Medium	38.2	6.5	35,282
High	18.2	22	15,727
Total	35.6	9.8	76,270

Source: NFHS - 2, 1998-99.

More than one third of women (36 percent) have a chronic energy deficiency. CED is particularly pronounced for rural women, illiterate women and women living in household with a low standard of living. Higher than average levels of CED also observed in women 15-29 years of age. Among the states that the level of CED are highest in Orrisa (41 percent) and West Bengal (39 percent), followed by Maharashtra (36 percent), Bihar (45 percent).women who consume milk or curd everyday are less likely than other women to have CED, even after the household's standard of living is controlled for (Data not shown). Similarly women who eat While the focus of attention in the field of nutrition continues to be on the substantial proportion of women with a chronic energy deficiency, the NFHS-2 findings on the percentage of overweight and obese women clearly demonstrate that this problem cannot be ignored. This phenomenon is becoming a well recognized aspect of the nutrition transition, with changes in dietary patterns and levels of physical activity leading to an increase in overweight and obesity. The substantial proportion of overweight or obese persons, together with continuing high overall levels of under nutrition produces a dual burden of nutritional disorders for the country.

Influence of Socio-economic Characteristics on Pregnancy Complications

It has been highlighted in the above discussion that most of the health problems experienced by pregnant women in Uttar Pradesh are mainly due to her nutritional status and to some extent they are because of physiological reasons. Nutritional status of woman is influenced by her socio-economic backgrounds while certain demographic factors influence the physiological problems. Therefore a set of such variables are considered and problems during pregnancy are analyzed against these variables for a better understanding. The demographic variables include age of mother at time of childbirth, birth order of the child and birth interval with the preceding child. Among the socio-economic variables are considered place of residence of the woman, her religion and caste, educational status of woman, woman's work status, standard of living of the household and woman's exposure to mass-media. The influences of socio-economic characteristics on pregnancy problems are shown in Table 2. Maternal age affects the frequency of complications during pregnancy and childbirth (Pebley et al., 1996). This is so because the woman's age may be related to her attitude about health care provisions. Young women who become pregnant are often at risk of obstructed labour if they have not yet grown to their full height or pelvic size. Obstructed labour causes death when adequate emergency obstetric care is unavailable. Also young women are more likely to suffer from eclampsia, which can be life-threatening to mother and baby. Pregnancies at older ages are not free from complications. The health risks of childbearing increase after age 39. From the table it is seen that across age groups excessive fatigue and anaemia are the two major problems women experience during pregnancy. However, these problems are more acute for women in the older age groups. This is because older women may have accumulated various health problems during their lives, such as, hypertension and diabetes, which can cause problems during pregnancy.

Birth order of the child also influences problems during pregnancy. The high birth orders (birth order of four and above) of the child takes a heavy toll on the mother's health. It is noticed from the table that 50.2 per cent of the women with high birth order experiences excessive fatigue during pregnancy and about 34 per cent of them suffer from anaemia and blurred vision. Moreover, the proportion of such women suffering from swelling (28 per cent) and convulsions (20 per cent) are also high. Apart from birth order it is also the interval between two births that exert a great influence on the woman's health. A review of literature suggests that if the birth interval between two births is shorter than 24 months then it has a negative impact on the health of the woman, especially during pregnancy. This fact is proved from the analysis, which shows that women with shorter birth intervals (less than 24 months) are more likely to suffer from various problems during pregnancy. It is so because these women do not get proper time to recover from the strains of the previous pregnancy and hence fall easy victims to problems such as

Table 2
Percentage Distribution of Pregnancy Complications According to Socio-economic Background of Women, Uttar Pradesh, NFHS-2 Data

	Pregnancy Complications						
Background Characteristics	*Night blindness Excessive fatigue*	*Blurred Vision*	*Convul-sions*	*Swelling*	*Excessive fatigue*	*Anemia*	*Vaginal Bleeding*
Age of Mother							
< 24	14.1	26.4	16.3	22.5	43.2	29.4	4.5
25 - 34	14.2	29.2	16.9	26.5	46.9	31.4	4.6
35 +	17.5	34.6	18.3	27.1	46.6	37.3	4.6
Birth Order							
Less than 4	12.4	24.4	14.6	22.5	41.8	28.7	4.3
4 and more	17.5	34.4	20.0	28.0	50.2	34.5	5.0
Birth Interval							
< 24 months	14.5	33.0	17.7	26.2	46.2	31.5	5.8
24 months & more	16.1	29.9	17.4	25.5	49.5	32.2	4.5
Residence							
Rural	15.7	28.5	17.3	23.9	44.5	30.9	4.6
Urban	8.3	28.8	14.1	29.0	49.3	32.1	4.6
Education							
Illiterate	16.4	30.0	17.3	25.1	44.0	29.9	4.5
Primary	14.1	30.3	18.3	25.4	47.7	35.2	6.1
Middle	11.8	26.3	14.9	19.6	49.8	33.7	5.1
High School+	3.4	17.5	12.5	25.1	48.3	33.2	2.9
Work Status							
Working	20.4	29.6	19.1	26.1	45.5	33.8	5.8
Not working	13.1	28.3	16.2	24.4	45.2	30.4	4.3
Std. Of Living							
Low	19.1	30.2	18.7	25.7	43.2	30.9	5.3
Medium	13.4	28.6	16.2	23.9	4 4.7	31.7	4.1
High	7.5	24.0	14.5	25.7	52.5	29.5	5.1

excessive fatigue and swelling in the following pregnancy. Place of residence also bears an impact on a woman's health status during pregnancy. Nonetheless, the pattern of problems during pregnancy does not vary with place of residence. Excessive fatigue and anaemia are the two major problems that women experience during pregnancy irrespective of place of residence. Interestingly the proportion of urban women experiencing pregnancy problems are more compared to their rural counterparts. A plausible cause for such situation is that in urban areas due to more awareness of health women's reporting of their problems is better. Educational level of woman is another vital factor whose influence on pregnancy cannot be overemphasized. Educated women are more aware about the problems that might occur during pregnancy and they are in a better position to take care of such problems.

The Table 2 reveals some of interesting results as the educated women are more likely to experience excessive fatigue and anaemia compared to their illiterate counterparts. This is perhaps because of the fact that most of these women might be engaged in economic activities outside the house, which demands a considerable amount of their time and energy and prevent them from taking adequate rest. Another reason might be that women being more conscious about their health reporting of their health might be better. But with an increase in educational level of women there is a decrease in their proportion suffering from night blindness and blurred vision. There is a positive relationship between education of women and standard of living of the household. Since these educated women belong to higher income households their diet is generally better. Though very less proportion of women reported vaginal bleeding during pregnancy there is an inverse relationship with level of education. Economic independence of women is one of the pre-requisite of women's empowerment that increases her decision making power in the family and enhances her position in the household. The nature of women's work bears an impact on their health status. If women are engaged in work that requires professional skill and educational qualifications then they have higher chances of interacting with the outside world and are therefore more aware about their health problems and its precautions. In Uttar Pradesh, most of the women work as agricultural labourer and it does not require any educational skill and hence does not widen their outlook rather it has an adverse effect on their health as their strenuous work is not supplemented with proper diet leaving them malnourished and prey to various problems during pregnancy.

The household's standard of living is used as a proxy variable to determine the income of the household. With an improvement in the economic status of the household there is also an improvement in the nutritional status of women and it has a positive effect on her health, especially during pregnancy. The figures also confirm to this association. There is an overall decrease in the proportion of women suffering from various problems during pregnancy as the standard of living increases. In addition there is little variation in case of excessive fatigue, which tends to rise with an increase in the standard of living. The reason for this is not clear. To summarize, it is observed that irrespective of socio-economic backgrounds, excessive fatigue and anaemia continues to be two major problems during pregnancy among women in Uttar Pradesh. But in general, lower age of mother, lower birth order, longer birth interval coupled with higher education of women, urban residence and higher standard of living of household act in favour of improving health of women during pregnancy.

Health-seeking Behaviour Among Pregnant Women in Uttar Pradesh

After having analyzed the pattern of health problems among pregnant women in Uttar Pradesh the health-seeking behaviour of these women during pregnancy are examined. For this purpose their utilization of antenatal care (ANC) services has been selected. ANC is one of the four most important pillars of safe motherhood along with family planning, safe delivery and essential obstetric care (WHO 1996). The Safe Motherhood Initiative proclaims that all pregnant women must receive basic, professional antenatal care. The package of ANC apart from physical treatment of checking, vaccinations and prescribing medicines also includes dietary advice and counseling on safe motherhood. Women receiving proper ANC are assured of undergoing safe pregnancies without posing much risk to the life of both mother and child. A woman may receive ANC either from a health worker visiting at home or from clinic. The Reproductive and

Child Health Programme recommends that as part of antenatal care, women receive two doses of tetanus toxoid vaccine, adequate amounts of iron and folic acid tablets or syrup to prevent and treat anaemia, and at least three antenatal check-ups that include blood pressure checks and other procedures to detect pregnancy complications (Ministry of Health and Family Welfare, 1997). The health-seeking behaviour varies according to source of ANC and is hence examined separately. In Uttar Pradesh according to NFHS-2 only 34.6 per cent of women receive any type of ANC and this figure is the lowest in the country. Table 3 shows the influence of ANC coverage on problems during pregnancy. It is noticed from the table that women are more likely to experience problems during pregnancy if they have not received any type of ANC checkups. The proportion of women suffering from various problems during pregnancy is very low if a health worker visits them during pregnancy for ANC checkups. But there is an increase in the proportion of women experiencing problems during pregnancy if they receive ANC from a clinic. When a woman visits a clinic for ANC she might not feel free to discuss all her problems if there is a male doctor. On the other hand when a health worker (who is always a lady) visits her at home she perhaps develops a rapport with the health worker and takes her into confidence to discuss all her problems. This might be one of the reasons explaining the drastic change in proportion of women suffering from pregnancy problems if they receive ANC from different sources. Moreover, a member of the family (mainly some member from her in-laws) generally accompanies a woman when she goes to a clinic for ANC checkups. This perhaps prevents her from discussing all her problems with the doctor. If she complaints too much about her health it might portray her weak health to the in-laws and in turn it might hamper her status in the household, especially in a state like Uttar Pradesh where society is not very liberal. In order to avoid such a situation she might prefer not to disclose her problems to the doctor. However, not much change is noticed in the figures of pregnancy problems if women have had any type of ANC checkups (it includes either by health worker or visiting a clinic).

When we analyse the pattern of pregnancy problems according to source of ANC it is observed that if health worker does not visit women they are more prone to suffer from anaemia and excessive fatigue, though for all problems figures exceed 90 per cent. More women suffer from night blindness, blurred vision and convulsions if they do not visit a clinic for ANC checkups. The scenario remains the same (though the figures change) if a woman does not receive ANC from either of the sources. Thus in brief it might be stated that ANC plays an important role in improving the health of women during pregnancy. Apart from these above mentioned criteria health-seeking behaviour of these women are also influenced to a large extent by the socio-economic and demographic variables, respectively. Grover et al (2001) observe that with increasing age proportion of women receiving antenatal care (ANC) services during pregnancy declines. It is due to the fact that over time there has been an increase in realization of importance of ANC services along with improvement in availability of ANC services. The younger women today are at an advantageous position in contrast to the older women, who had their last pregnancy, some time back, and had lesser access to ANC services and were less aware of their availability. Place of residence influences spousal communication, and exposure to mass media, which in turn increase women's awareness and likelihood of availing ANC services. In India the proportion of urban women utilizing the maternal care services is more than two-times as compared to rural women (Govindasamy and Ramesh, 1997). This is because the urban women are at a beneficial position regarding accessibility to the maternal care services. There exist a social distance between the caste groups and the lower castes cannot avail of the health care services (Kopparty, 1991). Grover et al. (2001) have concluded that higher the caste status (scheduled castes as against OBC and higher castes) of women improves, there is an increase in the proportion of women receiving the package of medical checkups and tetanus toxoid injections and iron folic tablets during pregnancy.

Govindasamy and Ramesh (1997) observe that women of lower castes are less likely to avail of the maternal care services compared with the higher caste women. This is mainly because caste status influences the educational status of women and their attitude about health care provisions. When the influences of other intervening factors are controlled, education emerges as the single most important determinant of maternal health care utilization in India (Govindasamy and Ramesh 1997). Educated women with at least middle schooling are nearly eight times as likely to receive antenatal care for their births as illiterate women and literate women with less than middle schooling are more than three times likely. The pattern is similar for utilization of the other maternal care services. Education increases ANC awareness and brings about changes in health seeking behaviour for better.

Conclusions

In Uttar Pradesh a majority of women experience various problems during pregnancy and in most of the cases they suffer from more than one problem. These problems are usually related to nutritional deficiencies, which results from women's low status in the household along with her poor socio-economic backgrounds. The study also reveals that religion plays a vital role in influencing the woman's health problems during pregnancy. From this study it can be concluded that the health-seeking behaviour of women has an important influence on problems experienced during pregnancy. Therefore, attention should be given to improve the ANC coverage by health workers, especially in a state like Uttar Pradesh, which records the lowest ANC coverage in India. But ANC coverage alone cannot reduce the plight of pregnant women. The status of women has to improve so that they are not discriminated against in matters of food. It should be realized that women should not be looked upon only as potential mothers rather she should be given all opportunities to grow up as a healthy child and then develop to a healthy adult. Then only can she become a healthy mother capable to bear a healthy child. This requires change in the attitude of the whole society.

References

Doll, R. (1992), "Health and the Environment in the 1990's", *American Journal of Public Health* 82: 933-941.

Govindasamy, Pallavi and B. M. Ramesh (1997), *Maternal Education and Utilization of Maternal and Child Health Services in India.* National Family Health Survey Subject Reports, No.5, Mumbai: IIPS.

Government of India (1997), *Report of the Sub-committee on Reproductive Health Research Needs Assessment (RHRNA).* New Delhi: National Committee on Research in Human Reproduction, India Ministry of Health and Family Welfare.

– –(1997), *Reproductive and Child Health Program: Scheme for Implementation.* New Delhi: Ministry of Family Welfare, Department of Family Welfare.

Grover, Deepak, Reena Singh, Keshav C. Kaishtha, Rita Gawari, Sawarn Singh, and Gurrdarshan Singh (2001), "RCH- the Role of ANM", Paper presented at *24th Annual Conference of IASP,* Visakhapatnam.

International Institute of Population Sciences (2000), *National Family Health Survey-2, Key Findings, (1998-99).* Mumbai: IIPS.

Kopparty, S.N.M. (1991), "Caste and Utilisation of Health Resources", *Eastern Anthropologist* 21(4): 365-84.

Pebley, Anne R., Noreen Goldman, and German Rodriguez (1996), "Prenatal and Delivery Care and Childhood Immunization in Guetemala: Do Family and Community Matter?", *Demography* 33(2): 231-246.

Saracci, Rodolfo (1997), "The World Health Organization Needs to Reconsider Its Definition of Health", *British Medical Journal* 314: 1409-10.

World Health Organization (1992), *Basic Document,* Geneva: WHO.

World Health Organization (1996), *Regional Health Report, 1996.* New Delhi: WHO Regional office for South East Asia. .

8

Does Illiteracy Increases Reproductive Tract Infections Among Women in a Slum Setting of Greater Mumbai?

V. M. Sarode

Introduction

Absence of reproductive tract infections (RTIs) is essential for a healthy life for both women and men and is critical for their ability to meet their reproductive goals. There are three different types of reproductive tract infections for women: endogenous infections that are caused by the multiplying of organisms normally present in the vagina; iatrogenic infections caused by the introduction of bacteria or other infection-causing micro-organisms through medical procedures such as an IUD insertion; and sexually transmitted infections (STIs). Endogenous infections and several of the iatrogenic and sexually transmitted infections are often easily cured if detected early and given proper treatment. If left untreated, RTIs can cause pregnancy-related complications, congenital infections, infertility, and chronic pain. They are also a risk factor for pelvic inflammatory disease and HIV (Population Council, 1999). This paper focuses on reproductive tract infections and discusses the awareness of reproductive health of women in slums, RTIs and its prevalence. This paper also discusses the health personnel's visits to the respondents.

A community-based study was carried out (Monika et al., 2007; Kamal et al., 2004) to assess the prevalence of reproductive tract infections (RTIs) among ever married rural women aged 15 -45 years at village Naila during 2002. At least one symptom related to RTIs was found in 55 percent sample women. Out of 263 clinically examined, 43 percent had cervicitis, 26 percent had bacterial vaginitis, 14 percent had fungal infection, 8 peercent had trichomonas vaginitis, 22 percent had pelvic inflammatory disease and 19 percent had cervical erosion. Prevalence of RTI was significantly associated with age, personal hygiene, material used for menstrual blood, gravida status, type of attendance at child birth, invasive contraceptives, gynaecological surgery but caste, literacy status and place of deliveries were not significantly associated with RTI status in the study.

A study carried out by Srivastava et al. (2004) with an aim to find out perception of women about Reproductive Tract Infection and comparison was done in rural. The results revealed that the perception about Reproductive Tract Infection was responded correctly by 74.78 percent in urban, 28.69 percent in rural and 45.22 in urban slum women and difference was found to be significant ($P<0.05$) in all three areas. The occurrence of vaginal discharge was found 54.78 percent in rural 43.48 percent in urban and 43.48 percent in urban slums.

Syndrome approach was used (Singh et al., 2001; Phanindra and Prakasam, 1998; Sarode, 2007) to identify reproductive tract infections (RTIs) by a trained public health nurse among 130 ever-married women aged 15-45 years in a resettlement colony, Chandigarh and observed that majority of women suffering from vaginitis (52.1 percent), followed by cervicitis, pelvic inflammatory disease and urinary tract infections.

Large survey data analysis (NFHS-2) carried out by Prakasam (2004) revealed that at least 31.4 percent women suffer from one or the more complications of reproductive health. Analysis shows that reproductive morbidity problems were found to be more for the study women in Andhra

Pradesh than in Tamil Nadu. Similarly the women who delivered within 14 years of age and got married over 14 years of age were found to have higher odds than reference category in reporting RTI problems.

In slums of Bangalore, it was observed that every fourth person (The Times of India, 2003) was contracted with sexually transmitted disease (STD) or reproductive tract infection (KSAPS). Some 24.5 per cent of slum-dwellers, who attended the camp, suffer from STD and RTI. Among women, it was 26.3 per cent and men 17.3 percent. Ulcers, discharge, wound, infection and pain in reproductive tract were the symptoms of the diseases. One of the reasons for poor reproductive health condition found to be poverty unaware of the existing health facilities available in the area.

Objectives

Keeping above points in view an attempt was made with the following objectives:

(i) To study the perception about reproductive tract infection among reproductive women in the age group 15-49 in a slum community in Greater Mumbai.

(ii) Utilization of health services available in the study area by the women.

Data and Methodology

For the present investigation, two stage sampling procedure has been adopted. In the first stage, the slums in the Greater Mumbai according to their population size were listed using the "Directory of Slums" published by office of the additional collector (ENC), Mumbai and Mumbai Sub-District Two lists were prepared, one for plain area slums and other for hilly area slums. From plain area slum list, one slum was selected at random. This plain area slum was Rafi Nagar slum located at Deonar, Mumbai which comes under M-ward of Brihan Mumbai Municipal Corporation. The populations of this slum (study area) were 5000 respectively.

In the second stage of sampling, from this selected slum area, using cluster sampling, two clusters were selected at random. From these two clusters of Rafi Nagar slum area 433 households were selected, thus represents slum population in Greater Mumbai. This survey was conducted from June to August, 2005.In the survey, the data were collected from the study women on some common symptoms of RTIs, namely problems with abnormal vaginal discharge, urinary tract infections and intercourse-related pain in the three months preceding the survey. Specifically, the prevalence of reproductive health problems among currently married women is estimated from women's self-reported experience with each of the following problems: vaginal discharge accompanied by itching, by irritation around the vaginal area, by bad odour, by severe lower abdominal pain, or by any other problem; pain or burning while urinating; and painful intercourse. The study Women who experience one or more of these reproductive health problems could either have or be at risk of getting an RTI/STI. However, since information on health problems is based on self reports rather than clinical tests or examinations, the results were interpreted with caution.

Results

Reproductive Health Problems of Study Women in Slum

The prevalence of different reproductive health problems among women in slum area (Table 1) by education level of women shows that three percent of the study women reported at least one type of problem related to vaginal discharge, and 15 percent of the study women reported symptoms of a urinary tract infection. Overall, 18 percent study women reported either problems with vaginal discharge or symptoms of a urinary tract infection. Pus in urine was 10 percent in among the study women. Among problems related to vaginal discharge, itching or irritation was mentioned most frequently (17 percent) in Rafi nagar slum area, followed by severe lower abdominal pain (29 percent), and bad odour (23 percent). Low

Table 1

Percentage of Women Reporting Reproductive Health Problems Across their Education, in a Slum (Rafi Nagar), Mumbai

Reproductive Health Problems		*Education of Women*							
		Illiterate		1- 6 Std.		> 6 Std.		Total	
White Discharge	Yes	141	(49.5)	35	(48.6)	30	(39.5)	206	(47.6)
	No	144	(50.5)	37	(51.4)	46	(60.5)	227	(52.4)
Abnormal Vaginal Discharge	Yes	11	(3.9)	1	(1.4)	1	(1.3)	13	(3.0)
	No	274	(96.1)	71	(98.6)	75	(98.7)	420	(97.0)
Itching around Vagina	Yes	50	(17.5)	13	(18.1)	12	(15.8)	75	(17.3)
	No	235	(82.5)	59	(81.9)	64	(84.2)	358	(82.7)
Pain in Lower Abdomen	Yes	83	(29.1)	20	(27.8)	22	(28.9)	125	(28.9)
	No	202	(70.9)	52	(72.2)	54	(71.1)	308	(71.1)
Pain during Abdomen	Yes	24	(8.4)	5	(6.9)	4	(5.3)	33	(7.6)
	No	261	(91.6)	67	(93.1)	72	(94.7)	400	(92.4)
Frequent Urination	Yes	43	(15.1)	7	(9.7)	14	(18.4)	64	(14.8)
	No	242	(84.9)	65	(90.3)	62	(81.6)	369	(85.2)
Genital Ulcer/Rash	Yes	42	(14.7)	7	(9.7)	14	(18.4)	63	(14.5)
	No	243	(85.3)	65	(90.3)	62	(81.6)	370	(85.5)
Pain during Intercourse	Yes	31	(10.9)	7	(9.7)	7	(9.2)	45	(10.4)
	No	254	(89.1)	65	(90.3)	69	(90.8)	388	(89.6)
Low backache	Yes	148	(51.9)	29	(40.3)	41	(53.9)	218	(50.3)
	No	137	(48.1)	43	(59.7)	35	(46.1)	215	(49.7)
Foul Smelling	Yes	72	(25.3)	14	(19.4)	14	(18.4)	100	(23.1)
	No	213	(74.7)	58	(80.6)	62	(81.6)	333	(76.9)
Pus in Urine	Yes	34	(11.9)	6	(8.3)	4	(5.3)	44	(10.2)
	No	251	(88.1)	66	(91.7)	72	(94.7)	389	(89.8)

backache was 50 percent reported by the respondents of Rafi nagar slum area. Ten percent reported painful intercourse in Rafi nagar slum area.

From the Table 1 it was evident that reproductive were found maximum among the illiterate women except fequent Urination and Genital ulcer/rash when compared with women having education up to 6th standard and women having education more than 6th standard. Thus it can be concluded that the illiterate women suffer more due to reproductive health problems compared with the literate women.

Table 2 shows that about 65 per cent of study women in Rafi Nagar slum have delayed in reporting the RTI symptoms. Sixty five percent of respondents from the area had given opinion that they were not serious where as sixty eight percent of illiterate women compared with the other two categories of education were the maximum and were not serious about reporting of their RTI problems to the health personnel.

Fifty eight percent of study women from Rafi nagar slum area had taken treatment from government health facility, where as 13 percent have taken treatment from private health facility and 28 percent did not go for treatment where as 38 percent of illiterate women did not go for treatment at all. Seventy two percent from Rafi nagar slum area were not found satisfactory with the treatment availed where as only 68 percent of illiterate women satisfactory with the treatment availed.

A reason was asked, for not availing treatment, 42 percent of study women from Rafi nagar slum area told that they were not serious about the gravity of problems. Thirty three percent of study women from Rafi nagar slum area told that they felt shy to talk about the problems. Twenty four percent of study women told that they had no money for treatment. Thus it can be concluded that the respondents of Rafi nagar slum area did not availed treatment.

The opinion of the respondents were taken about development of this problem, 64 percent of study women from Rafi nagar slum area told that they had unclean delivery

Table 2
Percentage of Women Reporting Reasons for Delay in Reporting, Treatment Availed, Reasons for Not Availing Treatment and the Development of RTI in Rafi Nagar Slum, Mumbai

Opinion	*Education of Women*			
	Illiterate	*1-6 std*	*>6 std*	*Total*
Have You Delayed in Reporting these Problems?				
Yes	139 (65.0)	32 (68.1)	37 (62.7)	208 (65.0)
No	75 (35.0)	15 (31.9)	22 (37.3)	112 (35.0)
If Yes, Do You Feel that these Problems are not Serious?				
Yes	95 (68.3)	19 (59.4)	22 (59.5)	136 (65.4)
No	44 (31.7)	13 (40.6)	15(40.5)	72 (34.6)
Where Did You Avail the Treatment to Cure these Problems?				
Govt. health facility	121 (56.5)	32 (68.1)	34 (57.6)	187 (58.4)
Private health hospital	26 (12.1)	6 (12.8)	9 (15.3)	41 (12.8)
Applying home remedies	1 (0.5)	29 (4.3)	1 (1.7)	4 (1.3)
No treatment	66 (30.8)	7 (14.9)	15 (25.4)	88 (27.5)
Were You Satisfied with the Treatment?				
Yes	101 (68.2)	31 (77.5)	35 (79.5)	167 (72.0)
No	47 (31.8)	9 (22.5)	9 (20.5)	65 (28.0)
Please Tell Reason for No Treatment				
Did not think its seriousness	25 (37.9)	5 (71.4)	7 (46.7)	37 (42.0)
Felt shy to talk about	22 (33.3)	1 (14.3)	6 (40.0)	29 (33.0)
No idea where to take treatment	1 (1.5)	0	0	1 (1.1)
No money	18 (27.3)	1(14.3)	2(13,3)	21 (23.9)
In Your Opinion How Did Develop this Problem?				
After unclean delivery	40 (60.6)	5 (71.4)	11 (73.3)	56 (63.6)
After unclean abortion	8 (12.1)	2 (28.6)	0	10 (11.4)
From husband	8 (12.1)	0	1 (6.7)	9 (10.2)
After inserting IUD	1 (1.5)	0	0	1 (1.1)
After pelvic examination	9 (13.6)	0	3 (20.0)	12 (13.6)
Was Your Husband also Given Treatment due to these Problems You had?				
Yes	9 (13.6)	0	1 (6.7)	10 (11.4)
No	57 (86.4)	7(100.0)	14 (93.3)	78 (88.6)

where as just 61 percent of illiterate women said that RTI was due to unclean delivery. This indicates that other two educated groups have more knowledge about development of RTI. 11 percent of study women from Rafi nagar slum area told that RTI was developed due to unclean abortion.

12 percent of illiterate women expressed their opinion that RTI was developed from their husband where as Ten percent of the study women from Rafi nagar slum area told

that they developed the problems from their husband. 14 percent of study women from Rafi nagar slum area and told that they developed the problems after pelvic examinations. Thus, it can be concluded that the illiterate category of study women of Rafi nagar slum were unaware about the development of RTI they had.

ANOVA Table and Discussion

The variations of the degree of awareness of reproductive morbidity diseases is same in different age groups, was tested using ANOVA test (Table 3). The symptoms reported by study

Table 3
ANOVA Table for Symptoms of Reproductive Health Problems of Study Women from Rafi Nagar Slum Area, Mumbai

Symptoms of Reproductive Health Problems	*Sum of Squares*	*df*	*Mean Square*	*F*	*Sig.*
White Discharge					
Between Groups	.846	2	.423	1.698	.184
Within Groups	107.149	430	.249		
Total	107.995	432			
Abnormal Vaginal Discharge					
Between Groups	.164	2	.082	2.827	.060
Within Groups	12.446	430	.029		
Total	12.610	432			
Itching around Vagina					
Between Groups	.919	2	.459	3.233*	.040
Within Groups	61.091	430	.142		
Total	62.009	432			
Pain in Lower Abdomen					
Between Groups	1.716	2	.858	4.231*	.015
Within Groups	87.198	430	.203		
Total	88.915	432			
Pain during Urination					
Between Groups	.091	2	.045	.643	.526
Within Groups	30.394	430	.071		
Total	30.485	432			
Frequent Urination					
Between Groups	1.719	2	.859	6.996**	.001
Within Groups	52.822	430	.123		
Total	54.540	432			
Genital Ulcer / Rash					
Between Groups	2.226	2	1.113	9.274**	.000
Within Groups	51.608	430	.120		
Total	53.834	432			

Contd.

Symptoms of Reproductive Health Problems	*Sum of Squares*	*df*	*Mean Square*	*F*	*Sig.*
Pain during Intercourse					
Between Groups	1.236	2	.618	6.797**	.001
Within Groups	39.088	430	.091		
Total	40.323	432			
Low Backache					
Between Groups	.828	2	.414	1.658	.192
Within Groups	107.417	430	.250		
Total	108.245	432			
Foul Smelling					
Between Groups	1.845	2	.922	5.285**	.005
Within Groups	75.060	430	.175		
Total	76.905	432			
Pus in Urine					
Between Groups	.947	2	.474	5.279**	.005
Within Groups	38.582	430	.090		
Total	39.529	432			

*P< 0.05, ** P<0.01

women were white discharge, abnormal vaginal discharge, itching around vagina, pain in lower abdomen, pain during urination, frequent urination, genital ulcer / rash, pain during intercourse, low backache, foul smelling, pus in urine. Symptoms except white discharge, abnormal vaginal discharge, pain during urination, low backache was significant where as symptom, pain during intercourse showed significant from Ramabai nagar slum area. Here we can say that the symptom, pain during intercourse probably leads to dyspareunia. This can be a sign of infection, most commonly a yeast infection and the other, frequent urination leads to menstruation problem. This can be a sign of urination tract infection.

Awareness of Reproductive health problems between different age groups in Rafi nagar Slum, Mumbai

Table 4 shows that 46 percent of study women from Rafi nagar have abnormal vaginal discharge problem among the age group of 30-49. It clearly indicates that Rafi nagar slum respondents have more RTI problems in the later age which is quite serious.

Table 4
Percent Women Experiencing Reproductive Health Problems in Rafi Nagar Slum, Mumbai by Age Group

Reproductive Health Problems	15-24	25-29	30-49
Abnormal Vaginal discharge			
Yes (Percentage)	23.1	30.8	46.2
Frequent Urination			
Yes (Percentage)	45.3	20.3	34.4

Utilization of Health Services for the Reproductive Morbidity

Respondents were asked about the discussion held with the health personnel when visited their house about visiting the

Table 5
Percentage of Women Who have Availed the Health Facilities, Rafi Nagar, Mumbai

Utilisation of Health Facilities	Yes	Per cent
Did any health personnel ever visited to you?	241	55.7
If yes, please name the Clinic/Hospital they Belonged		
Government/Municipal Hospital	145	60.2
UHC/UHP/UFWC	92	38.2
Government Mobile Clinic	1	0.4
Private Hospital	2	0.8
Others	1	0.4
What did they Discussed with You?		
Immunization	140	58.1
Breast feeding	23	9.5
Personal health and hygiene	10	4.1
RTI/STD/HIV/AIDS	16	6.6
Family planning	40	16.6
Small family size	11	4.6
Income generating activities	1	0.4
Whether Any Meeting was Arranged by them during the Last Three Months?	165	68.5
If yes, what issues were discussed during the meeting		
Immunization	90	54.5
Breast feeding	16	9.7
Personal health and hygiene	12	7.3
RTI/STD/HIV/AIDS	12	7.3
Family planning	29	17.6
Small family size	4	2.4
Income generating activities	2	1.2
Total	165	100.0

hospitals, to take care of personnel and child health etc. Fifty six percent of respondents (Table 5) from Rafi nagar slum area told that health personnel had visited their residence.

Sixty percent of respondents from Rafi nagar slum area told that health personnel were from Government / Municipal hospital. Similarly, 38 were from UHC/UHP. 58 percent of respondents from Rafi nagar slum area said that health personnel discussed about immunization. Similarly 10 discussed about breast feeding and 17 discussed about family planning. Sixty nine percent of respondents respectively from Rafi nagar slum area said that the health personnel had organized meeting with them. 55 percent discussed about immunization and 18 percent discussed about family planning. Thus, it can be concluded that health personnel had played more role in discussing the problems of health in Rafi nagar slum area.

Summary and Conclusions

In this study the reproductive tract infection among the study women has been identified in the slum area of Rafi Nagar, Deonar, Mumbai. The primary data of sample size of 433 reproductive women who have given at least one live birth prior to the survey on the symptoms of RTI, such as white discharge, abnormal vaginal discharge, itching around vagina, pain in lower abdomen, pain during urination, frequent urination, genital ulcer/rash, pain during intercourse, low backache, foul smelling, pus in urine; delay in reporting of RTI problems, availing the treatments, whether satisfied with the treatment availed and the reasons for developing these problems was collected. This study revealed that the reproductive health problems of illiterate women were found to be quite serious compared with the other two categories of the women who had education up to 6th standard and above including delay in reporting of such RTI to the health personnel. The illiterate category of study women of Rafi nagar slum were unaware about the development of RTI they had.

Seventy two percent of the study women from Rafi nagar slum area were of the opinion that they were not found satisfactory with the treatment availed where as only 68 percent of illiterate women were found satisfactory with the treatment availed. 46 percent of study women from Rafi nagar have abnormal vaginal discharge problem among the age group of 30-49. It clearly indicates that Rafi nagar slum respondents will suffer more with RTI problems in the later age which is quite serious. Respondents were asked about the discussions held with the health personnel when visited their house about visiting the hospitals, to take care of personnel and child health etc. Fifty six percent of respondents from Rafi nagar slum area told that health personnel had visited their residence.

The variations of the degree of awareness of reproductive morbidity diseases is same in different age groups, was tested using ANOVA test (Table 3). Symptoms except white discharge, abnormal vaginal discharge, pain during urination, low backache was significant where as symptom, pain during intercourse showed significant from Rafi Nagar slum area. Here we can say that the symptom, pain during intercourse probably leads to dyspareunia. This can be a sign of infection, most commonly a yeast infection and the other, frequent urination leads to menstruation problem. This can be a sign of urination tract infection.

Thus, it is suggested that training of nurses, health workers, dais, *anganwadi* workers regarding RTI identification and referral using syndromic approach and promotion of menstrual hygiene, genital hygiene and health care seeking behaviour would help in reducing the burden of RTI in the community. Indigenous methods of sanitary pads like clean, sundried domestic cloths can be promoted during menstrual periods so that their economic conditions do not act as a barrier in the maintenance of hygiene. Emphasis should be given for psychosocial and physical development of girl child so that she may become a healthy, future mother of the community. Govt. sector of health services should be strengthened and widely approachable especially in the field of family welfare. For this involvement of health workers in family planning programmers should be intensified in such slum areas and similarly the cooperation and involvement of Non Governmental Organization (NGOs) should also be sought.

References

Srivastava, A.D. Nandan, A.K. Mehrotra, B.B. Maheshwari, and S.K. Mishra (2004), "A Comparative Study of Perception about Reproductive Tract Infections Among Married Women in Rural Urban and Urban Slum Areas", *Indian Journal of Community Medicine* 29(2) 4-6.

Monica, Rathore, Leela Vyas, and A.K. Bhardwaj (2007), "Prevalence of Reproductive Tract Infections Amongst Ever Married Women and Socio Cultural Factors Associated with It", *Journal of Indian Medical Association* 105: 71-4 & 78.

Kamal, Nashid, and Rumana Rashid (2004), "Environmental Risk Factors Associated with RTI/STD Symptoms Among Women in the Urban Slums", *The Journal of Developing Areas* 38(1).

International Institute for Population Sciences and ORC Macro (2000), *National Family Health Survey (NFHS-2), 1998-1999,* India, *IIPS,* Mumbai.

Phanindra, N., Prakasam, C.P. (1998), "Quality of Health Care Delivery in Rural Gujarat, India: Evidence from NFHS Data", *Proceedings of the International Geographical Conference,* Vadodara, India, 21-23 January.

Population Council (1999), *Reproductive Tract Infections: A Set of Fact Sheet.* Bangkok: Population Council.

Prakasam C.P. (2004), "Reproductive Morbidity Among Adolescent Women in Andhra Pradesh and Tamil Nadu: Evidences from NFHS-2 Data", In: P.J. Reddy, (ed.), *Women, Health and Development.* Tirupati: Department of Population Studies Sri Venkateswara University.

Sarode, V.M. (2007), "Health-Seeking Behaviour Among Reproductive Women in Slums in Greater Mumbai", *The International Journal of Interdisciplinary Social Sciences* 2(4): 115-130.

Singh, M.M, Devi, R, Garg, S., Mehra, M. (2001), "Effectiveness of Syndromic Approach in Management of Reproductive Tract Infections in Women", *Indian Journal of Medical Science* 55:209-214.

9

Women Empowerment and its Consequences on Reproductive Health in Selected States: NFHS-3 Data Analysis

C. P. Prakasam

Introduction

The World Bank has suggested that empowerment of women should be a key aspect of all social development programs (World Bank, 2001). Since then researchers examined "empowerment of women" by defining in different domains viz: political, economic, social, family and individual level. Amin et al. (1998) split the concept of women's empowerment into three components each measured separately: Inter-spouse consultation index, which seeks to represent the extent to which husbands consult their wives in household affairs; Individual autonomy index, which represents women's self-reported autonomy of physical movement outside the house and in matters of spending money; and the Authority index, which reports on actual decision-making power (which is traditionally in the hands of the patriarch of the family). Hashemi (1996) in his study identifies women empowerment in eight components viz: mobility, economic security, ability to make small purchases, ability to make larger purchases, involvement in major decisions, relative freedom from domination by the family. World Bank's Sourcebook on Empowerment and Poverty Reduction (Narayan, 2002), clearly indicates empowerment as "expansion of freedom of choice and action.., *women's* empowerment encompasses some unique additional elements". For assessing women's "empowerment", researchers have measured as "autonomy" (Dyson and Moore, 1983; Basu and Basu, 1991; Jejeebhoy and Sathar, 2001), as "women's land rights", as "domestic economic power" as "gender equality" (World Bank, 2000; 2001), or "gender discrimination".

It is a complex phenomenon to define empowerment. However, Batliwala (1994) defines it as "the process by which the powerless gain greater control over the circumstances of their lives. It includes both control over resources (physical, human, intellectual, financial) and over ideology (beliefs, values and attitudes)... means greater extrinsic control, but also a growing intrinsic capability, greater self-confidence, and an inner transformation of one's consciousness that enables one to overcome external barriers to access resources or changing traditional ideology". According to Kishor (2000) women's empowerment means "women's increased control over their own lives, bodies, and environment", further "women's decision-making roles, their economic self-reliance, and their legal rights to equal treatment, inheritance and protection against all forms of discrimination". Operationalization of empowerment is another complex phenomenon.

It is a fact that measurement of women's empowerment is a complex phenomenon because the set of variables are different for different societies, geographical areas and to different ethnic regions. However, a broader category of variables, which are derived from the large survey: the National Family Health Survey-3 (NFHS-3) forms the base for the analysis of this study.

Objectives

Keeping in view of the aforesaid points in view this study aims:

- To examine the influence of socio-economic variables on women's empowerment among currently married women in five selected states viz: Bihar, Madhya Pradesh, Gujarat, Andhra Pradesh and Kerala.
- Consequences (risk) of Reproductive health problems due to different empowerment status.

Conceptualization and Measurement of Empowerment

In this study women's empowerment is focused on her decision-making role, control over their own lives, bodies and protection against all forms of discrimination. A fundamental element of empowerment is the rejection of a normatively prescribed power of men *over* women and of unequal rights and privileges on the basis of the sex of an individual. This normatively ascribed right of husband on wives' body and behavior leads to physical and sexual violence. Hence, women who believe that husbands' control over them (physical) is justified can be considered as less empowered than women who think otherwise. Considering this concept, women's low or high empowerment is measured in terms of "acceptance of men's exercise of power over women", which is measured as: *Agreement* with the (selected) reasons justifying wife beating and *disagreement* with the (selected) reasons justifying a wife's refusal to have sex with her husband as "low empower (LM)" otherwise "empower (EM)" status. Further, to understand the influences of women empowerment on reproductive health problems information about "had any STD in last twelve months, had genital sore/ulcer in last twelvemonths and had genital discharge in last twelve months" have been analyzed.

Data and Methodology

Data for the present study has been drawn from National Family Health Survey-3 (NFHS-3) conducted during 2005-06 (IIPS and Macro International, 2007). NFHS-3 collected data from currently married women in the age group 15-49 years by asking questions that a husband was justified in hitting or beating if she goes out without telling him, if she neglects the house or children, if she argues with him, if she does no cook food properly (Physical violence). Further information about wife is justified in refusing to have sex with her husband when she knows her husband has sexually transmitted disease and when she knows her husband has sex with other women (refusal to sex), has been collected and analyzed. Considering these two aspects viz: Wife beating (Physical violence) and refusal to sex and access to health care, empowerment index has been derived.

Empowerment index has been calculated by considering: women access to health care, agree/disagree for husband beating (Physical) for selected reasons, and accept/refuse for sex (sexual) knowing her husband with STD or affairs with another women. Physical and sexual items considered for measurement is listed in Table 1. List of variables considered for analysis and scoring pattering is given in Table 1. Agreement for husband beating is given low score as Agree=1, and disagreeing=1 to refusal for sex. Further access to health care for self is given high score and to others as low score. The score range for the empowerment index would 11 to 22. Hence considering composite score between 11-16 as low empower (LM) and 17-22 as empower (EM) has been derived.

To achieve the objectives, data were collected from NHFS-3 for the five selected states viz: Bihar, Madhya Pradesh, Gujarat, Andhra Pradesh and Kerala (IIPS and Macro International, 2007). These five states have been selected with a view that Bihar represents one of the developing states with high physical violence, low status of women. Madhya Pradesh with low age at marriage and child marriages with low status of women and Gujarat with high dowry deaths, Andhra Pradesh being developing state with high acceptance of family planning at low age with 35.2 percent of currently married women experiencing physical and sexual violence and Kerala with high age at marriage and high status of women .Further these Five states have different socio-economic and cultural setting. Hence, analysing the data for these states with different socio economic conditions may reveal true picture in different cultural settings. List of variables considered for analysis is given in Table 1.

Table 1

List of Variables Selected for Analysis in Determining the Influence of Reproductive Health Variables on Empowerment of Currently Married Women in Selected States, NFHS - 3 data

Category of Variables	*Variables*		
Background Variables	Socio-economic Variables		
	Current Age (in 5 years group)	Marital Duration	
	Type of Place of Residence	Religion	
	Wealth Index	Work Status	
	Partner's Education	Partner Occupation	
	Husband Living with the Respondent		
Empowerment Variables	Access to Resources:		
	1. Own health care		Score
	2. Making large household purchase		Self=2, Other=1
	3. visiting family or relatives		Self=2, Other=1
	4. Deciding what to do with money husband earns		Self=2, Other=1
	Physical:		Self=2, Other=1
	Agrees husband beating for reasons		
	1. 'if wife goes without telling husband'		Agree: 1 Disagree: 2
	2. 'neglects house or children'		Agree: 1 Disagree: 2
	3. 'argues with husband'		Agree: 1 Disagree: 2
	4. 'refuse to have sex with husband'		Agree: 1 Disagree: 2
	5. 'does not cook food properly'		Agree: 1 Disagree: 2
	Sexual:		
	Refuse to have sex if she knows husband is having		
	1. sexually transmitted disease		Agree: 2 Disagree: 1
	2. affairs with other women		Agree: 2 Disagree: 1
Empowerment Index	Low Empower, Score 11 to16 **(LE)**		
	Empower, Score 17 to 22 **(EM)**		
Sexual Reproductive Health Variables	Had STD in last 12 months		Yes/No
	Had genital sore ulcer in last 12 months		Yes/No
	Had abnormal genital discharge in last 12 months		Yes/No

The analysis carried out in three stages. Initially, the reasons for justifying husband beating for physical and sexual reasons with the background variable have been analyzed to know the attitude of currently married women towards "empowerment" in selected five states. In the second stage the influence of major predictors (determinants) of currently married women determining Empowerment index (low empowered (LE), Empower (EM)) in the selected five states have been analyzed by applying stepwise Logit regression analysis and risk ratio of Sexual Reproductive health problems among low empower, Empower women has been calculated which gives the influences of empowerment on reproductive health problems.

Results and Discussion

Attitude towards Wife Beating - Physical and Sexual Reasons

Agreement with the reasons of wife beating gives an indication of low empowerment of women. Hence the attitude towards wife beating and socio economic variables for the five selected states has been analyzed and results are given in Table 2. It has been observed that highest percent (57.9) of women in Andhra Pradesh followed by Kerala (56.6) agrees husband is justified in hitting or beating with at least one reason (Table 2) contribute towards low empowerment status. The developing states Bihar (46.5) and Madhya Pradesh (33.2), less percentage of women agrees that a husband is justified in hitting or beating. Analysis done on the bases of attitude towards wife beating (Physical) many not reveal true picture of "empowerment" of currently married women. Hence the response towards "refusal" to sex has been analysed.

Currently married women who believe that a wife is justified in refusing to have sexual intercourse with her husband when she knows that he (husband) has a STD or affairs with other women reveal status of "empowerment" towards her own body. The percentage of women who agrees of "refusing sex" with one reason found to be high in Madhya

Pradesh (Table 3) followed by Bihar (93.3) and least Kerala (81.7) and in Andhra Pradesh (81.4). Among the two reasons, majority of women agrees to "refuse" sex with husband when they know he has a STD than he has a sex with other women, in all these five states.

On the basis of the variables listed in Table 1, respective scores have been given to Access to Health care, attitude towards wife beating and refusal to sex and empowerment index has been calculated. Index values between 11and 16 considered as "low empower (LM)" and between 17 and 22

Table 2
Percentage of Currently Married Women Who Agrees that a Husband is Justified in Hitting or Beating Wife for Specific Reasons Across Selected States, NFHS-3 data

	Percentage who agree with specific reasons						
States	*Percentage who agree with atleast one reason*	*Wife goes with out telling husband*	*Wife neglects house or children*	*Wife argues with husband*	*Refuse to have sex with husband*	*Wife does not cook food properly*	*Number of Currently Married Women*
Bihar	46.5	22.4	20.0	30.8	11.0	16.3	2992
Madhya Pradesh	33.2	16.9	19.1	20.9	9.5	14.5	4923
Gujarat	52.6	32.3	39.6	38.5	19.9	27.5	2829
Andhra Pradesh	57.9	43.4	50.5	37.6	23.1	25.9	5149
Kerala	56.6	37.0	43.2	25.8	14.7	20.6	2616

Table 3
Percentage of Currently Married Women Who Believes that a Wife is Justified in Refusing to have Sexual Intercourse with her Husband in Specific Circumstances Across Selected States, NFHS-3 Data

	Agrees that a wife is justified in refusing to have sex with her husband when she:					
States	*Knows husband has a sexually transmitted disease*	*Knows husband has a sex with other women*	*Percent Women who agree with one reason*	*Percent Women who agree with two reasons*	*Percent Women who agree with none of the reason*	*Number of Women*
Bihar	90.3	86.6	93.3	83.6	6.0	2992
Madhya Pradesh	91.0	93.2	96.7	87.5	2.6	4923
Gujarat	77.8	80.2	86.0	71.9	10.3	2829
Andhra Pradesh	77.0	75.0	81.4	70.6	13.8	5148
Kerala	73.7	75.7	81.7	67.7	15.6	2616

considered as "Empowered (EM)". Percentage of currently married women according to the empowerment index is listed in Table 4. Currently married women in Madhya Pradesh were more empowered than women in other states. Among these five states currently married women in Andhra Pradesh were in low empowerment category (Table 4). This may be due to Physical and sexual violence against women and may be "women acceptance" towards husband behavior. To understand further, the influence of Socio economic factors on women empowerment has been analyzed by using Logit analysis.

Table 4
Percentage of Currently Married Women According to Empowerment Index in Selected States: NFHS-3 Data

	Empowerment index					
States	*Low Empower (LE)*		*Empowered (EM)*		*Total No. of Women*	
Bihar	1293	(43.2)	1697	(56.8)	2990	(100.0)
Madhya Pradesh	1550	(31.5)	3373	(68.5)	4923	(100.0)
Gujarat	1301	(46.0)	1528	(54.0)	2829	(100.0)
Andhra Pradesh	2603	(50.6)	2545	(49.4)	5148	(100.0)
Kerala	1274	(48.7)	1340	(51.3)	2614	(100.0)

Influence of Socio Economic Variables in Determining Women Empowerment: Results of Logit Regression analysis

Logit regression technique was applied to examine the effect of Socio economic variables (independent variables) on women empowerment index (dependent dichotomous variable-Less empowered (LE) or Empowered (EM)). The Step wise logistic regression results for the five states are presented in Table 5. Out of eight background variables marital duration wealth index, partner occupation, respondent women working for cash have show significant contribution in determining "women empowerment" in Bihar. In Bihar, women with 10 or more years marital duration (odds 1.479), partner's occupation with white collar job (odds 3.027) and women working for cash (odds 1.462) shows high empowerment than other categories (Table 5). Type of place of residence, wealth index, partner education, women working for cash shows significant effect in determining women empowerment in Madhya Pradesh. Women in rural areas (odds 1.672) when compare to urban (as reference category) exhibits more at risk of achieving empowerment than urban women (Table 5).

In Gujarat, Marital duration, religion, wealth index showed significant impact in determining women empowerment. Among these variables women with marital duration more than 5 years, belong to Hindu religion and poor wealth strata are more at risk of attaining empowerment than other category (Table 5). Similarly, in Andhra Pradesh, variables viz., type of place of residence, wealth index, partner's occupation and working for cash show significant influence in determining empowerment index. In Kerala, out of eight socio economic variables only partner's occupation showed significant influence on low empowerment of currently married women.

Odds refer to the probability of achievement in dependent variable (empowerment-LE) decreases with improving position of women according to socio-economic variables. For example, when compare to wealth index in Bihar State, the probability of women empowerment (LE) was much less among middle (.267) and rich people (.359) when compare to poor. This explains that in Bihar currently married women belong to poor strata are at more risk (nearly 4 to 5 times) than middle and rich class women in achieving empowerment. Similarly, in Gujarat state, currently married women belongs to poor strata is more risk than middle and rich category. In Madhya Pradesh state, women residing in rural areas (odds ratio: 1.672) increases the risk in achieving empowerment than urban women and similarly with wealth index.

The states Andhra Pradesh and Kerala revealed different results. In Andhra Pradesh currently married women belongs to rural areas twice at risk (2.046) than urban women. Further in respect of marital duration, when compared to less than five years group (reference group), the women in longer marital duration were (1.521 and 1.144 times) at risk of

Table 5
Results of STEP-WISE Logistic Regression Analysis of Socio Economic Variables Influencing Women Empowerment Index in Selected States: NFHS-3 Data

Socio-economic Variables	*States*				
	Bihar	*Madhya Pradesh*	*Gujarat*	*Andhra Pradesh*	*Kerala*
Age Group					
15-19 years **(ref)**					
20-29 years					
30-39 years					
40-49 years					
Type of Placeof Residence					
Urban(ref)		1.000		1.000	
Rural		1.672		2.046	
Marital Duration					
<5 Years **(ref)**	1.000		1.000		
5-10 Years	.624		1.521		
10+ Years	1.479		1.144		
Religion					
Hindu **(ref)**			1.000		
Non-Hindu			.663		
Wealth index					
Poor (ref)	1.000	1.000	1.000	1.000	
Middle	.267	.574	**.630**	.681	
Rich	.267	.805	**.575**	.724	
Partner's Education					
No Education **(ref)**		1.000			
Educated		.662			
Partner's Occupation					
Unemployed **(ref)**	1.000			1.000	1.000
White Collar Job	3.027			.677	1.897
Blue Collar Job	.723			1.451	**2.090**
Respondent Working for Cash					
No **(ref)**	1.000	1.000		1.000	
Yes	1.462	.776		**.548**	
Constant	3.291	2.695	1.685	.631	.762
-2 Log likelihood	1211.41	3009.67	1998.60	2777.56	1028.32
100 * R^2	7.10	9.30	3.10	10.7	3.90

Variables entered in to Step-wise Logit :
Bihar State: Marital Duration, Wealth index, Partners occupation, Respondent Working for cash (4); **Madhya Pradesh**: Type of Place of residence, Wealth index, Partner education, Respondent working for cash (4); **Gujarat**: Marital Duration, Religion, Wealth index (3); **Andhra Pradesh**: Type of place of residence, wealth index, partner occupation, respondent working for cash (4) ;**Kerala**: Partner occupation (1)

achieving empowerment. In Kerala state only partner's occupation showed significant odds with white collar and blue collar jobs.

Relative Risk of Reproductive Health Problems due to Women Empowerment

From the foregoing data analysis (Table 5) it has been observed influence of socio economic variables determining women's empowerment. But comparison of reproductive health problems among women who are Low Empowered (LE) and Empowered (EM), will give clear understanding about the risk due to Empowerment index. Hence relative risk has been computed as:

$$\frac{\text{Incidence of Reproductive Health Problem among currently married women with Low empowerment (LE)}}{\text{Incidence of Reproductive Health Problem among currently married women with empowerment (EM)}}$$

Relative risk gives incidence of reproductive health problem among women with LE with respect to women who is EM. Relative risk ratio equals to "one" indicates when incidence of Reproductive health problems are same among women with LE and EM status. Table 6 gives the relative risk of Reproductive Health problems due to women empowerment.

Table 6
Relative Risk of Reproductive Health Problems Among Low Empower Women (LE) in Relation to Empowered (EM) Women in the Selected States

	Reproductive Health problems during last 12 Months		
Selected States	*Genital Sore Ulcer*	*Abnormal Genital Discharge*	*STD*
Bihar	0.941	1.077	1.478
Madhya Pradesh	0.862	1.388	1.643
Gujarat	1.821	1.471	1.656
Andhra Pradesh	1.457	3.807	1.562
Kerala	1.336	1.578	2.791

From the Table 6, it is evident that women with Low empowerment (LE) are experiencing reproductive health problem more than Empowered women (EM). In case of abnormal genital discharge this ratio was 3.8 times higher among low empowered women when compared to empowered women. It was evident that risk of STD among currently married women found to be more than 1.5 times more among low empowered women than empowered women. The results also clearly indicate that risk of experiencing reproductive health problems (Abnormal Genital Discharge, STD and Genital Sore Ulcer) among currently married women is within the range of 1.07 to 3.8 times among Low empowered women than empowered women.

Conclusions

Identification of women's empowerment variables is a complex phenomenon because it encompasses political, economic, social, family and individual level domains. In this research paper women's empowerment has been examined by considering her belief that husbands' control over her physical and sexual behavior. Agreement with the (selected) reasons justifying wife beating and disagreement with the (selected) reasons justifying a wife's refusal to have sex with her husband as "low empower (LM)" otherwise "empower (EM)" status. A composite index of women empowerment has been calculated by considering access to resources, agreement with husband beating (Physical) and sexual refusal (Sexual). The calculated index value less than 16 considered as low empower (LM) and more than 16 as Empower (EM). The influence of major predicators of currently married women determining Empowerment index in selected five states have been analyzed by using stepwise Logit regression analysis.

It has been observed that:

- Highest percent women in Andhra Pradesh and Kerala agree husband justified in hitting or beating contributes towards low empowerment status.

- Currently married women who believe that a wife is justified in refusing to have sexual intercourse with her Husband when she knows that he has a STD or affairs with other women reveal status of "empowerment" towards her own body. Highest percent currently married women in Bihar and Madhya Pradesh exhibit more empowered than other states related to refusal to sex.
- The empowerment index calculated by considering access to resources, physical, sexual variables shows that more than 50 percent currently married women are empowered in the states Bihar, Madhya Pradesh and Gujarat.

Based on the Step-wise Logistic regression analysis (Table 5) the following conclusions have been derived:

- Out of eight socio-economic determinants in Bihar State marital duration, wealth index, partner's occupation and respondent working for cash (4 variables); in Madhya Pradesh, type of place of residence, wealth index, partner's education and respondent working for cash (4 variables); in Gujarat, marital duration, religion and wealth index (3 variables); in Andhra Pradesh, type of place of residence, wealth index, partner occupation and respondent working for cash (4 variables); and in Kerala, partner's occupation alone have showed significant net effects on empowerment index.
- Currently married women with 10 or more years of marital duration, belongs to poor strata, partner's occupation as white collar job and respondent working for cash showed higher odds of "low empowered" in Bihar than other category of variables.
- In Kerala, only partner's occupation exhibited significant influence on women empowerment among the selected eight socio economic variables. Currently married women whose partner with blue collar job

had twice the risk of low empowered than unemployed women. This may be due to lack of inter personal communication between wife and husband and male want to dominate in terms of her body and economic status.

- Low empower women are more than 1.4 times at risk in getting STD than women who are empowered in all selected five states.
- Low empower women exhibited high risk of getting abnormal genital discharge than empowered women in all these states.

The consequences of women empowerment on reproductive health showed that low empowered women are at risk of getting reproductive health problems than empowered women in all these study states. Hence, to enhance currently married women's empowerment, it is necessary to educate women (wife) and men (husband). Planners have to aim at improving women's education and her work participation by providing self-employment. Further, providing health facilities at the doorstep will enhance her access to health care and enhance empowerment status at household level.

References

Amin Rahul, Becker Stan and Byes Abdul (1998), "NGO-Promoted Micro credit Programs and Women's Empowerment in Rural Bangladesh: Quantitative and Qualitative Evidence", *The Journal of Developing Areas* 32: 221-236.

Basu, Alaka Malwade and Kaushik Basu (1991), "Women's Economic Roles and Child Survival: Case of India", *Health Transition Review* 1(1):

Batliwala, Srilatha (1994), "The Meaning of Women's Empowerment: New Concepts from Action" In: Gita Sen, Adrienne Germain and Lincoln Chen (eds.), *Population Policies Reconsidered: Health Empowerment and Rights*. Cambridge, Mass: Harvard University Press pp.127-138.

Hashemi Syed, Sydney Ruth Schuler and Ann Riley (1996), "Rural Credit Programs and Women's Empowerment in Bangladesh", *World Development* 24(4): 635-653.

Narayan, Deepa (Ed.), (2002), *Empowerment and Poverty Reduction: A Source Book.* Washington: World Bank.

Dyson Tim and Mick Moore (1983), "On Kinship Structure, Female Autonomy, and Demographic Behavior in India", *Population and Development Review* 9(1): 35-60.

International Institute for Population Sciences (IIPS) and Macro International (2007), *National Family Health Survey (NFHS-3), 2005-06: India.* Mumbai: IIPS.

Jejeebhoy, Shireen J. (1995), *Women's Education, Autonomy, and Reproductive Behaviour: Experience from Four Developing Countries.* International Studies in Demography. IUSSP, Oxford: Clarendon Press.

Jejeebhoy, Shireen, J. (2000), "Women's Autonomy in Rural India: Its Dimensions, Determinants, and the Influence of Context", In: Harriet Presser and Gita Sen, (eds.), *Women's Empowerment and Demographic Processes: Moving Beyond Cairo.* New York: Oxford University Press.

Jejeebhoy, Shireen J, and Zeba A. Sathar (2001), "Women's Autonomy in India and Pakistan: The Influence of Religion and Region", *Population and Development Review* 27(4): 687-712.

Kishor, Sunita (2000), "Empowerment of Women in Egypt and Links to the Survival and Health of Their Infants", In: Harriet Presser and Gita Sen, (eds.), *Women's Empowerment and Demographic Processes: Moving Beyond Cairo.* New York: Oxford University Press pp.119-155.

World Bank (2000), *Engendering Development: Through Gender Equality in Rights, Resources, and Voice.* World Bank Policy Research Report, Oxford: Oxford University Press.

World Bank (2001), *World Development Report 2001: Attacking Poverty.* New York: Oxford University Press.

10

Autonomy of Women and Ante Natal Care: A Comparative Study of Two Indian States Evidence from NFHS-3

Deepshikha Tarai

Introduction

Every minute a women dies in the developing world as a result of pregnancy and childbirth. These young women in the prime of their lives die from causes, which can be prevented or treated. But it is a question of how much the life of women is considered to be worth. When societies invest less in girls and underestimate the economic contribution of women and when few women are in decision making positions, it should be of no surprise, in resource-poor settings, that a low priority is for to saving for the lives of mothers. Societies have an obligation to protest women's right to life when they go through the risky process of giving us life. Safe motherhood is a human right issue for which countries should be held accountable.

The Government of India had established several programmers to improve the maternal health in all over the states. Like the Child Survival and Save Motherhood (CSSM) Programmer was launched in India in August 1992 with the objective to improve health status of women and children and reduction of maternal, infant and child morbidity and mortality rate. The Safe motherhood component by and large aimed to reduce maternal morbidity and mortality rate (WHO, 1996). The National Population Policy 2000 also aims at reducing MMR to below 100 per 100 000 live birth and IMR to below 30 per 1000 live births by 2010.Howere, till today maternal mortality and infant mortality rate in India is very high in almost all the states. As per the National Family Health Survey-2, MMR in India is 540 per 100 000 live birth and IMR is 70 per thousand live births (SRS 2001). In Orissa IMR are 71, which is one of the highest in the country (SRS 2007). This is due to the low autonomy of women which restraint them from availing proper and timely health care. Whereas in AP the IMR rate is very low it may because for its particular culture. According to the Government, the major causes of death under pregnancy and childbirth include bleeding during pregnancy and puerperal, abortion and anemia (MOHFW, 1999).Many of theses deaths could have been avoided if the pregnant women take full antenatal are timely. Actually the main purposes of Ante Natal Care are to prevent certain complications such as anaemia, to ensure that the mother is physically and psychologically healthy or healthier, to detect factors occurring during pregnancy which may adversely affect the healthy growth and development of the baby; to educate the mother about the process of pregnancy and child birth and to provide information about nutrition, breast feeding, adjustment to parenthood, sexuality and other matters which may affect both the parents and their baby.

NFHS–2, 1998-99 (IIPS and ORC Macro, 2000) found that about one third (34 percent) of women in India did not receive any ANC and the reasons cited for not receiving are not necessary (59.5 percent) followed by too much costs (14.7 percent).At that time more than 90 percent mothers received antenatal check-ups in A.P. which very much higher than Orissa (74 percent). In Orissa more than 12 percent of women especially received ANC from *anganwadi.*

In A.P. 87 percent or more of all literate mothers received ante checkups for their births, where as only 72 percent of illiterate mothers received ante natal checkups. The proportion of births whose mother received ante natal checkups from a doctor increases steadily with education, from 42 percent for illiterate mothers to 96 percent among who have completed at least high school. Conversely the prevalence of only home visit from a health worker decreases with mother's education.

Women's Autonomy and Ante Natal Care

Much of the relevant demographic literature that has addressed the links between gender inequality and fertility regulation has also focused on antenatal care. The concept of autonomy is multidimensional. Alternative terms such as women's status, women's position in a society and in a household, control over resources and female prestige are all frequently used in the literature interchangeably to define women's autonomy. Each and every author is used different dimension to measure the women's autonomy or women's status. Like in most of the articles, involvements in decision making, freedom of movement and access to resources are used as a direct indicator of women's autonomy (Jejeebhoy, 2000; Roy and Niranjan, 2004) were as employment, education, occupation, age difference between spouses, education difference between spouses Standard of living, exposure to mass media parity of the women etc are taken as an indirect indicator of women's autonomy (Patel et al., 2002; Jejeebhoy, 1995; Roy and Niranjan, 2004). Some of the other studies concluded that autonomy has been defined as the degree of women access to material resources including food, income, land and other forms of wealth and to social resources including knowledge, power and prestige within the family, in the community and society at large. Proportion of females married in the age group 15-19 years, Singulate mean age at marriage for females, female work participation rate, female workers as a percentage of male workers, percentage of females in non-agricultural activities, female literates as a percentage of male literates all these dimension are used to address the women's status in most of developing countries (Vaidyanathan, 1998).

Female autonomy and antenatal care are the two sides of the coin. Women's autonomy greatly influences ante natal care, which is indispensable for pregnant women. Developing countries has shown that women who score greater autonomy are more concerned about fertility, desire family sizes, contraceptive use, antenatal care services etc. (Basu, 1992). A descriptive study in New Delhi, among two groups of immigrants from Uttar Pradesh and Tamil Nadu, found that Tamil women scored higher in all areas of autonomy and those who are highly educated they are more concern about antenatal care and facility-based delivery care for their last birth to a greater extent than women from Uttar Pradesh (Basu, 1992). High economic status, education, perceived problem during pregnancy and freedom of movement all have a strong and positive relation to the antenatal care (Bloom et al., 2001; Kishor and Parasuraman, 1998).

Objectives

The objective of the present study is to know the autonomy of women and its linkage with ante natal services in Orissa and Andhra Pradesh. The specific objectives of the present analysis are as follows:

1. To examine the impact of socio-economic factors on women's autonomy,
2. To explore the impact of women's autonomy on utilization of antenatal care services, and
3. To find out the impact of socio-economic factors on Antenatal care in two selected states viz: Orissa and Andhra Pradesh.

Data and Methodology

For the present study, NFHS-3, 2005-2006 (IIPS and Macro International, 2007) data has been used. This National Family Health survey covered representative sample of total 124385 married women in the age group 15-49 years. Here we have selected two states 1) ORISSA and 2) ANDHRA PRADESH. Autonomy Index (high, medium and low) has been calculated

Table 1
Variables Included in Construction of Index on Autonomy of Women by Categories NFHS-3 Data

Variables	*Responses*	*Scores*
	Final say on:	
Own health care	Respondent alone	4
	Respondent & husband	3
	Respondent & other partner	3
	Husband	2
	Some one else	1
Making large household purchases	Respondent alone	4
	Respondent & husband	3
	Respondent & other partner	3
	Husband	2
	Some one else	1
Making household purchases for daily needs	Respondent alone	4
	Respondent & husband	3
	Respondent & other partner	3
	Husband	2
	Some one else	1
Visit to family or relative	Respondent alone	4
	Respondent & husband	3
	Respondent & other partner	3
	Husband	2
	Some one else	1
Access to Money		
Deciding what to do with money husband earns	Respondent alone	4
	Respondent & husband	3
	Respondent & other partner	3
	Husband	2
	Some one else	1
Allow to Go to:		
Market	Alone	4
	With someone else only	1
	Not at all	0
Health Facilities	Alone	4
	With someone else only	1
	Not at all	0
Outside Place	Alone	4
	With someone else only	1
	Not at all	0

for all ever married women of women. To study the antenatal care aspects, only those women who have had become pregnant at least once in the last three years preceding the survey have been included.

Measure of Women's Autonomy

The degree of women's autonomy is assessed in three different areas: women's decision-making power in making large household and daily purchases etc, extent of freedom of movement and access to money. For computing a women's autonomy into three levels (low, medium and high), index has been computed by classifying the responses in to different categories. Scores considered for the index is listed in Table 1.

To know the situation of autonomy of women and factors associated with availing of ante natal care and linkage between autonomy of women, data have been cross tabulated and interpreted. Further to know the impact of socio-economic variables on autonomy of women multi nominal logistic regression analyses have been carried out.

Ante Natal Care indicators

From the NFHS-3 data information on whether the mother took IFA tablets or syrups, whether she received two or more tetanus taxoid/tetanus injection and whether she received ANC at home and outside home during her pregnancy (last pregnancy for the present study) has been collected. ANC is computing by taking three variables: Two or more tetanus taxoid injections during pregnancy, Received Iron Folic Acid (IFA) syrup or tablets for three months during pregnancy and Antenatal visits for pregnancy

Results

Level of Autonomy of Women

By considering the scores given in Table.1, women autonomy index have been calculated and classified in to Low, medium and high. Result given in Table 2 reveals that out of total sample women (3242) almost one third of women (35 percent) have low autonomy and same percentage with high autonomy in both the states. Nearly 34 percent of the women have medium autonomy in Andhra Pradesh (Table 2), which is slightly more than Orissa (30.7 percent). Combine the medium and high autonomy index, it has been can observed that in Andhra Pradesh nearly two third percentage of women (68 percent) have autonomy and in Orissa it was 65.5 percent. Its implies that, in compare to Orissa, Andhra Pradesh women's have taking more decision in household related matters, mobility and health care for themselves, which might have direct bearing on the decision making about her own health and particularly about availing ANC.

Table 2
Percent Distribution of Ever Married Women by Autonomy of Women in Orissa and Andhra Pradesh: NFHS-3 Data

	Orissa		*Andhra Pradesh*	
Women's Autonomy	*Frequency*	*Percent*	*Frequency*	*Percent*
Low	1120	34.5	1658	32.4
Medium	995	30.7	1689	33.4
High	1127	34.8	1770	34.6
Total	3242	100.0	5117	100.0

Impact of Socio-economic Characteristics on Autonomy of Women: Results of Multinomial Logistic Regression Analysis

To understand the impact of background variables on women autonomy index ("Medium", "High" index value) Multinomial Logistic regression has been applied and results are given in Table 3. The Regression results shows that control for the effect of other socio economic characteristics, place of residence has a significantly effect on the autonomy of women. Women who are from urban area in Orissa are 2.16 times and in Andhra Pradesh 3.29 times more likely to have high autonomy compare to rural women (reference category, Table 3).

Table 3
Impact of Socio-economic Characteristics on Autonomy of Women in Orissa and Andhra Pradesh: NFHS-3 Data Analysis

	ORISSA						*ANDHARA PRADESH*					
	Medium			*High*			*Medium*			*High*		
Background Characteristics	*B*	*Sig.*	*Exp(B)*	*B*	*Sig.*	*Exp(B)*	*B*	*Sig.*	*Exp(B)*	*B*	*Sig.*	*Exp(B)*
Place of Residence												
Urban	.376	.002	1.457	.772	.000	2.164	.754	.000	2.126	1.193	.000	3.298
Rural®			1.000			1.000			1.000			1.000
Religion												
Hindu	-.531	.311	.588	-1.434	.002	.238	.015	.935	1.015	-.105	.553	.901
Muslim	-1.112	.089	.329	-3.301	.000	.037	-.523	.011	.593	-1.130	.000	.323
Others®			1.000			1.000			1.000			1.000
Resp.'s Education												
Illiterate	.277	.448	1.319	-.675	.030	.509	-.293	.141	.746	-.394	.046	.674
Primary	.193	.592	1.213	-.484	.110	.617	-.501	.014	.606	-.520	.010	.594
Secondary	.156	.643	1.169	-.451	.098	.637	-.446	.011	.640	-.802	.000	.449
Highest®			1.000			1.000			1.000			1.000
Husband Education												
Illiterate	.349	.168	1.418	.002	.993	1.002	.248	.125	1.281	.012	.942	1.012
Primary	.372	.117	1.450	-.331	.141	.718	.258	.120	1.294	-.009	.957	.991
Secondary	.141	.498	1.151	-.360	.055	.698	.136	.300	1.146	-.136	.315	.873
Highest®			1.000			1.000			1.000			1.000
Resp.'s Occupation												
Not working	-.491	.000	.612	-1.190	.000	.304	-.445	.000	.641	-1.064	.000	.345
Working®			1.000			1.000			1.000			1.000

Contd.

	ORISSA						ANDHARA PRADESH					
	Medium			*High*			*Medium*			*High*		
Background Characteristics	*B*	*Sig.*	*Exp(B)*	*B*	*Sig.*	*Exp(B)*	*B*	*Sig.*	*Exp(B)*	*B*	*Sig.*	*Exp(B)*
Husband occupation												
Not working	-.678	.169	.508	-.093	.819	.911	-.048	.893	.953	.832	.009	2.298
Working®			1.000			1.000			1.000			1.000
Mass Media												
No Exposed	-.288	.023	.750	-.624	.000	.536	-.161	.184	.851	-.114	.343	.892
Have Exposure®			1.000			1.000			1.000			1.000
Caste												
Backward	-.227	.042	.797	-.266	.018	.767	-.117	.216	.890	-.045	.642	.956
Advance®			1.000			1.000			1.000			1.000
Standard of living												
Low	.322	.045	1 380	.567	.001	1.763	.018	.891	1.018	-.153	.233	.853
Medium	.152	.274	1.165	.298	.036	1.347	-.143	.125	.866	-.038	.690	.963
High ®			1.000			1.000			1.000			1.000

Education is an important variable for the determination of women's autonomy. Level of Education enhances the autonomy on women. But here the result reveals that in compare to highly educated women, those women who are illiterate .509 times; women who completed primary education .617 and for secondary education .637 times less likely to have high autonomy in Orissa. Whereas in case of Andhra Pradesh same pattern of trend we can observed.

It has been observed that Husband's occupation determines the autonomy of women, especially in the joint family. It is assumed that if husband is working, wife is likely to enjoy better status. In the present analysis (Table 3) it has been observed that after controlling the effect of other characteristics, husband working status has positively and significantly effect on autonomy of women in Andhra Pradesh. But in case of Orissa the effect is totally opposite means in Orissa if husband occupation doesn't give much effect on autonomy of women, whereas its effect very much positive in Andhra Pradesh.

In compare to other caste (reference category), women who are Muslim are .037 times and Hindu women .002 times are less likely to have high autonomy in Orissa. Whereas in Andhra Pradesh Muslim women .323 times and Hindu .901 times less likely to have high autonomy. Here also the result is highly significant (Table 3).As compare to the women who are exposed to mass media, women who are not exposed .538 times in Orissa and .892 times in A.P. are less likely to enjoy high autonomy. On the other way, exposures to mass media women are more likely to have higher autonomy.

Standard of living is also an indicator for the determination of autonomy women. In the present analysis medium and high autonomy is in increasing trend in case of all type of household. Data reveals that in compare to higher standard of living, the household of medium standard of living women 1.347 times and low standard of women 1.763 times more likely to have high autonomy in Orissa. But in case of Andhra Pradesh the .963 times medium standard of living and .853 times low standard of living women are less likely to have high autonomy. It indicates that in Andhra Pradesh the standard of living doesn't give much effect on autonomy of women.

The above analysis reveals that women's autonomy is positively and significantly affected by place of residence and standard of living in both the states (Table 3).

Ante Natal Care

National Family Health Survey-3 Data reveals that total 1321 women become pregnant at least once during the last five years preceding the survey in Orissa and 1672 in Andhra Pradesh. Out of these women in Orissa 83 percent women who have received ANC partially and only 10 percentage

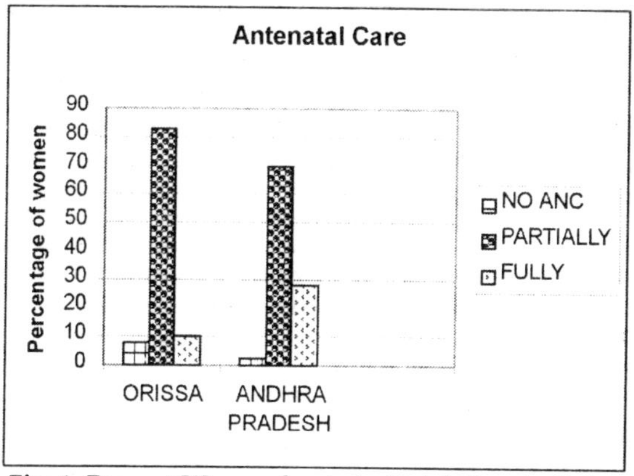

Fig: 1: Percent Women by Ante Natal Care in Orissa and Andhra Pradesh: NFHS-3 Data

women received full ANC (Fig:1). On the other hand in Andhra Pradesh the percentage of fully received ANC is higher (28 percent) when compare to Orissa (9.9 percent). In other words A.P. women comparatively better status than Orissa currently married women. Results revealed that 2.3 percent women in Andhra Pradesh and 7.5 percent in Orissa did not receive any antenatal care or not utilized ANC(not received IFA Tablets , tetanus injection etc) .

Women's Autonomy and Ante Natal Care

Women's autonomy and Anti natal care has been cross classified and the results are given in Table 4.The percentage of women who received Fully ANC among the low autonomy women is higher than those women who have medium autonomy. So it implies that even women have low autonomy but they are more conscious about ANC in both the states. In Andhra Pradesh among the low autonomy one third (32 percent) women had reported that they had received full ANC which is much higher in compare to Orissa (10.1 percent). Analysis also reveals that there is no difference in percentage of women who received fully ANC among low (10.1 percent) and high (10.7 percent) autonomy of women in Orissa. On the other side the difference is less among the medium and high autonomy women. It also implies that autonomy of women do not play significant role in availing of ANC. But when compare between two states, result indicates that Andhra Pradesh women are more conscious about ANC than Orissa women.

Table 4
Percent Women in Orissa and Andhra Pradesh by Women's Autonomy and Ante Natal Care, NFHS-3 Data

	ORISSA				*ANDHRA PRADESH*			
Women's Autonomy	*No ANC*	*Partially*	*Fully*	*Total Cases*	*No ANC*	*Partially*	*Fully*	*Total Cases*
Low	5.9	84.0	10.1	524	2.7	65.4	32.0	679
Medium	8.5	82.2	9.3	399	2.0	72.5	25.5	545
High	8.3	81.0	10.7	374	2.0	73.6	24.4	401
Total ANC Cases	96	1071	130	1297	37	1134	454	1625

Impact of Socio-economic Characteristics on Ante Natal Care

Result in Table 5 shows that level of education, husband's education, husband's occupation, mass media, castes and standard of living has positive impact on availing ANC in both the states. Utilization of ANC was high among the urban areas women in both the states. In Orissa nearly 15 percent women who are from urban area taking full ANC, whereas in A.P. more than one fourth women (28.3 percent) receiving full ANC and also even very less difference in cases of rural area.

Among different religious groups (Table 5), the proportion of women receiving full ANC was 10.0 percent among Hindu, 5.6 percent among Muslim and 11.8 percent among the remaining religious groups in Orissa. On the other hand in A.P. 27.1 percent among Hindu, 31.5 percent among Muslim and 22.1 percent among the remaining religious group women receiving full ANC. So it indicate that in Orissa other castes women and in A.P. Muslim women's are more conscious about full ANC.

Summary and Conclusions

An attempt has been made in this paper to understand the relationship between women's autonomy and Ante Natal Care of two Indian states. The analyses shows that, Andhra Pradesh women have greater autonomy in making decision regarding their own health care, freedom of movement and access to money, compare to Orissa. Place of residence is found to have the most extensive impact for both the states, those women who are from urban area their autonomy is higher in compared to rural area. Among the other indicators, standard of living gives positive impact on autonomy of women in Orissa. But in Andhra Pradesh, husband occupation played a major role to determine the autonomy of women.

In context to ANC, some factors such as place of residence, respondent's education, husband's occupation, exposed to mass media, caste and better standard of living showed positive impact on received ANC, whereas mother's involvement in labour force showed less impact on received ANC. After that according to this study, autonomy of women do not play significant role in availing ANC in both the states. But still in compare to Orissa, Andhra Pradesh women's are more conscious about Ante Natal Care.

Table 5

Percent Women Utilising ANC by Background Characteristics in Orissa and Andhra Pradesh: NFHS-3 Data

	ORISSA				*ANDHARA PRADESH*			
Background Characteristics	*No ANC*	*Partially*	*Fully*	*Total Cases*	*No ANC*	*Partially*	*Fully*	*Total Cases*
Place of Residence								
Urban	4.9	80.8	14.3	349	1.8	69.9	28.3	1040
Rural	8.4	83.2	8.3	972	3.0	69.9	27.1	632
Religion								
Hindu	7.3	82.7	10.0	1262	2.8	70.1	27.1	1242
Muslim	5.6	88.9	5.6	18	0.8	67.7	31.5	362
Others	11.8	76.5	11.8	34	.0.0	77.9	22.1	68
Resp.'s Education								
Illiterate	13.6	81.2	5.2	553	5.8	70.7	23.5	553
Primary	6.4	84.7	8.9	235	1.7	71.6	26.6	229
Secondary	1.9	83.5	14.6	466	0.3	70.1	29.7	708
Highest	0.0	80.6	19.4	67	0.0	64.8	35.2	182
Husband Education								
Illiterate	16.4	76.3	7.3	371	4.7	70.9	24.4	426
Primary	3.1	90.8	6.1	261	2.9	67.5	29.7	209
Secondary	4.6	83.2	12.2	501	1.5	10.9	27.6	742
Highest	0.6	84.5	14.9	161	0.0	66.1	33.9	277
Resp.'s Occupation								
Not working	4.9	83.3	11.7	912	1.3	69.7	29.0	1119
Working	13.2	80.9	5.9	409	4.3	70.3	25.3	553

Contd.

Background Characteristics	ORISSA				ANDHARA PRADESH			
	No ANC	Partially	Fully	Total Cases	No ANC	Partially	Fully	Total Cases
Husband occupation								
Not working	0.0	93.3	6.7	15	0.0	90.0	10.0	10
Working	7.5	82.6	10.0	1302	2.3	69.7	28.0	1655
Mass media								
No Exposure	15.9	77.7	6.4	346	7.3	74.1	18.6	247
Have Exposure	4.5	84.3	11.2	973	1.4	69.2	29.3	1421
Caste								
Backward	9.0	83.2	7.8	912	3.0	70.7	26.3	1094
Advance	4.3	80.8	14.9	395	0.9	68.8	30.3	574
Standard of living								
Low	12.2	82.2	5.7	510	5.3	73.4	21.3	263
Medium	5.3	83.5	11.2	339	2.4	71.7	25.8	534
High	1.1	84.0	14.9	281	0.9	66.4	32.7	703

Education is considered to have greater effect on any aspect of demography; thereby it is also expected to have great role in fertility behavior. Thus, this result highlights that in both the states with increases in level of women's education, the proportion of receiving ANC also increases. Research studies carried out in developing countries support the above findings that the education level of women is one of the most significant factor which positively effect on ANC. In low fertility countries like, Bangladesh, Malaysia, Philippine and other regions of India, the relationship between utilization of maternal care services and the education attainment has show positive relation (Mason, 1984; Mason et al., 2000; Jejeebhoy, 2000).

In the present study it is found that level of husband's education has a significant bearing in women receiving ANC. Wife of highest educated husband 19.4 percent more receive ANC compared to those women whose husband is illiterate (7.3 %). And on the other side same type of result we can find in case of A.P. Thus it may be said that in order to increase the percentage of women receiving ANC, education of both female and male up to certain level is quite essential.

In case of women work status, here the pattern shows that receiving antenatal care has been batter among the non-working women than the working women. Supported by Yesudian (2004) in his article impact of women's empowerment, autonomy and attitude on maternal health care utilization in India summarized non-working mothers are receiving more antenatal and natal care utilization than working mothers. From this type of conclusion we can say that work fertility relationship cannot be always negative.

In context to relationship between husband's occupation and receiving antenatal care, figure shows that only 8 percent women receiving full ANC in case of, if husband is not working. But there percentage is increased with change in the status of husband occupation (working husband) i.e.11.2 percent women receiving full ANC in Orissa if there husband is in working status. On the other hand in A.P. more than 30 percent a woman's receiving full ANC, which is much higher than Orissa women's. So over all figure reveals that if husband is in working status then wife are more conscious about ANC compare to not working husband.

It is found that exposure to mass media play a significant role in fertility decision and taking proper ANC. It is found that fully exposed mass media women are more aware about ANC, compare to less exposed women. Data shows that among the women who are more exposed to mass media, around 11 percent women's are taking full ANC in Orissa and 29.3 percent in A.P.

Result shows that out of total cases advance caste women receiving more ANC in compare to backward caste in both the states.

There is a positive relationship between standard of living and receiving Full ANC. With the increase in standard of living, percentage of receiving full ANC among the women is gradually increases. In Andhra Pradesh too similar pattern is apparent. To enhance the women autonomy work participation of women and literacy level should be increased by organizing suitable programs.

References

Basu, A.M. (1992), *Cultural the Status of Women and Demography Behaviour,* Oxford: Claredon Press.

Bloom, S.S, Wypij D., and Das Gupta M. (2001), "Dimensions of Women's Autonomy and the Influence on Maternal Health Care Utilization in a North Indian City", *Demography* 38(1): 67-78.

Jejeebhoy, Shireen, J. (2000), "Women Autonomy in Rural India: Its Dimensions, Determinants and Influence of Context" In: Harriet Presser and Gita Sen, (eds.) *Women's Empowerment and Demographic Processes: Moving beyond Cairo.* New York: Oxford Press.

Jejeebhoy, S.J, and Sathar Zeba (2001), "Women's Autonomy in India and Pakistan: The Influence of Religion and Region", *Population and Development Review* 27(4): 687-712.

Jejeebhoy, S. (1995), *"Women's Education, Autonomy and Reproductive Behaviour: Experience from Development Countries.* Oxford: Claredon Press.

Kishor Sunita and Sulabha Parasuraman (1998), *Mother's Employment and Infant and Child Mortality in India.* NFHS subject Report No 8. Mumbai: IIPS.

Mason, Karen Oppenheim (1984), *The Status of Women: A Review of Its Relationship to Fertility and Mortality.* New York The Rockefeller Foundation.

Mason, Karen Oppenheim and Herbert L. Smith (Aug, 2000), "Husband versus Wives Fertility Goals and Use of Contraception: The Influence of Gender Context in Five Asian Countries", *Population Association of America* 37(3): 299-311.

International Institute for Population Sciences and ORC Macro, (2000), *National Family Health Survey (NFHS-2), 1998-1999, India.* Mumbai: IIPS.

International Institute for Population Sciences (IIPS) and Macro International (2007), *National Family Health Survey (NFHS-3), 2005-06: India: Volume I.* Mumbai: IIPS.

Patel, M. Rajnikant and Dey. D. (2002), "Impact of Women's Education on Fertility: Evidences from NFHS-II Data", Paper presented in 25th *Annual Conference of the India Association for the Study of Population* held at IIPS, Mumbai.

Roy, T.K., and S. Niranjan (2004), "Indicators of Women's Empowerment in India", *Asia-Pacific Journal of Population* 19(2):

Vaidyanathan, K.E. (1998), "Status of Women and Family Planning: The Indian Case", *Asia-Pacific Population Journal* 14(2):

Yesudian P. (2004), "Impact of Women's Empowerment, Autonomy and Attitude on Maternal Health Care Utilization in India", Paper presented at *Global Forum for Health Research 8,* Mexico.

SECTION – 3

Maternal Health

11

Maternal and Child Health of Urban Poor in India: Implications for Achieving the MDGs

Siddharth Agarwal, Aradhana Srivastava, Monisha Vaid

Background

India is committed to achieving the Millennium Development Goals (MDGs) set by the UN Millennium Declaration in 2000. MDGs ably summarize crucial global development concerns, encompassing multiple dimensions of economic and social poverty. As a result, they have been incorporated smoothly into the five-year planning framework of the country. Specifically with regard to health, the Eleventh Five Year Plan is optimistic about achieving the MDG targets for infant and maternal mortality rate (IMR and MMR) by the end of the plan period. The plan also acknowledges the need for action on many fronts to achieve this, including improved access to health centres, institutional deliveries, nutritional supplementation, and clean drinking water and sanitation. However, attainment of these goals within the given time frame is possible only through targeted focus on vulnerable groups that significantly account for the country's burden of poverty and deprivation, and lag far behind in the country's march towards development.

India's Urban Transition

India is currently on the threshold of an urban transition, witnessing unprecedented urbanization in recent years. During the decade 1991-2001 India's urban population grew by 31.2 per cent while the rural population grew at a much slower rate of 17.9 per cent. It is estimated to number about 336 million in 2008 (RG of India, 2006). It is projected that by the year 2030, 41 percent of the country's population, numbering around 600 million, will live in cities and by the year 2050, this proportion is expected to increase to 55 percent of the total population (UNDESF, 2008).

Increasing Share of Urban Poverty

Growing urbanization in India has led to an increase in the share of poverty in urban areas. Urban poor are in fact the fastest growing segment of Indian population, owing to migration, expansion of city limits and natural growth, and are expected to increase from the estimated 80-100 (NSSO, 2007; MOHFW, 2000) million in 2005 to 202 million in less than 15 years (UN-HABITAT, 2006). They also constitute a major socially excluded group, suffering severe deprivation. Most of the urban poor reside in slums, many of which are unlisted in official records. These unlisted or hidden slums suffer greater vulnerability and exclusion owing to their inability to access basic services and government programmes for the poor.

Even within slums there are pockets of more vulnerable groups such as scavengers, construction site workers, workers of local industries, those residing along large drains or temporary migrants amidst older settlers. Such groups are left out of the social fabric and therefore suffer from lack of confidence to express their requirements and very low negotiating power.

Urban Poor and the MDGs: Where do they Stand?

The urban poor are vulnerable to many health risks as a consequence of living in conditions characterized by cramped, low-quality housing with limited sanitation, limited access to affordable quality health care, widespread illiteracy, social isolation, and a lack of negotiating capacity to demand improved public services. This is reflected in their health outcomes. Health indicators among urban poor are worse than urban averages and exhibit sharp disparity between poor and non-poor. Women and children are the most vulnerable to slum environments and urban poverty. Slums are fertile breeding grounds for a number of diseases such as diarrhea, fever, respiratory infections, tuberculosis, jaundice and malaria. Children have little immunity against their onslaught. Women suffer from poor maternal health on account of early pregnancies, which are multiple and closely spaced, undernutrition, home deliveries, largely unsafe and without trained assistance, besides denial of rights, domestic violence and crime. These deprivations directly impact the MDGs 1, 4, and 5 relating to maternal and child health and nutrition.

Objective

There are several research studies available across the world showing a trend of poorer maternal and child health and nutrition leading to higher morbidity and mortality in urban slums. However, commonly available large-scale statistical data does not highlight these intra-urban inequities. The objective of the paper is to analyse maternal and child health status of urban poor in India vis-à-vis that of the non-poor, especially relating to targets set by the MDGs.

Data and Methodology

Analysis of the National Family Health Survey NFHS-3, 2005-06 (IIPS and Macro International, 2007) data disaggregated by economic status was conducted to determine the health indicators of the urban poor and its comparison with other population groups. NFHS-3 used the wealth index based on 33 assets and household characteristics for categorising population into economic group quintiles. The same cut-offs were used irrespective of rural or urban residence. As a result, the urban population was concentrated in the upper quintiles. In fact, the cumulative share of urban population in the bottom two wealth index quintiles was only 9.4 percent. This did not realistically capture intra-urban economic disparity.

In this study, the urban sample population was taken separately and divided into wealth index quartiles. The lowest quartile was selected as representative of the urban poor and the three upper quartiles were merged to represent the non poor. The lowest quartile is estimated to be reasonably representative of urban poverty; in view of the latest Planning Commission estimates put the number of urban poor in India at about 80.8 million or 25.7 percent of the total urban population.

This methodology was developed by Urban Health Resource Centre (UHRC). The results show that it has brought out the extent of deprivation suffered by the urban poor vis-à-vis the non-poor in relation to maternal and child health indicators, as well as indicators like access to water supply and sanitation.

Results and Discussion

A number of indicators derived from the NFHS-3 data relating to maternal and child health of the urban poor are relevant in the context of the MDGs. While some of the indicators are also MDG indicators, some others relate to them and are equally significant in assessing where the urban poor stand vis-à-vis the MDGs. This section presents some key indicators for the urban poor gauging their status on specific MDG targets as well as related indicators.

MDG 1: Eradicate Extreme Poverty and Hunger

Besides poverty reduction, MDG 1 also aims to halve, by 2015, the proportion of people who suffer from hunger. Child undernutrition is one of the key indicators to assess the progress on this front. It is, however, also a grim reality among the urban poor in India.

MDG Indicator 1.8: Prevalence of underweight children under-five years of age

- About half (47.1 percent) of the children below five years of age among the urban poor (Fig. 1) were underweight (-2 SD weight for height). The non-poor, on the other hand, have a lower prevalence of undernutrition with 26.2 percent children below five years of age being underweight.

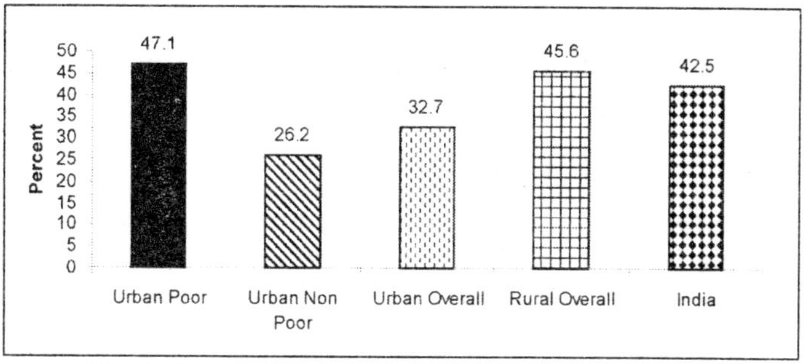

Fig. 1: Proportion of Underweight Children, 2005-06 (% Children aged below 5 years who were underweight)

High prevalence of undernutrition among young children is the result of a combination of several factors including faulty infant feeding practices, poor dietary intake as a consequence of food insecurity, lack of hygiene, food contamination and lack of proper child care practices. Frequent occurrence of infections which deplete the body of nutrients and impede their proper absorption is also a major problem (Ghosh and Shah, 2004).

Insecurity of income and livelihood along with absence of social support networks implies that cash availability with the urban poor is not uniform, thereby leading to irregular food consumption and poor nutrition outcomes, especially among children and women.

MDG 4: Reduce Child Mortality

MDG 4 aims to reduce child mortality by two thirds by 2015. However, every year about 2.5 million children in India die due to illnesses, most of which are easily preventable through immunization (World Bank, 2007).

The poor health and survival of children among the urban poor vis-à-vis the non-poor is quite visibly reflected in neonatal, infant and under-five mortality. Neonatal mortality among the urban poor was 34.9 per thousand live births, much higher than the non-poor average of 25.5 per thousand.

MDG Indicator 4.1: Under-five Mortality Rate

- Under-five mortality among the urban poor was 72.7 per thousand, substantially higher than that of the non-poor (41.8) or the overall urban average (51.9).

MDG Indicator 4.2: Infant Mortality Rate

- The urban poor have an infant mortality rate of 54.6 in comparison to 35.5 among the non-poor and the urban average of 41.7 (Fig. 2).

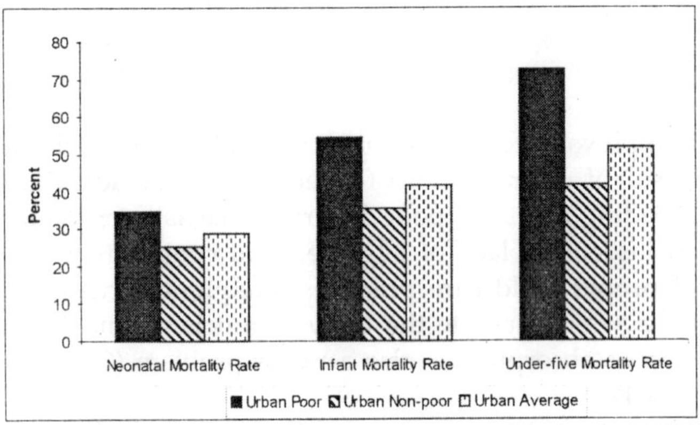

Fig. 2: Neonatal, Infant and Under-five Mortality Rates, 2005-06

Vaccination of children against six serious yet preventable diseases, namely tuberculosis, measles, diphtheria, whooping cough, tetanus and polio, is the cornerstone of child health programmes in India. Children of the urban poor suffer accentuated vulnerability to such illnesses, as outbreaks of vaccine preventable diseases are more common in urban slums owing to high population density and continuous influx of new pool of infective agents with immigrating population (Loening and Coovadia, 1983; Lal and Vashisht, 2003; AFP Alert, 2002; Awasthi and Agarwal, 2003; Agarwal et al., 2005). The overcrowding results in prolonged exposure to infections and greater severity of infections in such cases (Lodha et al., 2000; Aaby et al., 2005).

MDG Indicator 4.3: Proportion of 1 year-old children immunized against measles

- 52.6percent urban poor children 12-23 months of age had received measles immunization as compared to 80percent among the non-poor and the urban average of 72percent.
- Only 40 percent children among the urban poor received complete immunization as per NFHS-3, which is much lower than 65.4 percent coverage among the non-poor. 29.5 percent children among the urban poor were left out from Universal Immunization Programme. In spite of facing equal or even greater risk of infections, immunization benefits have not been able to reach all urban poor children, in spite of comparatively easier geographical access.

MDG 5: Improve Maternal Health

The fifth MDG aims to reduce maternal mortality ratio by three quarters and achieve universal access to reproductive health by 2015. Maternal health is a serious concern in India, with the country reporting the largest number of maternal deaths in the world (WHO et al., 2007). NFHS-3 data indicates that the urban poor are a high-risk group in terms of access to maternity care and suffer from poor access to reproductive healthcare.

MDG Indicator 5.2: Proportion of births attended by skilled health personnel

- Despite proximity to specialty hospitals, 56percent of slum children are born at home, possibly without skilled birth attendance. This is much higher than 21.5 percent among the non-poor and the urban average of 33 percent.

MDG Indicator 5.3: Contraceptive prevalence rate

- About half (49percent) of the urban poor use any modern method of family planning as compared to 58percent among the non-poor and the urban average of 56 percent. The use of spacing methods among the urban poor is limited to only 8 percent.

- Urban poor populations are characterized by low levels of acceptance of family planning methods, owing to lack of awareness, non-compliance as well as non-availability of such facilities (Mamdani, 1993; Joshi and Patil, 2007). Preference for large family size also is a possible reason for non-acceptance or delayed acceptance of family planning methods. This is indicated by the finding that 71.4 percent women opting for sterilization among the urban poor did so after 3 or more births in the family.

MDG Indicator 5.5: Antenatal care coverage (at least 1 visit & at least 4 visits)

- Only about 54percent mothers had at least 3 antenatal care visits among the urban poor, much lower as compared to the urban average (75 percent) and that of the non-poor (83 percent) (Fig. 3).

Prevalence of anemia is another key indicator for maternal health and has a bearing on birth outcomes as well. 58.8 percent urban poor women aged 15-49 years suffered from anemia as compared to 45.3 percent of the non-poor women. Consumption of IFA tablets for 90 days or more (as recommended in the Reproductive and Child Health programme RCH-II) was 18.5 percent among urban poor mothers as compared to 41.8 percent mothers among the non-poor.

Tetanus toxoid (TT) vaccination is the third component of antenatal care in RCH-II, which recommends two TT vaccinations for pregnant women. NFHS-3 data shows that three fourths (75.8 percent) of pregnant women among urban poor got TT vaccinations, though the figure was lower than the urban non-poor average of 90.7 percent.

On the whole, only 11 percent mothers received complete antenatal care (which includes at least 3 ANC visits, IFA supplementation for 90 days and 2 TT vaccinations) among the urban poor. This is much lower than the non-poor average of 29.5 percent.

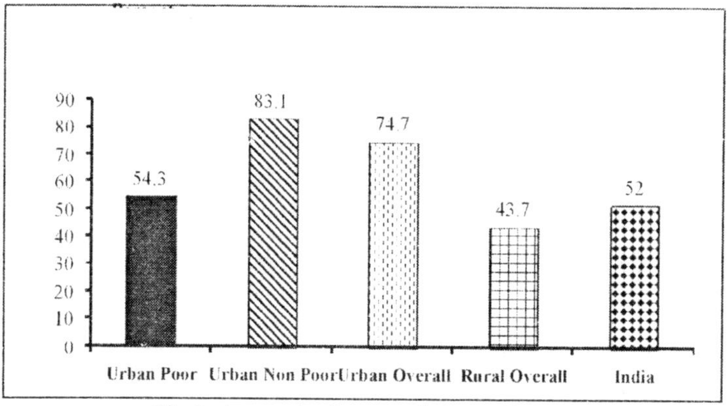

Fig.3: Access to Antenatal Care, 2005-06
(% Mothers who had at least 3 antenatal care visits)

MDG Indicator 5.6: Unmet need for family planning

- Unmet need for family planning among the urban poor was 14 percent as compared to 8.3percent among the non-poor and an urban average of 10 percent.

Unmet need is a critical and programmatically most relevant aspect of family planning. It points to the gap between women's reproductive intentions and actual contraceptive behavior, and poses a challenge for the family planning programme of reaching and serving such women (Singh, 2004). Some common reasons for unmet need among the urban poor include difficulty of access and poor quality of family planning services, concern about side effects of contraceptives, son preference and opposition from spouse/family members (Puri et al., 2004).

MDG 7: Ensure Environmental Sustainability

A crucial target of MDG 7 is to halve by 2015, the proportion of people without sustainable access to safe drinking water and basic sanitation. Environmental sanitation is especially relevant in the context of child health, since poor sanitation accounts for a number of common infections among children, such as diarrhea, jaundice and typhoid.

MDG Indicator 7.8: Proportion of population using an improved drinking water source

- Only 18.5 percent urban poor households have access to piped water supply at home, which is much less than the urban average of 50.7 percent households and even lower than that among the non-poor (62.2 percent).

MDG Indicator 7.9: Proportion of population using an improved sanitation facility

- Only 47.2 percent urban poor have access to toilet facilities as compared to the urban average of 83.2 percent and 96 percent among the non-poor.

Most slums and urban poor habitations are encroachments on public or private lands, under constant threat of eviction. Since they are unauthorized occupations, slums are also not served by any civic amenities, including water supply, drainage and sanitation. This adds to the poor living environment and higher prevalence of infections among slum dwellers, especially children.

Challenges in Improving Maternal and Child Health Among the Urban Poor

The above discussed statistics highlight the situation of the urban poor in India as a highly vulnerable group, suffering similar gaps in maternal and child health indicators as other vulnerable groups in the country. Targeting the urban poor is essential for achieving all-round improvement in maternal, child health and nutrition in order to effectively achieve MDGs within the timeframe of 2015.

There are several challenges associated with the access of maternal and child healthcare among the urban poor.

Community level Challenges

1. *Poverty and Poor Living Conditions*: Poverty is an over-arching factor which intervenes through poor nutrition, compromised ability to seek health care and poor living conditions resulting in poor health outcomes among slum

communities. It compels urban poor communities to live in crowded, closely packed slums that lack access to basic services. Such an environment is ideal breeding ground for many infections which are a grave threat to child health.

2. *Lack of Community Awareness and Culturally Influenced Behaviors*: Slum residents often have no/limited knowledge on appropriate behaviors with respect to maternal and reproductive health, child and newborn care, hygiene and prevention of infections among children. Religious and traditional beliefs also sometimes promote harmful practices and hamper the acceptance of recommended behaviors. Slum dwellers are also often not aware of the schemes and services being provided for them, including health or immunization camps. Ignorance is also a reason for non-recognition or delayed recognition of symptoms regarding newborn and child diseases, often leading to complications and even fatality on account of delayed action.

3. *Weak Social Cohesion and Poor Negotiating* Capacity: Slums communities are socially excluded from the urban mainstream. They also suffer from weak social cohesion internally. This is a hindrance to organized community collective efforts among them and prevents them from raising a strong demand for essential services and thereby influencing public action.

Legality and Exclusion

4. *Illegality and Social Exclusion*: Slums are almost always initially informal settlements with no land tenure rights. The illegal nature of occupied land prevents their inclusion in official slum lists (Ramanathan, 2004). Owing to long delays in updating of official slum lists in most cities, slums may remain unrecognized for years (Taneja and Agarwal, 2003). Civic and health services usually do not reach such hidden and missing pockets of urban poor that are not a part of official records. They are also deprived of the

benefits of public schemes like ICDS and PDS, which are crucial for the welfare of the poor.

Weak Health Services

5. *Inadequate and Ineffective Public Health Services*: Unlike rural areas which have a dedicated primary health infrastructure, such structure is absent in urban areas. Moreover, the rapidly growing urban population especially of the urban poor renders the already scarce urban health infrastructure further inadequate. One primary health care facility in an urban area therefore caters to a much higher population compared to the norm of 1 center for every 50,000 population (Shekhar and Ram, 2005). Initiatives like the World Bank funded India Population Project (IPP- VIII) (1993 to 2002) have helped augment urban health facilities in larger cities like Bangalore, Delhi, Hyderabad and Kolkata, but largely remain absent from other cities.
6. *Expensive Private Facilities*: Though health facilities in the private sector have a wide presence in urban areas, they are often not accessible to the poor because of the high cost. The poor are therefore forced to fall back on the largely unqualified private providers practicing in slum areas who provide poor quality services. Moreover, these informal providers do not provide preventive health services such as immunization, antenatal care, health education and family planning since these services are not profitable.

Weak Linkages and Coordination

7. *Weak Community-provider Linkages and Low Demand for Services*: Owing to poor linkage between slum communities and health providers, slum residents are likely to be unaware of the location and services provided by health facilities, out-reach visits of health workers etc. This results in poor demand and utilization of health services. This problem is exacerbated in the case of recent or temporary migrants with little social support. Similarly, from the

providers' perspective health service delivery in slums is an enormous challenge, given the large and rapidly mobile population.

8. *Unclear Accountability and Weak Coordination Among Different Stakeholders*: In addition to limited infrastructure, there is lack of clarity of roles, coordination and accountability for providing services to the urban poor by the agencies responsible for providing health services in urban areas. These include state health department, municipal bodies, ICDS, NGOs, charitable organizations etc. There is little coordination between these agencies leading to both overlapping service areas and large un-served pockets.

How do the Urban Poor Progress Ahead on the MDG Path?

In order to overcome the challenges in addressing maternal and child health issues among urban poor communities, any programmatic intervention needs to focus on the "supply" of health services as well as the "demand" side. All slums are not equal and therefore effective programming entails the need to target resources and efforts at the more vulnerable slums. This section outlines possible measures which can impact both the demand and supply aspects of maternal and child healthcare among the urban poor.

Supply Side Measures

City specific planning for healthcare

City-specific planning for healthcare is crucial to effectively address health needs of the urban poor, especially reaching out to excluded and un-served clusters. This can be most effectively achieved through city-specific slum situation analysis, mapping and planning on the basis of the exercise. It is also essential to build the capacity of municipal bodies in management of health services at the local level through various means such as trainings, orientations and exposure visits of elected representatives as well as officials to well-managed urban health programmes.

Augment Public Sector Urban Health Services Including Outreach Activities with Focus on Vulnerable Urban Settlements

Primary health care facilities have not grown systematically to cater to the explosive growth of urban population especially the poor (Agarwal et al., 2007). Therefore facilities for the poor are not evenly distributed across the city and not necessarily in physical proximity to urban slum clusters. Location of primary health facilities in urban areas on the basis of slum identification and mapping is essential to maximize reach and coverage of such facilities.

Promote Pro-poor Public Private Partnership for Health Service Delivery

Given the large presence of the private sector (both profit and non-profit) in providing health services even to the disadvantaged sections, partnerships with the sector helps expand reach and coverage of health facilities to urban poor communities. Such partnerships can also help improve the quality of health services provided to the urban poor. Several examples of such partnerships are available from corporate as well as civil society initiatives (UHRC, 2007). Such initiatives need to be scaled up and replicated to achieve larger coverage of urban poor population who can benefit from them.

Strengthen Program Management Capacity (including financial management)

A number of programmes such as JNNURM, SJSRY and IHSDP aim at improving livelihood and providing better infrastructure and services for the urban poor, which will ultimately also have a positive impact on their health status. Ensuring an effective programme management setup at all levels, especially the district and ULB level, which includes efficient financial management, will help maximize the programme benefits to slum populations.

Capacity Building of Health Workers

Motivational training should be provided to health providers (ANMs, Supervisors, MOs) working in slum areas to i) understand the unique problems and complexities relating to health in slum communities; ii) be more sensitive towards disadvantaged communities, and ii) recognize and coordinate with community health workers, slum-based community organizations and other agencies working for healthcare among urban poor.

Demand Side Measures

Increase Awareness about Optimal Behaviors, Services and Provisions

One of the main reasons accounting for the gap in utilization of antenatal care and institutional deliveries between the urban poor and non poor is lack of awareness on maternal health issues among the slum dwellers (Agarwal and Bharti, 2006; Agarwal et al., 2007). Promotion of safe delivery practices and optimal care of newborns during the neonatal period are vital for addressing high neonatal mortality among the urban poor. Post-neonatal mortality needs to be targeted through extended immunization coverage along with programmes for hygiene promotion and prevention of undernutrition (UHRC, 2007).

Ensure that Demand is met with Increased Availability

Ensuring linkages between the community and providers, as well as involvement of the community in the programmes are essential for their effectiveness as well as sustainability. Linkages and coordination between community and providers and among the providers themselves is also crucial for regularity and improved coverage of services (UHRC, 2006). Slum women can be trained to serve as the crucial link between community and health services and for assisting others in accessing maternal and child health services and in counselling to raise demand for services (Agarwal, 2006; Agarwal, 2007).

Enhance Peoples' Capacity to Improve Behavior and Negotiate for Services

Empowered slum communities can ensure better accessibility and supply of services. Collective voice has greater strength and ability to influence change. Therefore, organizing slum communities into CBOs and raising their awareness on health issues, services and entitlements helps empower them to negotiate for better services and access to entitlements. Building linkages between the service providers CBOs also ensures increased demand for services at slum level as well provision of quality services at the providers' level.

Conclusions

The MDGs have, as one of their targets, achieving a significant improvement in the lives of at least 100 million slum dwellers by 2020. This reflects the growing realization of the need to impact urban poverty. The effort, however, is not sufficient to make a significant impact on the lives of the urban poor at the global level. Since urban poor constitute about a tenth of India's population and are also the fastest growing segment, it is essential to address their needs in order to substantially impact overall achievement of MDGs in the country.

- Impacting maternal and child health among urban poor warrants increased policy measures and energetic implementation on multiple aspects including housing, basic services, livelihoods, food security besides healthcare. Such measures have been initiated through a number of policies and programmes. Recent Indian Government initiatives for the urban poor, including the Jawaharlal Nehru National Urban Renewal Mission, efforts to universalize the ICDS and the forthcoming National Urban Health Mission offer apt opportunity for accelerated efforts to make slums healthier environments for their inhabitants.
- Existing policies at all levels can also be made more urban poor friendly, practical and measurable. Participatory implementation of programmes and efficient programme management is essential for the many public policy efforts to have an effective impact on the urban poor. Another important requirement for energetic policy implementation is training of

officers and increased information flow to urban poor, to activate and reinforce demand-supply linkages.

- Slums have some inherent advantages such as greater accessibility, concentrated population, presence of NGOs and less intense scarcity of health facilities, which can be leveraged to facilitate effective impact of interventions. Successful innovative approaches available in civil society and PPP initiatives can be scaled up and replicated to achieve larger coverage of urban poor population who can benefit from them.
- Coordinated interventions from all concerned sectors are required for improvement in the health of mothers and children in urban slums. Multi-stakeholder coordination meetings at city and ward level of coordination committees at each level would help achieve a synergistic impact through – i) convergence of related schemes to achieve common goals, ii) integrated planning and pooling of resources and iii) jointly reviewing progress and taking remedial actions.

In the absence of such efforts, indeed, achieving the MDGs on time will remain a distant dream.

References

Aaby, P. et al., (2005). "Non-specific Effects of Measles Vaccination on All-cause Child Mortality: Revisited", *Indian Pediatrics*, 42(2): 541-44.

AFP Alert, (2002): "National Polio Surveillance Project: A Govt. of India - WHO Initiative", 6(3): Jul-Dec.

Agarwal, S., (2006). "To Catch a Virus and Miss the Disease", *The Indian Express*, September 16: p 9.

Agarwal, S., (2007). "Feel the Pulse of Poverty", *Hindustan Times*, Thursday, May 3.

Agarwal, S., and B. M. Bharti, (2006). "Reproductive Health in Urban Slums", *The Journal of Obstetrics and Gynaecology of India* 56 (3): 255-257.

Agarwal, S., A. Bhanot, and G. Goindi, (2005). "Understanding and Addressing Childhood Immunization Coverage in Urban Slums", *Indian Pediatrics* 42: 653-63.

Agarwal, P., M. M. Singh, and S. Garg, (2007). "Maternal Health Care Utilization among Women in an Urban Slum in Delhi", *Indian Journal of Community Medicine* 32(3): 203-205.

Agarwal, S. et al., (2007). "Urbanization, Urban Poverty and Health of the Urban Poor: Status, Challenges and the Way Forward", *Demography India* 36(1): 121-134.

Awasthi, S., and S. Agarwal, (2003). "Determinants of Childhood Mortality and Morbidity in Urban Slums in India", *Indian Pediatrics* 40: 1145-61.

Ghosh, S., and D. Shah, (2004). "Nutritional Problems in Urban Slum Children", *Indian Pediatrics* 41(7): 682-96.

International Institute for Population Sciences (IIPS) and Macro International, (2007). *National Family Health Survey (NFHS-3), 2005-06: India: Volume I.* Mumbai: IIPS.

Joshi, S. M., and S. B. Patil, (2007). "Knowledge and Practices of Family Planning in an Urban Slum of Mumbai", *Indian Journal of Preventive and Social Medicine* 38(1 & 2): 1-4.

Lal, S., and B. M. Vashisht, (2003). "Innovative Approaches to Universalize Immunization in Rural Areas", *Indian Journal of Community Medicine* 28(2): 51-56.

Lodha, R. et al., (2000). "Diptheria in Urban Slums of North India", *The Lancet* 355: 204.

Loening, W., and H. Coovadia, (1983). "Age-specific Occurrence Rates of Measles in Urban, Peri-urban, and Rural Environment: Implications for Time of Vaccination", *The Lancet* 322: 324-26.

Mamdani, M., (1993). "Fertility and Contraceptive use in Poor Urban Areas of Developing Countries", *Health Policy and Planning* 8(1): 1-18.

Ministry of Health and Family Welfare, (2000). *National Population Policy, 2000.* New Delhi: MOHFW.

National Sample Survey Organization, (2007): Poverty Estimates based on 61st round, 2005-06. New Delhi: NSSO.

Puri, A., S. Garg, and M. Mehra, (2004). "Assessment of Unmet Need for Contraception in an Urban Slum of Delhi", *Indian Journal of Community Medicine* 29(3): 139-40.

Ramanathan, U., (2004). *Illegality and Exclusion.* International Environmental Law Research Centre Working Paper No. 2. Switzerland: IELRC.

Registrar General of India, (2006). *Population Projections for India and the States 2001-26.* New Delhi: Office of the Registrar General and Census Commissioner.

Shekhar, C., and F. Ram, (2005). *National Report on Evaluation of Functioning of Urban Health Posts/Urban Family Centres in India.* Mumbai: IIPS.

Singh, P., (2004). *Trends in Fertility, Mortality, Nutrition and Health Indicators.* Background paper for Vision 2020. New Delhi: Planning Commission, Government of India.

Taneja, S., and S. Agarwal, (2003). *Situational Analysis for Guiding USAID/India and EHP/India: Technical Assistance Efforts in Indore, Madhya Pradesh, India.* Virginia: USAID-EHP.

UHRC, (2007). "Public-Private Partnership for Improving Health of the Urban Poor", *UHRC Newsletter* Dec. 2007.

UN Department of Economic and Social Affairs, (2008). *World Urbanization Prospects: The 2007 Revision-Highlights.* New York: United Nations.

UN-HABITAT, (2006). *State of the World's Cities Report 2006/2007.* London: Earth Scan.

World Bank, (2007). *Improving Conditions of the Urban Poor and Increasing Access to Basic Services.* Washington: The World Bank.

WHO, UNICEF, UNFPA and The World Bank, (2007). *Maternal Mortality in 2005: Estimates by WHO, UNICEF, UNFPA and The World Bank.* Geneva: World Health Organization.

12

Cause of Maternal Mortality and Morbidity in Tamil Nadu 2007-2008

A. Krishnamurthy, P. Muniappan

Introduction

Maternal death is an important indicator of the reach of effective clinical health services to the poor and is regarded as one of the composite measures to assess the country's progress. The international conference on population and development in 1994 had recommended reduction in maternal mortality by atleast 50 percent of the 1990 levels by the year 2000 and further one half by the year 2015. The Millennium Development goals (MDG) have set the target of achieving 200 maternal deaths per one lakh live births by 2007 and 109 by 2015.

The maternal mortality ratio (MMR) varies from 820 per one lakh live births in African countries to just 9 in the developed countries. It is estimated in the year 2000 that 5.29 lakh women die due to maternal causes all over the world. Among these deaths, 95percent of maternal deaths shared by Asian and African countries. Particularly in India more than one lakh women die every year due to maternal causes. Hence India accounts for 20percent of all maternal deaths world-wide.

The past estimates for India by using indirect methods suggested that MMR had declined from over 750 in the 1960s to about 400 in the 1990s. The National Family Health Survey-1 (NFHS-1) provided a national estimate of 424 in 1992-93. The NFHS-2 suggested that the MMR had not changed significantly from 424 in 1992-93 to 540 in 1998-99.

In India it has been observed that calculation of MMR in Tamil Nadu found to be reliable because of the procedure adopted and initiation collectively taken by the Ministry of Health and Family planning, Government of Tamil Nadu (Dept. of Family Welfare, Chennai, 2008). In Tamil Nadu the district level MMR has been calculated by direct method every year since 1994 onwards district level MMR has been estimated from the vital events survey (VES) conducted for the year 1995, 1997, 1998, 1999 and 2003. Around 1100 maternal deaths occur every year which is about 1percent of maternal deaths occurring in India and 0.2 percent of maternal deaths in the world. This gives estimates of 100. The sample Registration system (SRS), the official source of information on vital rates publishes an estimate of 301 and 134 (2001-2003) for India and Tamil Nadu, respectively.

Objective

The objectives of this research paper are:

1. To analyse the maternal deaths occurred in Tamil Nadu for the year 2007-2008,
2. To examine the maternal deaths by age, religion, community parity and period of death,
3. To look into the maternal deaths by place of delivery and place of death, and
4. To observe the maternal deaths by cause.

Results and Discussion

Method of Collection of Maternal Deaths by Districts

Recognising the importance of maternal deaths, in Tamil Nadu an innovative reporting system for collecting the maternal deaths both from rural and urban areas has been evolved. On the instructions of the Project Director, the MIES of the Project Directorate has been collecting the details on maternal deaths from the field staff by telegram within 24 hours of occurrence followed by a detailed medical audit report. At this juncture, it is worthwhile to mention that the MIES has also been collecting the Primary Health Centre (PHC) wise information on sex ratio, sex ratio at birth, infant deaths (gender wise and component wise) and infanticide and publishing the block wise report (district wise) every year from 1994. It has been observed 1059 maternal deaths for 1120727 births during 2007-2008 in Tamil Nadu (Dept. of Family Welfare, Chennai, 2008). The district wise MMR for the year 2007-2008 is given in Table 1. Maternal Mortality Ratio (MMR) is defined as the number of women dying from causes related to pregnancy and delivery complications (Maternal Deaths) per one lakh live births in a year. Maternal Mortality Rate is defined as number of maternal deaths per one lakh women in the reproductive age groups of 15-49 years.

Table 1
District Wise Maternal Mortality Ratio in Tamil Nadu, 2007-08

Name of the District	*No. of Live Births*	*No. of Maternal Deaths*	*MMR*
Chennai	80243	26	32
Kanyakumari	24693	11	45
Coimbatore	76270	39	51
Kancheepuram	55121	34	62
Tiruvallur	54112	42	78
Theni	20295	17	84
Cuddalore	36135	31	86
Thanjavur	42170	37	88
Thoothukudi	24994	22	88
Vellore	59668	53	89
Salem	57831	55	95
Sivagangai	22115	21	95
Virudhunagar	30590	31	101
Villupuram	58585	76	103
Nagapattinam	24170	25	103

Contd.

Name of the District	*No. of Live Births*	*No. of Maternal Deaths*	*MMR*
Madurai	52910	57	104
Namakkal	23134	24	104
Tirunelveli	247933	51	106
Erode	39036	42	108
Karur	15700	17	108
Dindigul	34592	39	113
Thiruvarur	20415	23	113
Pudukottai	26854	32	115
Ramanathapuram	22228	26	117
Krishnagiri	29829	37	124
Tiruvannamalai	39787	50	126
Dharmapuri	27749	35	126
Tiruchirapalli	41777	53	127
Perambalur	21193	29	137
The Nilgiris	10598	24	226
Tamil Nadu	1120727	1059	95

Among the 30 districts, 17 districts (Table 1) have reported more than the state level MMR of 95. The Nilgiris district has reported the highest MMR of 226 and Chennai district has reported the lowest MMR of 32. Thus a great variation is observed among the 30 districts from 32 to 226. The highest MMR of Nilgiris district is followed by Perambalur (137), Villupuram (130), Trichirapalli (127), Thiruvannamalai (126) and Ramanathapuram (117). The lowest MMR of Chennai district is followed by Kanniyakumari (45), Coimbatore (51), Kancheepuram (62), Theni (84) and Cuddalore (86).

Maternal Deaths by Age of Mother

Though the legal age at marriage is 18 years, still 4 percent of deaths reported from adolescent girls. More than 10 percent of maternal deaths from adolescent women are reported from Krishnagiri (16.2%) and Theni (11.8%). The maternal deaths in the age group 35+ years are high in Thirunelveli (15.7%), Thanjavur (13.5%), and Krishnagiri (13.5%) and in Chennai (11.5%).

Since more number of deliveries are conducted for the women in the age group of 20-29 years more than three fourth of the deaths occur in this fertile age group. Hence this table has to be analysed by MMR of each age group. The age of the mother and the risk of dying due to pregnancy and delivery related causes are positively correlated. In other words when the age of mother increases, the MMR also increases. It is clear from table 2, that MMR in the lower age group is lower than the higher age group of 35+years. The risk of dying in 35+ year's women is more than 3 times in the lower age group.

Table 2
Number and Percentage Maternal Deaths and Maternal Mortality Rate by Age of women in Tamil Nadu 2007-08

Age of Women	*No. and % of Maternal Deaths*		*Estimated No. of Live Births*	*Maternal Deaths*	*MMR*
15-19	42	(4.0)	55,000	42	76
20-24	431	(40.7)	5,61,700	431	77
25-29	375	(35.4)	3,65,900	375	102
30-34	126	(11.9)	1,03,200	126	122
35-39	70	(6.6)	28,800	70	243
40+	15	(1.4)	6,000	15	250
Total	1059	(100.0)	11,20,600	1059	95

Maternal Deaths by Religion

India is one of the most religiously diverse nations in the world. Religion plays a central and definite role in the life of the country and most of its people. Of the 1059 maternal deaths reported, 985 (93.5%) mothers are Hindus, 43 (4.1%) are Muslims and the remaining 25 mothers (2.4%t) are Christians. As per 2001 census, Hindu population constitutes 88.1 percent, Muslims 5.6 percent and Christians 6.1 percent. This clearly shows that more number of maternal deaths reported from Hindus and less number of maternal deaths reported from Christians.

Maternal Deaths by Community

The community details are available for 1027 cases only. Among these mothers, 353 maternal deaths (34.4%) reported from scheduled caste and 42 mothers (4.1%) from scheduled tribe. As per 2001 census, 19 percent of Tamil Nadu population was scheduled caste, one percent was schedule tribe and the remaining 80percent was other communities. The maternal deaths from the two communities constitute 38.5percent where as their share in total population is 20 percent only. Hence, more number of maternal deaths are reported from SC and ST than other communities.

Maternal Deaths by Gravida

Maternal deaths by gravida are available for 1008 cases. 408 mothers (38.9percent) are with first gravida 293 (29.1%t) are with second gravida 158 (15.7%) are with 3rd gravida and the remaining 149 (14.7%) are with 4+ gravida (Table 3). The first gravida deaths are high in Karur (52.9%), Nilgris (58.3%), Tiruvallur (54.8%), Sivagangai (52.3%) and Tiruvarur (52.2%) 4+ gravida deaths are high in Cuddalore (22.5%) and Madurai (20.7%). Like, age of the mother, the gravida and MMR is also positively correlated. If the gravida increases the MMR also increases. From the table 3, the MMR for primi and second gravida are less than the state average. The MMR for the 4+ gravida is highest. It is five times higher than the first and second gravida.

Table 3
Number and Percentage of Maternal Deaths and MMR by Gravida in Tamil Nadu, 2007-2008

Gravida	*No. and % of Maternal Deaths*	*Estimated No. of Live Births*	*Maternal Mortality Rate*
1	408 (38.9)	5,46,900	75
2	293 (29.1)	4,15,700	71
3	158 (15.7)	1,18,800	133
4+	149 (14.7)	39,200	380

Maternal Deaths by Period of Death

The maternal period starts from the day of conception and ends on 42 days of child birth. The above period is subdivided into Ante-natal (A.N), Natal and Postnatal (P.N). The maternal deaths are analysed by period of death 23 percent deaths occur during A.N period, 5percent during the process of delivery and the remaining 72percent occur during P.N. period High variation in A.N. deaths is observed among 30 districts. The A.N. deaths are high in Madurai (39%), Erode (36%) and Tiruvallur (36%) and Kancheepuram (32%t). The A.N. deaths are low in Kanyakumari (9%), Thoothukudi (9%) Karur (12%t), Nagapattinam (12%) and Coimbatore (13%). No death during natal period is reported from Dindigul, Kancheepuram, Karur, Krishnagiri, Madurai, Perambalur and Sivagangai.

Maternal Deaths by Place of Delivery and Place of Death

Place of delivery plays a vital role for safe delivery of mother and child. Primary Health centres (PHCs) and Health Sub-centre (HSCs) situated very nearer to the community is suited for normal deliveries. Nearly 2 lakh normal deliveries take place every year in PHCs and HSCs. HSC deliveries are not conducted in any state in India except Tamil Nadu. In Tamil Nadu normal deliveries are conducted in all PHCs where as normal deliveries are conducted not in all PHCs, only in main PHCs in Kerala. For complicated and risk pregnancies the community should prefer the tertiary institutions. The details on the place of delivery and place of death are available for 730 cases (excluding the A.N deaths). The two way table for place of delivery and place of birth is furnished in Table 4. Among the 171 mothers delivered in teaching institutions, 147 mothers died in the same institution, one in head quarters hospital 10 in private hospitals, 8 during transit and five in home. For the 72 deliveries in the head quarters hospitals, 37 died in the same hospital, 14 in teaching institutions, 1 in HSC, 9 in private hospitals and 7 during transit. Out of 237 mothers delivered in private hospitals, 156 died in the private hospitals, 17 in teaching institutions, 4 in headquarters hospitals, one each in taluk hospital and PHC, 13 in home and 45 during transit. Since the teaching institutions are provided with round the clock service, availability of blood bank, equipments and life saving drugs, the mothers with critical condition are

Table 4
Distribution Mothers by Place of Delivery and Place of Deaths During 2007-08

	Place of Death of Mother								
Name of Hospital (*Place of Delivery*)	*Teaching Hosp.*	*HQ Hosp.*	*Taluk Hosp.*	*PHC*	*HSC*	*Home*	*Private Hospital*	*Transit*	*Total*
Teaching Hosp.	147	1	0	0	0	5	10	8	171
HQ Hospital	14	37	0	0	1	4	9	7	72
Taluk Hospital	23	1	28	0	0	7	5	13	77
PHC	9	3	1	5	0	7	6	27	58
HSC	4	1	0	0	2	5	2	7	21
Home	13	7	2	0	0	38	6	21	87
Private Hospital	17	4	1	1	0	13	156	45	237
Transit	2	0	1	0	0	1	0	3	7
Total	229	54	33	6	3	80	194	131	730

referred to these hospitals. Hence more number of deaths reported from medical college hospitals (Table 4).

Maternal Deaths within 24 hours of Delivery

Medical attention within 24 hours to the delivered mothers is a crucial period for the survival of mother and infant. Though the institutional deliveries is more than 90 percent, more than two fifth (342 deaths) of the maternal deaths reported within 24 hours of delivery. Comparison between the maternal deaths on the first day of life and average number of maternal deaths per day for the remaining period is furnished in Fig 1. Of the 817 deaths (excluding A.N. deaths), 342 deaths reported within 24 hours of delivery and at an average of 11 deaths per day during the remaining days (41 days) of the P.N. period.

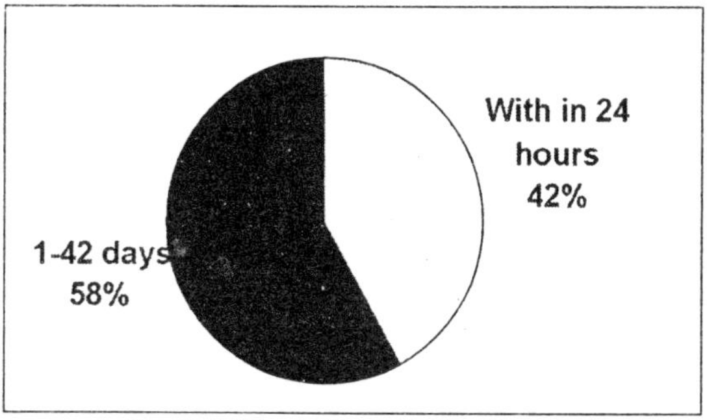

Fig. 1: Maternal Deaths by Duration

This clearly shows that medical attention immediately after delivery is essential for the survival of the mother. More number of one day deaths are reported in Tirunelveli (60%), Pudukottai (63%), Ramnad (58%), Trichy (56%), Thoothududi (55%) and Madurai (51%). It is least in Virudhunagar (17%), Dindugal (18%) and Chennai (20%). If these deaths are prevented, the MMR would be reduced by one third.

Maternal Deaths on Sundays

In all hospitals the service delivery is normally poor on Sundays. For comparing the quality of treatment provided between working days and Sundays, the maternal deaths reported on Sundays are analysed. There are 165 maternal deaths reported in 52 Sundays and 894 maternal deaths reported in remaining 314 working days. Average number of maternal deaths reported is 2.8 and 3.2 in working days and Sundays respectively. Non availability of the required number of doctors in Sundays may be the reason for more number of cases reported on Sundays. Hence the quality of medical services provided on Sundays and working days in the all hospitals are not equal and there exists quality difference.

Maternal Deaths during Transit

The maternal death in tribal and remote villages is usually high due to transportation problems especially at night. The pregnant mothers should admit the needy hospitals according to their complications when labour pain starts. The non medical cause of maternal deaths includes three types of delays: i) Delay in decision making to arrive at a hospital when labour pain starts, ii) Delay in reaching the hospitals, and iii) Delay in initiating treatment in the hospitals. The first two delays resulted in transit deaths. There are 170 (18%) maternal deaths reported during transit. If the ambulance services are available in time, these 190 deaths could be prevented. Kanniyakumari is the only district, where there is no transit death. Maternal death during transit is very high in Madurai (30%), Perambalur (28%), Thanjavur (27%), Villupuram (26%) and Nilgiris (25%).

Sterilization Deaths

Annually three lakh female sterilizations are performed in Tamil Nadu. During the process of sterilization and after sterilization about 40 sterilization deaths are reported every year. These deaths which are LSCS with sterilization and pup sterilization which happens during postnatal period are also included in maternal deaths. During the reported year, there are 39 sterilization deaths in which 22 are pup sterilization deaths 13 deaths are LSCS with sterilization two are laparoscopic deaths and another two are M.T.P. with sterilization deaths. Details on community are available for 28 mothers. Of the 28 deaths, 12 mothers (43%) are from scheduled community. The death of scheduled caste mothers are high compared to their population size.

Maternal Deaths for Home Deliveries

It is obvious that the risk of dying is high for the deliveries conducted at home where there is no proper medical care. There are 87 maternal deaths reported for whom the deliveries take place at home. These deaths are high in Krishnagiri (11%), Tiruvannamalai (11%), Villupuram (8%) and Vellore (7%). Considering the fact that most of these deaths are higher order pregnancies and in higher age of women, counseling pregnant women of the higher gravida and higher age, about not planning for a home delivery and planning for a delivery in an appropriate facility is an important step in reducing maternal deaths. Of the 87 deaths, 38 died at home, 21 during transit, 6 in private hospitals and 22 in govt. hospitals. Among these 87 deaths, more than 50percent of deaths are from scheduled caste and scheduled tribe.

Maternal Deaths at Home

Among the maternal deaths, 101 maternal deaths are at home 170 maternal deaths are during transit as place of death. Nearly 27 percent of women died at home or transit without appropriate care. More number of home deaths are reported from Villupuram (15%), Tiruvannamalai (10%), Tiruvallur (9%) and Virudhunagar (9%). Of the 101 maternal deaths at home, the place of delivery takes place at home for 87 deaths. Among these 87 deaths, 38 deaths are at home. Educating the community on the importance of proper planning for delivery place and immediate referral, along with provision of appropriate mode of transport could prevent more than one fourth of the maternal deaths.

Maternal Deaths by Cause

Though there are many causes for maternal deaths, majority of maternal deaths reported due to few major causes. The cause of maternal deaths is available only for 921 deaths out of 1059 maternal deaths. The major causes for maternal deaths are furnished in Table 5. The major causes for maternal deaths are haemorrhage (23%), pulmonary embolism (11%), heart

Table 5
Causes of Maternal Deaths in Tamil Nadu 2007-08

Causes of Deaths	*Antenatal Deaths*	*Natal Deaths*	*Post natal Deaths*	*Total*
Hemorrhage	6	8	196	210
Pulmonary Embolism	4	2	91	97
Heart Disease Complicating Pregnancy	2	2	85	89
Anaemia and Malnutrition	26	3	27	56
Pregnancy Induced Hypertension	13	2	39	54
Cardiac Arrest	49	1	0	50
Thrombus Phlebitis	2	1	46	49
Sepsis and Septicemia	6	0	40	46
Eclampsia	11	2	31	44
Jaundice Complicated Pregnancy	7	1	16	24
Pulmonary Edema	18	1	4	23
Post Operative Complications	0	1	20	21
Suicide and Social Complication	14	0	12	26
Renal Complications	0	1	12	13
Bad Obstetric History	3	0	0	3
Rupture Uterus	2	3	1	6
Abortion and Related Complication	3	0	0	3
Prolonged / Obstructed Labour	0	1	0	1
Card around Neck	0	0	1	1
Entopic Pregnancy	1	0	0	1
Diabetic Complicated Pregnancy	0	0	1	1
Spontaneous Expulsion	0	1	0	1
STD / HIV / AIDS	0	0	3	3
Others	27	13	59	99
Total	194	43	684	921

disease complicating pregnancy (10%), Anaemia and malnutrition (6%) and pregnancy induced hypertension (6%). An analysis of the causes of maternal deaths in Tamil Nadu brings out the fact that a large number of these are preventable. The reduction of MMR therefore lies in reducing maternal death due to hemorrhage. Availability of blood in time in government hospitals is to be ensured by Govt.

As per National Family Health Survey-2 in Tamil Nadu 57 percent of women have some degree of anaemia. Among these women, 37 percent of women are with mild anaemia 16percent are with moderate anaemia, and 4percent are severely anaemia. The prevalence of anaemia is higher for rural women than urban women in Tamil Nadu. The prevalence of anaemia is much higher for women belonging to scheduled castes and scheduled tribes, illiterate women and women with low standard of living. Further, it is also important to start dealing with anaemia in adolescent girls rather than address the issue only when a woman becomes pregnant.

"Anemia may have detrimental effects on the health of women and child and may be the underling cause of maternal mortality and infant mortality" In coincidence with the above statement, among the maternal deaths from anaemia, 38.5percent are from scheduled community, 41.3percent are from most back ward community. All together 80percent of the maternal deaths are from most economically backward communities. Due to poor economic conditions of the rural women and due to higher percentage of anaemia pregnancy complications maternal deaths are higher among the mothers of scheduled community and backward community.

Maternal Morbidity

Maternal morbidity is another major cause for concern. More than 10,000 maternal complications are reported in I.O.G. Hospital Chennai where highest number of deliveries conducted in Tamil Nadu. The major complications include CPD (27percent), P.I.H (21percent), Rh factor (7percent), heart disease complications pregnancy (2.3percent) and APH

(2percent). A larger number of women suffer acute complications that can lead to death, life long pain, illness and infertility. Public health programmes should address these problems.

Important Findings

1. Though the MMR of Tamil Nadu is 95, high variation between districts is observed from 32 to 226.
2. 4 percent of maternal deaths are from the adolescent girls and 20 percent are from women more than 30 years.
3. MMR increases when age of the mother increases.
4. MMR increases when gravida increases.
5. Maternal deaths are high in SC/ST community (39%).
6. More than two third of maternal deaths reported during postnatal period.
7. During P.N. period, more than two fifth of maternal deaths reported within 24 hours of delivery.
8. Maternal deaths are high on Sundays when compared to working days.
9. 18 percent of maternal deaths reported during transit.
10. Nearly 10 percent of women died at home.
11. Major cause of maternal death is hemorrhage (23percent)

Action Taken by Government of Tamil Nadu to Reduce MMR

Government of Tamil Nadu has taken many steps to reduce MMR. The important steps include the following:

1. Established 125 CEMONC centres to provide round the clock service ensure blood bank facilities life saving drugs and equipments.
2. In each revenue district, four or five centres are established. There centres are located in such a way that any patient can reach this centre within in one hour. There should not be any re-referal from these centres.

3. Established free ambulance services from the residence to these centres by using the unique toll free telephone number of 108.
4. Medical audit for all maternal deaths is conducted by the district collector to find out the gaps in the health delivery system. The relatives of the deceased and the district officials attended the meeting.
5. Counseling the mothers and the family members on the various issues regarding the delivery such as birth preparedness and planning the place of delivery.
6. Ensured safe abortion for higher order and unwanted pregnancies. Improving access to safe abortion should be a priority if maternal mortality and morbidity rates are to be reduced.

Reference

Department of Family Welfare, Chennai (2008), *Tamil Nadu Vital Statistics Records, 2007-08*. Chennai: Department of FW, Government of Tamil Nadu.

13

Early Childhood Mortality in South Indian States: A Study of Levels, Differentials, Trends and Changes from NFHS and SRS

M.V. Vaithilingam

Introduction

The significance of research on infant mortality resides in the fact that the few human experiences are more tragic or emotionally devastating as the death of an infant or child. The infant mortality has been employed world wide as a key social indicator (World Bank, 1998). In demography, there is a growing recognition that 'studies of biology of death, mortality, longevity, and life are all informed by biological processes that demographers can not to ignore' (Frank, 2001). It has been considered as a critical test for identifying countries as superior health achievers (Caldwell, 1986), as an inverse proxy measure of development (Pattnayak and Shai, 1995) and as a synoptic indicator of the health and social condition of a population (Gortmaker and Wise, 1997). Integral to demographic research on infant mortality are studies of three birth outcome dimensions: birth weight, gestational age, and maturity[1], not only as risk factors typically viewed as having the most powerful and proximate impact on infant mortality, but also as pregnancy outcomes of interest in their own right (Cramer 1987; 1995; Frisbie et al., 1996; Kiely and Susser, 1992; Kline et al., 1989). Among surviving infants, low birth weight, pre-maturity, and/or immaturity are associated with great risk of congenital anomalies, neuro-developmental and behavioural disorders, lower levels of educational achievement, and problems of family functioning (Hack et al., 1995; McCormick 1985). Historical research on infant mortality and perhaps more frequently, child mortality has long had a prominent place in the demographic literature (McKowen, 1976; Preston, 1976; Preston and Haines, 1991). Demographers are well acquainted with the epidemiological transition which denotes the shift from acute and infectious diseases to chronic and degenerative conditions as leading causes of death (Omran, 1971; 1977).

Objectives

Keeping in view the importance of knowledge of early childhood mortality, this study intends to examine the levels, differentials, and change of early childhood mortality, i.e., neonatal mortality[2] post-neonatal morality[3], infant mortality[4], and under-five mortality[5] by using the data from National Family Health Surveys (IIPS, 1995; IIPS and ORC Macro, 2000; IIPS and Macro International, 2007) and Sample Registration System (1992-93, 1998-99 and 2005-06).

Results and Discussion

Neonatal Mortality

Specifically neonatal mortality has been used to approximate deaths due to endogenous causes, i.e., conditions that are related to genetic makeup or that are 'a consequence of circumstances occurring during the prenatal period and/or birth process ' (Frisbie et al., 1992). The causes of neonatal mortality are multifactor - low-birth weight, birth injury and difficult labour, congenital anomalies, haemolytic diseases of new born, conditions of placenta and cord, diarrhoeal diseases, acute respiratory infections and tetanus. Neonatal mortality is a measure of the intensity with which 'endogenous factors' (low birth weight, birth injuries) affect infant life. The neonatal mortality is directly related to the birth weight and gestational age; the lighter or more immature the baby, the higher the death rate. The high concentration of infant deaths in the early neonatal period with endogamous causes suggests the need to improve the antenatal and post-neonatal services to expectant mothers. However, neonatal mortality is the most difficult part of infant mortality to alter, because of the endogenous factors which are not sensitive to improvements in environmental conditions. Neonatal mortality is greater in boys throughout the world, because newborn boys are biologically more fragile than girls.

Post-neonatal Mortality

The causes of post-neonatal mortality are: diarrhoeal diseases, acute respiratory infections, other communicable diseases, malnutrition, congenital anomalies and accidents. Whereas neonatal mortality is dominated by endogenous factors, post-neonatal mortality is dominated by exogenous (environmental and social) factors (Park, 2002). Diarrhoea and respiratory infections are the main causes of death during the post-neonatal period. Malnutrition is an additional factor, reinforcing the adverse effects of the infections. In the developed countries, the main cause of post-neonatal mortality is congenial anomalies. Studies show that post-neonatal mortality increases steadily with birth order, and that infants born into already large families run a higher risk of death from infectious diseases. In some areas of South East Asia (including India), during the post-neonatal period girls die more frequently than boys. This is attributed to neglect of the female children in terms of nutrition and health care.

Infant Mortality

Infant mortality rate is universally regarded not only as a most important indicator of the health status of a community but also of the level of living of people in general, and effectiveness of MCH services in particular. IMR is given a separate treatment by demographers, because: (a) infant mortality is the largest single age category of mortality; (b) deaths at this age are due to a peculiar set of diseases and conditions to which the adult population is less exposed or less vulnerable; (c) infant mortality is affected rather quickly and directly by specific health programmes and hence may change more rapidly than the general death rate. The developed world had a much greater reduction in infant mortality rate compared to child mortality; while in the developing world the situation was reverse (UNICEF, 2007). The social demography of infant mortality has drawn heavily on the proximate determinants approach advanced by Mosley and Chen (1984). Infant mortality rate reflects the socio-economic development of a country. Deaths during the first four weeks are largely preventable by good health care. Much of the variations between developed and developing world in death among new born can be explained by differences in antenatal care- about half of all pregnant women in the least developed countries have no antenatal care and 7 out of 10 babes are born without the help of a trained birth attendant. The other major factors being malnutrition and high parity of the mother, low birth weight of the baby, and congenital anomalies. The principal causes of infant mortality in India are low birth weight, respiratory infections, diarrhoeal diseases, congenital malformations, and cord infection. Neonatal deaths make a major contribution (70%) to infant mortality. The decline in infant mortality has been attributed to: (a) improved obstetric and perinatal care, e.g., availability of oxygen, foetal monitoring during labour, improved techniques for the induction of labour; (b) improvement in the quality of life, i.e., economic and social progress, (c) better control of communicable diseases, i.e., immunization and oral rehydration, (d) advances in chemotherapy, antibiotics and insecticides, (e) better nutrition, i.e., emphasis on breast feeding, and (f) family planning, i.e., birth spacing. There is also an important literature on the consequences of infant mortality- consequences for demographic change in general and for reproductive behaviour in particular (Palloni and Rafalimanana, 1999).

Child Mortality

The child death rate is more refined indicator of the social situation than infant mortality rate. It reflects the adverse environmental health hazards (e.g., malnutrition, poor hygiene, infections and accidents), including economic, educational and cultural characteristics of the family. Mortality in this age group no longer depends on perinatal hazards and other endogenous factors, which often cause loss of life during the first year of life. In the age group 1-4 years, the second year is the period when the young child runs the highest risk of dying. In the developing countries, death in the second year of life commonly accounts for 50 percent of all deaths between 1-4 years of age (WHO, 1971).

Levels of Early Childhood Mortality

According to NFHS 3 (2005-06), the neonatal mortality rate ranges between from a low of 12 in Kerala to 40 in Andhra Pradesh, infant mortality rate between 15 and 54, and child mortality rate between 1 and 10 in the same respective states. The SRS figures also portrait the same trend, except the post-neonatal mortality rate which is more in Karnataka (14) according to NFHS figures. It is remarkable that the figures of the states Kerala and Tamil Nadu on these four early childhood mortality measures lie below the south Indian averages, and more or less the figures of these four south Indian states lie below the national averages (Table 1).

Differentials of Early Childhood Mortality

The differentials of early childhood mortality measures are explained in terms of socio-economic characteristics such as religious groups, caste/tribe groups, mother's educational level, family's wealth index, and demographic characteristics such as residence type, sex of the child, mother's age, birth order, birth interval, and birth size. It is found that neonatal mortality rate has been pronounced more among Buddhists/ Neo-Buddhists (43) followed by Hindus (40) Sikhs (36), Muslims (34) and Christians (32). The post-neonatal mortality

Table 1
Different Early Childhood Mortality Rates in India and South Indian States, NFHS and SRS, 2005-06

India / South Indian States	*NFHS*				*SRS*			
	NNMR	*PNNMR*	*IMR*	*CMR*	*NNMR*	*PNNMR*	*IMR*	*CMR*
India	39.0	18.0	57.0	18.4	37.0	20.0	57.5	17.0
South India	25.0	10.6	35.6	7.2	24.4	14.8	39.3	10.0
Andhra Pradesh	40.3	13.2	53.5	10.2	34.0	22.5	56.5	15.0
Karnataka	28.9	14.3	43.2	12.1	28.0	20.5	49.0	13.0
Kerala	11.5	3.8	15.3	1.0	10.5	4.0	14.5	3.0
Tamil Nadu	19.1	11.2	30.4	5.3	25.0	12.0	37.0	9.0

Note: NNMR=Neonatal mortality rate; PNNMR=Post-neonatal mortality rate; IMR= Infant mortality rate; CMR= Child mortality rate.

rate, infant mortality rate and child mortality rate seem to be high among Hindus and Muslims and low among Sikhs and Christians. The neonatal mortality and infant mortality rates are high among women belonging to scheduled caste group and post-neonatal and child mortality rates are high among women belonging to scheduled tribe group. More or less the early childhood mortality measures visualise higher the educational level and family wealth index values and lower the early childhood mortality measures (Table 2a).

As expected the early childhood mortality measures are high in rural areas compared to urban areas. As far as sex of the child is concerned, the post-neonatal mortality rate, infant mortality rate and child mortality rate are high among female children, whereas neonatal mortality is more among male children. The early childhood mortality measures by mother's age reveal that mothers age less than 20 years have more incidence of early childhood mortality compared to the subsequent age-groups 20-29 and 30-39. But after 20 years of age the mothers seem to have more incidence of early childhood mortality. As far as the child mortality by birth order is concerned, it increases as the birth order increases. However, the other three measures show high level of incidence of mortality among mothers having first order birth which explain increasing trend only after second birth order

Table 2a
Different Early Childhood Mortality Rates by Socio-economic Characteristics in India and South Indian States, NFHS 2005-06

Socio-economic Characteristics	*Neonatal Mortality Rate*	*Post-neonatal Mortality Rate*	*Infant Mortality Rate*	*Child Mortality Rate*
Religion				
Hindu	40.3	18.2	58.5	18.5
Muslim	34.1	18.2	52.4	18.6
Christian	31.5	10.1	41.7	11.6
Sikh	35.9	9.7	45.6	6.8
Buddhist/Neo-Buddhist	43.0	9.8	52.8	17.1
Others	43.3	41.4	84.6	50.4
Caste / Tribe				
Scheduled caste	46.3	20.1	66.4	23.2
Scheduled tribe	39.9	22.3	62.1	35.8
Other backward class	38.3	18.3	56.6	17.3
Others	34.5	14.5	48.9	10.8
Education				
No education	45.7	24.0	69.7	26.9
<5 years complete	48.4	17.6	66.0	13.8
5-7 years complete	34.5	15.1	49.5	11.5
8-9 years complete	32.0	9.5	41.5	5.6
10-11 years complete	26.9	9.6	36.5	3.6
12 + years complete	19.6	6.3	25.9	3.9
Wealth Index				
Lowest	48.4	22.0	70.4	32.3
Second	44.6	24.0	68.5	22.6
Middle	39.3	19.1	58.3	14.4
Fourth	31.9	12.1	44.0	7.5
Highest	22.0	7.2	29.2	4.8

onwards. The child mortality decreases with the increase of birth interval between present and previous births. However, the mothers having two-year gap have high incidence of neonatal, post-neonatal and infant mortality rates. Mothers who had births in very small size have more chance and mothers with average or larger size of births have less chance of early childhood mortality (Table 2b).

Trends of Early Childhood Mortality

The state Kerala visualises the lowest position in all the early childhood mortality measures in all the three periods (1992-

Table 2b
Different Early Childhood Mortality Rates by Demographic Characteristics in India and South Indian States, NFHS 2005-06

Demographic Characteristics	*Neonatal Mortality*	*Post-neonatal Mortality*	*Infant Mortality*	*Child Mortality*
Total	39.0	18.0	57.0	18.4
Residence				
Rural	42.5	19.7	62.2	21.0
Urban	28.5	13.0	41.5	10.6
Sex				
Male	40.9	15.4	56.3	14.2
Female	36.8	20.9	57.7	22.9
Mother's age				
<20	54.2	22.3	76.5	20.1
20-29	34.2	16.3	50.4	15.9
30-39	37.9	18.5	56.4	25.7
40-49	42.9	29.2	72.1	37.3
Birth Order				
1	47.8	16.4	64.1	11.4
2-3	30.3	16.2	46.5	16.5
4-6	41.5	20.4	61.9	25.2
7 +	48.6	31.2	79.8	39.0
Previous Birth Interval				
<2 years	57.9	27.8	85.7	32.5
2 years	30.9	18.6	49.5	20.1
3 years	19.2	10.6	29.8	15.1
4 + years	24.2	12.8	37.0	8.6
Birth Size				
Very small	91.4	37.2	128.6	40.2
Small	42.1	19.8	61.9	14.3
Average or Larger	32.3	16.2	48.6	18.0

93, 1998-99, and 2005-06) of NFHS and SRS followed by Tamil Nadu, Karnataka and Andhra Pradesh. However, Andhra Pradesh and Karnataka occupy the third and fourth lowest positions in terms of infant mortality rate during NFHS (2005-06). It is also remarkable to note that mostly in all the early childhood mortality measures the two states Kerala and Tamil Nadu, and Karnataka in one or two measures fall below the south India average in all the three periods of NFHS and SRS. All the four early childhood mortality measures of three periods of NFHS show the decreasing trend during the three periods (1992-93, 1998-99, and 2005-06). However, the

Table 3
Different Early Childhood Mortality Rates in India and South Indian States, NFHS and SRS, 1992-93, 1998-99, 2005-06

	National Family Health Survey			*Sample Registration System*		
India/ States	*2005-06*	*1998-99*	*1992-93*	*2005-06*	*1998-99*	*1992-93*
	Neonatal Mortality Rate					
India	39.0	43.4	48.6	37.0	45	46.8
South India	25.0	35.8	41.6	24.4	36.3	37.3
Andhra Pradesh	40.3	47.5	47.7	34.0	56.0	43.5
Karnataka	28.9	44.4	50.1	28.0	42.5	50.5
Kerala	11.5	15.3	22.1	10.5	11.0	10.5
Tamil Nadu	19.1	35.9	46.3	25.0	35.5	44.5
	Post-neonatal Mortality Rate					
India	18.0	24.2	29.9	20.0	25.5	24.6
South India	13.2	23.4	25.6	22.5	20.5	25.1
Andhra Pradesh	13.2	23.4	25.6	22.5	20.5	25.1
Karnataka	14.3	17.9	25.0	20.5	16.0	17.7
Kerala	3.8	5.6	8.9	4.0	4.0	4.6
Tamil Nadu	11.2	15.0	24.3	12.0	17.5	13.1
	Infant Mortality Rate					
India	57.0	67.6	78.5	57.5	71.0	71.5
South India	35.6	51.3	62.5	39.3	47.9	52.4
Andhra Pradesh	53.5	70.8	73.2	56.5	66.0	67.5
Karnataka	43.2	62.3	75.1	49.0	58.0	70.0
Kerala	15.3	20.9	31.0	14.5	15.0	15.0
Tamil Nadu	30.4	51.0	70.7	37.0	52.5	57.0
	Child Mortality Rate					
India	18.4	29.3	33.4	17.0	21.0	NA
South India	7.2	16.0	22.5	10.0	12.5	NA
Andhra Pradesh	10.2	22.0	24.6	15.0	17.5	NA
Karnataka	12.1	22.4	29.4	13.0	16.0	NA
Kerala	1.0	5.3	9.7	3.0	3.5	NA
Tamil Nadu	5.3	14.3	26.1	9.0	13.0	NA

neonatal and post-neonatal mortality rates of SRS figures fluctuate between the periods 1992-93 and 1998-99, and 1998-99 and 2005-06 (Table 3).

Change of Early Childhood Mortality during 1992-93 to 2005-06

The neonatal mortality and infant mortality rate have declined more in Tamil Nadu (59% and 57%) followed by Kerala (48%

and 51%), Karnataka (42% and 43%) and Andhra Pradesh (40% and 27%) respectively during the period from 1992-92 to 2005-06 according to NFHS (Table 4). The state Kerala has more percentage of declines in post-neonatal and child mortality rates (57% and 88%) followed by Tamil Nadu (54% and 80%), Andhra Pradesh (48% and 59%) and Karnataka (43% and 59%) respectively, However, as found in the levels of early

Table 4
Percent Change in Different Early Childhood Mortality Rates in India and South Indian States, NFHS and SRS, 1992-93 to 2005-06

	National Family Health Survey			*Sample Registration System*		
India / South India / South Indian States	*1992 -93 to 2005-06*	*1998 -99 to 2005-06*	*1992 -93 to 1998-99*	*1992 -93 to 2005-06*	*1998 -99 to 2005-06*	*1992 -93 to 1998-99*
		Neonatal Mortality Rate				
India	-19.8	-10.1	-10.7	-20.9	-17.8	-3.8
South India	-39.9	-30.2	-13.9	-34.6	-32.8	-2.7
Andhra Pradesh	-15.5	-15.2	-0.4	-21.8	-39.3	28.7
Karnataka	-42.3	-34.9	-11.4	-44.6	-34.1	-15.8
Kerala	-48.0	-24.8	-30.8	0.0	-4.5	4.8
Tamil Nadu	-58.7	-46.8	-22.5	-43.8	-29.6	-20.2
		Post-neonatal Mortality Rate				
India	-39.8	-25.6	-19.1	-18.7	-21.6	3.7
South India	-49.5	-31.6	-26.2	-2.0	2.1	-4.0
Andhra Pradesh	-48.4	-43.6	-8.6	-10.4	9.8	-18.3
Karnataka	-42.8	-20.1	-28.4	15.8	28.1	-9.6
Kerala	-57.3	-32.1	-37.1	-13.0	0.0	-13.0
Tamil Nadu	-53.9	-25.3	-38.3	-8.4	-31.4	33.6
		Infant Mortality Rate				
India	-27.4	-15.7	-13.9	-19.6	-19.0	-0.7
South India	-43.0	-30.6	-17.9	-25.0	-18.0	-8.6
Andhra Pradesh	-26.9	-24.4	-3.3	-16.3	-14.4	-2.2
Karnataka	-42.5	-30.7	-17.0	-30.0	-15.5	-17.1
Kerala	-50.6	-26.8	-32.6	-3.3	-3.3	0.0
Tamil Nadu	-57.0	-40.4	-27.9	-35.1	-29.5	-7.9
		Child Mortality Rate				
India	-44.9	-37.2	-12.3	NA	-19.0	NA
South India	-68.0	-55.0	-28.9	NA	-20.0	NA
Andhra Pradesh	-58.5	-53.6	-10.6	NA	-14.3	NA
Karnataka	-58.8	-46.0	-23.8	NA	-18.8	NA
Kerala	-89.7	-81.1	-45.4	NA	-14.3	NA
Tamil Nadu	-79.7	-62.9	-45.2	NA	-30.8	NA

childhood mortality measures, the percent change in all these four measures during 1998-99 to 2005-06 in all the four states is higher compared to the previous period 1992-93 to 1998-99. Mostly all the four states in all these early childhood mortality rates stand above the national average, and Kerala and Tamil Nadu stand above the south Indian average (Table 4). More or less the same is revealed through the SRS data also, though there are slight fluctuations.

Conclusions

The state Kerala seems to be having lowest level of neonatal, post-neonatal, infant and child mortality rates followed by Tamil Nadu. All the four south Indian states fall below the national average, and Kerala and Tamil Nadu lie below the south Indian average with regard to these rates. It is found that these early childhood mortality rates seem to be higher among the mothers residing at rural areas, belonging to Buddhists/Neo-Buddhists, scheduled caste group, whose level of education and values of family wealth index are low, whose age is below 20 years, who have higher birth order, whose birth interval is low and who delivered very small size births and among female children, portraying higher the socio-economic and demographic desirable status and lower the early childhood mortality. Mostly all the four early childhood mortality rates during these periods of NFHS and SRS show a declining trend. The states Kerala and Tamil Nadu visualise mostly higher percentage of change in all the four early childhood mortality rates. All the four states in all these rates stand above the national average, and Kerala and Tamil Nadu stand above the south Indian average.

Endnotes

1. Lack of maturity refers to infants who are small for gestational age (SGA) or intrauterine growth retarded (IUGR).
2. Neonatal deaths are deaths occurring during the neonatal period, commencing at birth and ending 28 completed days after birth. Neonatal mortality rate = (Number of deaths of children under 28 days of age in a year) / (Total live births in the same year) * 1000.
3. Deaths occurring from 28 days of life to under one year are called 'post-neonatal deaths.' The post-neonatal death rate is the ratio of post-neonatal

deaths in a given year to the total number of live births in the same year; usually expressed as a rate per 1000. Post-neonatal mortality rate = (Number of deaths of children between 28 days and one year of age in a given year) / (Total live births in the same year) * 1000.

4. Infant mortality rate is defined as the ratio of infant deaths registered in a given year to the total number of live births registered in the same year; usually expressed as a rate per 1000 live births (Hogarh, 1978). Infant mortality rate= (Number of deaths of children less than one year of age in a year) / (Number of live births in the same year) * 1000.
5. Child death rate is the number of deaths of children aged 1-4 years per 1000 children in the same age group in a given year. Child death rate (1-4 year mortality rate) = (Number of deaths of children aged 1-4 years) during a year)/ (Total number of children aged 1-4 years at the middle of the year) * 1000.

References

Caldwell, J.C. (1986), "Routes to Low Mortality in Poor Countries", *Population and Development Review* 12: 171-220.

Cramer, J.C. (1987), "Social Factors and Infant Mortality: Identifying High-risk Groups and Proximate Causes", *Demography* 24: 299-322.

Cramer, J.C. (1995), "Racial and Ethnic Differences Birth Weight: The Role of Income and Financial Outcomes", *Demography* 32: 231-247.

Frank, R. (2001), "The Misuse of Biology in Demographic Research on Racial/Ethnic Differences: A Reply to Van Den Oord and Rowe", *Demography* 38: 563-567.

Frisbie, W.P., D. Forbes, and R.G. Rogers (1992), "Neonatal and Post-neonatal Mortality as Proxies for Cause of Death: Evidence from Ethnic and Longitudinal Comparisons", *Social Science Quarterly* 73: 535-549.

Frisbie, W.P., D. Forbes, and S.G. Pullum (1996), "Compromised Birth Outcomes and Infant Mortality among Racial and Ethnic Groups", *Demography* 33: 469-481.

Hack, M., N.K. Klein, and H.G. Taylor (1995), "Long-term Developmental Outcomes of Low Birth-weight Infants", *The Future of Children* 5: 176-196.

Hogarh, J. (1978), *Glossary of Health Care Terminology*. Copenhagen: WHO.

International Institute for Population Science (IIPS) and Macro International (2007), *National Family Health Survey (NFHS-3), 2005-06, India*. Mumbai: IIPS.

International Institute for Population Science (IIPS) and ORC Macro, (2000), *National Family Health Survey (NFHS-2), 1998-99, India.* Mumbai: IIPS.

International Institute for Population Science (IIPS) (1995), *National Family Health Survey (NFHS-1), 1992-93, India*. Mumbai: IIPS.

Kiely, J. and M. Susser (1992), "Preterm Birth, Intrauterine Growth Retardation, and Prenatal Mortality", *American Journal of Public Health* 82: 343-345.

Kline, J., Z. Stein, and M. Susser (1989), *Conception to Birth: Epidemiology of Prenatal Development.* New York: Oxford.

McCormick, M.C. (1985), "The Contribution of Low Birth-weight to Infant Mortality and Childhood Mortality", New *England Journal of Medicine* 312: 82-90.

McKowen, T. (1976), *The Rise of Modern Population.* New York: Academic Press.

Mosley, W.H., and L.C. Chen (1984), "An Analytical Framework for the Study of Child Survival in Developing Countries", *Population and Development Review* 10 (Supp.): 25-45.

Park, K. (2002), *Park's Preventive Text Book of Preventive and Social Medicine.* Jabalpur: Banarsidas Bhanot.

Palloni, A., and H. Rafalimanana (1999), "The Effects of Infant Mortality on Fertility Revisited: | New Evidence from Latin America", *Demography* 36: 46-58.

Pattnayak, S.R. and D. Shai (1995), "Mortality Rates as Indicators of Cross-cultural Development: Regional Variations in the Third World", *Journal of Development Studies* XI (2): 252-262.

Preston, S.H. (1976), *Mortality Patterns in National Populations.* | New York: Academic Press.

Preston, S.H. and M.R. Haines (1991), *Fatal Years: Child Mortality in the Late 19th Century*. Prinston N.J., Princeton University Press

Registrar General & Census Commissioner, India (2005), Sample Registration System: Special Fertility and Mortality Survey, 1998. New Delhi: Controller of Publications.

Registrar General & Census Commissioner, India (2006), Sample Registration System: Statistical Report 2005. New Delhi: Controller of Publications.

Registrar General, India (2003), Sample Registration System: Statistical Report 1999. New Delhi: Controller of Publications.

Registrar General, India (2003), Sample Registration System: Statistical Report 1999. New Delhi: Controller of Publications.

Registrar General, India (2000), Sample Registration System: Statistical Report 1998. New Delhi: Controller of Publications.

Registrar General, India (1994), Sample Registration System: Fertility and Mortality Indicators 1992. New Delhi: Controller of Publications.

World Bank (1998), *1998 World Development Indicators.* Washington, D. C: World Bank.

SECTION – 4

Gender Dimensions of Health

14

Gender and Mortality Indicators of Health in India

S. Ramachandran, A. Subbiah, A.K. Ravishankar

Introduction

Health is man's normal condition, his birth right. It is the result of living in accordance with the natural laws pertaining to the body, mind and environment. To the layman, health implies a sound mind in a sound body in a sound family in a sound environment. The widely accepted definition is that given by the World Health Organisation which states: Health is a state of complete physical, mental and social well-being, and not merely absence of disease or infirmity (World Health Organisation, 1948). The fourth dimension suggested to be incorporated is the Spiritual Health. Recently emerged concept in many countries is that of improving the overall quality of life resulting from a combination of the effect of complete range of indicators determining health, happiness, education, and social attainment, freedom of action, justice, and freedom from oppression. Of the multitude of indicators of health, mortality indictors could also be used to assess the health condition of the population indirectly, because mortality and morbidity are health related components. Morbidity and mortality are the biologically related phenomena. There are gender differences in pattern of morbidity and mortality.

Many studies relating to gender issues explained gender differences, particularly discrimination against women. Interestingly, there is a quite contrasting picture regarding health status, which is more favourable to females compared to males. The biological difference causes gender gap in health condition of population.

Objectives

Therefore, this paper intends to address the gender based-issue. The Primary objectives of the paper are to:

(i) Analyse health status differentials or health inequity between sexes in terms of certain mortality indicators in India,

(ii) Examine the future prospects of presently existing morbidity and mortality trend, and

(iii) Analyse this issue with reference to regional differences in India.

Methods and Materials

Data were collected from various sources, viz., (1) National Sample Survey published by the National Sample Survey Organisation, (2) National Population / Censuses published by the Office of the Registrar General of India (3) Vital Statistics, and (4) Health statistics published by Department of Health and Family Welfare.

Selection of Indicators: This study intends to assess the Health status between the sexes in terms of certain Mortality and Morbidity Indicators such as (1) Crude Birth Rate, (2) Age Specific Death Rate, (3) Lie Expectancy at birth, (4) Infant Mortality Rate, (5) Morbidity risk (6) Incidence or Prevalence of Morbidity and Mortality. The definitions of each of these and the calculated procedures are given in the appendix-I

Gender Differences (Gap): The difference (Gap) between the sexes in terms of selected mortality indictors. Such difference is positive sign refers to an advantage position for women and the negative sign referring to disadvantage position.

Results and Discussion

Crude Death Rate

Crude death rate (CDR), defined as the ratio between the number of deaths occurred in a year and the mid year population in a region, is commonly used measure to assess health status of population at macro level. But the major drawback of this measure is that it takes into account the total population (all are not supposed to have exactly equal mortality risk) in denominator.

Table 1
Trends in Crude Death Rate in India, 1901–2001

Census Year	*Crude Death Rate **	*Difference*	*Year*	*Projected CDR ***
1911	42.6	-		
1921	47.2	4.6	2001-2002	7.5
1931	36.3	0.9	2006-2010	7.3
1941	31.2	5.1	2011-2015	7.2
1951	27.4	3.8	2016-2020	7.1
1961	22.8	4.6	2021-2025	7.2
1971	19.0	3.8		
1981	15.0	4.0		
1991	11.4	4.6		
2001	8.9	2.5		
2008****	8.2	0.7		
Gender Difference**				
2006	Total	Male	Female	Gender Gap
Total	7.5	8.0	7.0	1.0
Rural	8.1	8.5	7.6	0.9
Urban	6.0	6.6	5.4	1.2

Note:

* Family Welfare Year Book 2005, 2006.

** Report of Technical Group on Population Projections, May 2006.

*** SRS Bulletin, October 2007.

**** United Nations, 2008 ECAP Population Data Sheet.

Table 1 show that in India the death rate declined from 42.6 in 1911 to 8.2 in 2008, indicating improvement in health condition of India's population. Projected CDRs range from 7.5 during 2001-2002 to 7.2 during 2021-2025. Since India has already achieved the low level CDR almost equal to developed counties, declining trend of CDRs does not show remarkable differences. Interestingly, CDRs for females and males are at low levels, but the rates for females are relatively low which indirectly indicates relatively better health condition for females. The information relating to gender gap in crude death rates between the two sexes confirms the advantage position in health status of women in terms of crude death rate. There is more gender gap in urban areas which have relatively low levels of CDR.

State wise results shows that (Table 2) in some Northern states and Eastern states, the levels of CDR are comparatively greater. In States like Jharkhand, Sikkim, Chandigarh, Lakshadweep, the gender gap is in negative value explaining excessive death rate for females.

Life Expectancy

Life expectancy is defined as a group of people who are supposed to live on average after beginning of the age interval. This is also called average life at birth. This is indirect mortality indicator of health. There is a close linkage between mortality and life expectancy of population. Life expectancy inversely varies (Table 3) with mortality conditions of population. Estimation of life expectancy requires construction of life table. It is interesting to observe in table that not only 100 years back, even today females have higher life expectancy compared to males (Table 3). An increasing trend of life expectancy of males and females separately is clearly evident. A clear cut situation of existence of gender gap resulting from excessive life expectancy for females over males is also evident. The trend of projected life expectancy for males and females clearly established women at better health status relative to men. A gender gap of 2.5 could be achieved (Table 4 and 5) by 2025. Data explain how females (72.3 years) have less incidence of mortality compared to males (69.8 years). Regional variation is also empirically evident. All the states have high life expectancy for females, but this seems to be comparatively high in Kerala, Tamil Nadu, Maharashtra,

Table 2
State/UT wise Death Rates in India 2006

India / State / UT	*Total*			*Rural*			*Urban*		
	Total	*Males*	*Females*	*Total*	*Males*	*Females*	*Total*	*Males*	*Females*
India	7.5	8.0	7.0	8.1	8.5	7.6	6.0	6.6	5.4
Andhra Pradesh	7.3	8.5	6.1	7.9	9.4	6.5	5.8	6.5	5.1
Arunachal Pradesh	5.0	5.1	4.9	5.5	5.7	5.3	2.8	2.4	3.2
Assam	8.7	9.2	8.1	9.2	9.7	8.7	5.8	6.7	4.8
Bihar	7.7	7.4	7.9	7.8	7.6	8.1	6.3	6.0	6.6
Chhattisgarh	8.1	8.7	7.5	8.5	9.0	8.1	6.3	7.4	5.2
Goa	7.4	8.1	6.7	8.2	9.0	7.4	6.9	7.5	6.3
Gujarat	7.3	7.8	6.8	8.2	8.8	7.6	5.9	6.2	5.6
Haryana	6.5	7.3	5.6	6.9	7.7	6.0	5.6	6.5	4.5
Himachal Pradesh	6.8	8.4	5.4	7.1	8.7	5.5	4.8	5.3	4.3
Jammu & Kashmir	5.9	6.4	5.2	6.1	6.7	5.4	5.0	5.3	4.7
Jharkhand	7.5	7.0	8.1	7.9	7.3	8.6	5.9	6.1	5.7
Karnataka	7.1	8.0	6.3	8.0	8.9	7.2	5.5	6.3	4.6
Kerala	6.7	7.5	5.9	6.8	7.7	5.9	6.5	7.0	6.0
Madhya Pradesh	8.9	9.1	8.6	9.6	9.8	9.5	6.3	6.7	5.8
Maharashtra	6.7	7.3	6.1	7.4	7.8	6.9	5.8	6.7	4.9
Manipur	4.5	5.3	3.6	4.4	5.4	3.4	4.6	5.0	4.1
Meghalaya	8.0	9.1	7.0	8.5	9.6	7.4	5.8	6.7	5.0
Mizoram	5.5	6.7	4.3	6.2	7.6	4.7	4.8	5.6	4.0
Nagaland	4.8	5.7	3.8	4.9	5.8	4.0	4.1	5.2	3.0
Orissa	9.3	9.8	8.8	9.7	10.2	9.2	6.9	7.5	6.2
Punjab	6.8	7.4	6.1	7.4	7.9	6.7	5.8	6.6	4.9
Rajasthan	6.9	7.4	6.5	7.2	7.7	6.7	6.1	6.2	5.9

Contd.

India / State / UT	Total			Rural			Urban		
	Total	Males	Females	Total	Males	Females	Total	Males	Females
Sikkim	5.6	5.3	5.8	5.7	5.4	6.0	4.7	5.0	4.3
Tamil Nadu	7.5	8.4	6.6	8.3	9.2	7.4	6.4	7.3	5.5
Tripura	6.3	7.1	5.5	6.2	7.0	5.4	6.8	7.4	6.1
Uttar Pradesh	8.6	8.8	8.5	9.1	9.2	8.9	6.6	6.8	6.4
Uttarakhand	6.7	7.6	5.8	7.0	7.9	6.1	5.5	6.5	4.5
West Bengal	6.2	6.8	5.6	6.2	6.7	5.7	6.3	7.2	5.3
A & N Islands	5.1	6.0	4.1	5.7	5.9	5.6	3.8	6.1	1.4
Chandigarh	4.1	4.3	3.8	3.1	3.0	3.2	4.2	4.4	3.9
D & N Haveli	4.8	5.4	4.1	5.3	6.0	4.5	3.1	3.3	2.8
Daman & Diu	5.5	5.9	5.1	5.0	5.5	4.5	6.1	6.4	5.8
Delhi	4.7	5.0	-	5.4	6.3	4.3	4.6	4.8	4.3
Lakshadweep	6.4	7.3	5.5	6.8	6.4	7.3	6.0	8.2	3.9
Puducherry	7.3	8.2	6.5	8.0.	8.9	7.1	7.0	7.9	6.2

Source: SRS Bulletin October 2007.

Punjab, Bihar, etc. Some Northern States and Eastern States have at disadvantage position.

Table 3
Expectation of Life at Birth: India, 1901 - 2016

Census Year	*Male*	*Female*	*Combined*
1901-10	22.6	23.3	22.9
1911-20	19.4	20.9	20.0
1921-30	26.9	26.6	26.8
1931-40	32.1	31.4	31.8
1941-50	32.4	31.7	32.1
1951-60	41.9	40.6	41.3
1961-70	46.4	44.7	45.6
1970-75	50.5	49.0	49.7
1976-80	52.5	52.1	52.3
1981-85	55.4	55.7	55.4
1986-90	57.7	58.1	57.7
1991- 96 (p)	60.6	61.7	61.2
1996-2001(p)	62.3	65.3	NA
2001-2006(p)	63.9	66.9	NA
2006-2011(p)	65.7	67.7	NA
2011-2016	67.0	69.2	NA

Source: Occasional Paper SRS No. 3 of 1995
Population Projections for India & States: 1996-2016.
(P) = Projected.

Infant Mortality Rate (IMR)

The study of infant mortality is of central importance in mortality analysis. All children under one years of age are considered infants and so the term infant mortality refers to mortality among children of less than one year age. The importance attached to the study of infant morality can be understood in terms of (a) infant mortality is high in India, (b) infant mortality rate is a sensitive index of health and it is considered one of the indicators of Physical Quality of Life Index, (c) infant morality influences the living condition, housing condition (environmental condition), nutrition intake of mothers and the amount of health care given to children, (d) infant mortality determines the levels of fertility and mortality and (e) infant mortality data are very useful to planners and policy makers for planning, implementing and

Table 4
Life Expectancy at Birth in India & Major States 1997- 2005

India & Major States	1997-2001		1998-2002		1999-2003		2000-04		2001-05*	
	Male	Female	Male	Female	Male	Female	Male	Female	Male	Female
1	2	3	4	5	6	7	8	9	10	11
India	61.3	63.0	61.6	63.3	61.8	63.5	62.1	63.7	62.3	63.9
Andhra Pradesh	61.9	64.4	62.0	64.6	62.2	64.8	62.4	65.0	62.7	65.2
Assam	57.6	57.8	57.7	58.1	57.8	58.3	58.0	58.6	58.3	59.0
Bihar*	61.1	59.3	61.4	59.5	61.6	59.7	61.8	59.9	62.0	60.1
Gujarat	62.3	64.2	62.4	64.4	62.5	64.6	62.7	64.8	62.8	65.0
Haryana	64.6	65.2	64.7	65.4	65.0	65.6	65.3	65.8	65.6	66.0
Himachal Pradesh	65.5	66.1	65.7	66.3	65.8	66.6	66.1	66.8	66.3	67.1
Karnataka	62.6	66.0	62.8	66.2	62.9	66.4	63.1	66.7	63.4	66.9
Kerala	70.8	76.2	70.8	75.9	70.9	76.0	71.0	76.1	71.3	76.3
Madhya Pradesh*	56.7	56.4	57.0	56.7	57.2	56.9	57.5	57.2	57.8	57.5
Maharashtra	64.8	67.3	65.0	67.4	65.2	67.6	65.5	67.8	65.8	68.1
Orissa	58.0	58.2	58.4	58.5	58.6	58.7	58.9	58.9	59.2	59.2
Punjab	67.2	69.3	67.4	69.5	67.6	69.6	67.8	69.8	68.1	70.1
Rajasthan	60.3	61.3	60.5	61.6	60.7	61.8	60.9	62.0	61.2	62.2
Tamil Nadu	64.1	66.1	64.2	66.3	64.3	66.5	64.6	66.8	64.8	67.1
Uttar Pradesh*	59.2	58.1	59.4	58.5	59.6	58.7	59.9	59.0	60.1	59.3
West Bengal	63.2	64.6	63.3	64.8	63.5	65.0	63.7	65.2	63.9	65.5

Note: *Bihar, Madhya Pradesh & Uttar Pradesh include Jharkhand, Chattisgarh & Uttarakhand, respectively.
Source: SRS, Registrar General of India, 2006.

Table 5
Projected Levels of Expectation of Life at Birth in India & Major States 2001 – 2025

India & Major States	2001-05		2006-10		2011-15		2016-20		2021-25	
	Male	Female	Male	Female	Male	Female	Male	Female	Male	Female
1	2	3	4	5	6	7	8	9	10	11
India	63.8	66.1	65.8	68.1	67.3	69.6	68.8	71.1	69.8	72.3
Andhra Pradesh	63.4	67.9	65.4	69.4	66.9	70.9	68.4	72.1	69.4	73.3
Assam	59.6	60.8	61.6	62.8	63.6	64.8	65.6	66.8	67.1	68.8
Bihar	65.6	64.7	67.1	66.7	68.6	68.7	69.6	70.2	70.6	71.4
Gujarat	64.9	69.0	67.2	71.0	69.2	72.5	70.7	73.7	71.9	74.9
Haryana	66.4	68.3	67.9	69.8	68.9	71.3	69.9	72.5	70.9	73.7
Karnataka	64.5	69.6	66.5	71.1	68.0	72.3	69.0	73.5	70.0	74.5
Kerala	70.8	76.0	72.0	76.8	73.2	77.6	74.2	78.1	75.2	78.6
Madhya Pradesh	60.5	61.3	62.5	63.3	64.5	65.3	66.5	67.3	68.0	69.3
Maharashtra	66.4	69.8	67.9	71.3	68.9	72.5	69.9	73.7	70.9	74.7
Orissa	60.3	62.3	62.3	64.8	64.3	67.3	66.3	69.6	67.8	71.6
Punjab	67.7	70.4	68.7	71.6	69.7	72.8	70.7	73.8	71.5	74.8
Rajashthan	64.1	67.2	66.1	69.2	67.6	70.7	68.6	71.9	69.6	73.1
Tamilnadu	66.1	69.1	67.6	70.6	68.6	71.8	69.6	73.0	70.6	74.0
Uttar Pradesh	62.0	61.9	64.0	64.4	66.0	66.9	67.5	69.2	68.7	71.2
West Bengal	66.7	69.4	68.2	70.9	69.2	72.1	70.2	73.3	71.0	74.3

Source: Report of the Technical Group on Population Projections May 2006.

evaluation of health programmes and schemes. Infant mortality is a sensitive index of health. Though crude death rate has reached very low level, IMR still remains to be high. Therefore further decline in CDR for total population in general and for females in particular depends on decline in IMR and MMR. Table 6 shows that infant mortality rate declined from 114 in 1980 to 72 in 1999, from 113 to 70 for males and from 115 to 71 for females. A declining trend of infant mortality is observed, but the present rate is comparatively high in India. It is obvious that female infants have little high mortality rate compared to male infants. Even though sex determination is a biological aspect, the incidence of morbidity and mortality for infants is influenced by socio-economic conditions of population. Therefore, in children age group females have disadvantage position. This aspect needs a detail examination. In rural India (Table 7) Infant mortality rate among male births is 61 as against 64 among female births. These respective rates are 37 and 40 per 1000 live births in urban India. Though the levels vary between rural and urban areas, the gender gap (about 3) explains comparatively high female infant mortality rate which remains constantly low. This observation is quite true in all the regions (States Table 7) in India. The gender gap (about 1) is relatively low

Table 6
Infant Mortality Rates By Sex 1980-99 - All India

Year	*Males*	*Females*	*Persons*
1980	113	115	114
1985	96	98	97
1990	78	81	80
1991	81	80	80
1992	79	80	79
1993	73	75	74
1994	75	73	74
1995	73	76	74
1996	71	73	72
1997	70	72	71
1998	70	73	72
1999	70	71	70

Source: Registrar General, India, Sample Registration

Table 7
State/UT Infant Mortality Rates by Sex & Residence in India 2006

	Total			Rural			Urban		
State/UT	*Total*	*Male*	*Female*	*Total*	*Male*	*Female*	*Total*	*Male*	*Female*
1	*2*	*3*	*4*	*5*	*6*	*7*	*8*	*9*	*10*
India	57	56	59	62	61	64	39	37	40
Andhra Pradesh	56	55	58	62	61	63	38	37	41
Arunachal Pradesh	38	43	-	-	-	-	-	-	
Assam	67	67	68	70	69	71	42	41	43
Bihar	60	58	63	62	59	64	45	43	47
Chhattisgarh	61	59	62	62	61	64	50	48	53
Goa	15	16	14	-	-	-	-	-	-
Gujarat	53	52	54	62	60	64	37	36	37
Haryana	57	57	58	62	61	62	45	45	45
Himachal Pradesh	50	45	55	-	-	-	-	-	-
Jammu & Kashmir	52	51	53	54	54	55	38	33	44
Jharkhand	49	46	52	52	49	55	32	32	33
Karnataka	48	46	50	53	50	57	36	36	35
Kerala	15	14	16	16	15	17	12	11	14
Madhya Pradesh	74	72	77	79	77	81	52	50	54
Maharashtra	35	35	36	42	41	42	26	25	27
Manipur	11	10	13	-	-	-	-	-	-
Meghalaya	53	53	52	-	-	-	-	-	-
Mizoram	25	24	25	-	-	-	-	-	-
Nagaland	20	17	23	-	-	-	-	-	-

Contd.

	Total			Rural			Urban		
State/UT	*Total*	*Male*	*Female*	*Total*	*Male*	*Female*	*Total*	*Male*	*Female*
1	*2*	*3*	*4*	*5*	*6*	*7*	*8*	*9*	*10*
Orissa	73	73	74	76	75	76	53	52	54
Punjab	44	39	50	48	41	57	36	34	38
Rajasthan	67	65	69	74	72	76	41	40	42
Sikkim	33	26	40	-	-	-	-	-	-
Tamil Nadu	37	36	37	39	38	41	33	33	33
Tripura	36	31	41	-	-	-	-	-	-
Uttar Pradesh	71	70	73	75	74	76	53	51	54
Uttarakhand	43	42	44	-	-	-	-	-	-
West Bengal	38	37	40	40	39	42	29	27	31
A & N Islands	31	27	36	-	-	-	-	-	-
Chandigarh	23	20	27	-	-	-	-	-	-
D & N Haveli	35	28	44	-	-	-	-	-	-
Daman & Diu	28	28	28	-	-	-	-	-	-
Delhi	37	36	39	42	40	44	36	35	38
Lakshadweep	25	29	21	-	-	-	-	-	-
Puducherry	28	20	36	-	-	-	-	-	-

Notes: Per 1000 live births Infant mortality rates for smaller States and Union territories are based on three-year period 2004-06. On account of wide year-to-year fluctuations due to inadequate sample size, the infant mortality rate by sex, separately for rural and urban areas is not given.

Source: SRS Bulletin, October 2007.

in Tamil Nadu and Orissa. Invariably, majority of Northern States, Central Indian States, Eastern states and Western States have high levels (50 and above) of IMR. In Meghalaya and Goa, not only low levels but also very low gender gap is registered. This is the area where females (female children) have disadvantage position.

Maternal Mortality

Maternal mortality refers to deaths of women due to puerperal causes. Females are only subjected to this mortality type. It is stated that infant mortality and maternal mortality are the major areas which need special attention in the context of analysis of female reproductive morbidity and mortality. Table 8 shows that maternal mortality ratio was 301 during 2001-2003. While Kerala, Tamil Nadu, Punjab, Haryana, Maharashtra have low maternal mortality ratio (below 200), the rest of the states, particularly Northern and central Indian States, have rates greater than 200. Under the condition of

Table 8
Maternal Mortality Ratio in India & Major States
1999-2001 & 2001-03

India/Major States	*1999-2001*	*2001-2003*
India	327	301
Andhra Pradesh	220	195
Assam	398	490
Bihar	400	371
Gujarat	202	172
Haryana	176	162
Karnataka	266	228
Kerala	149	110
Madhya Pradesh	407	379
Maharashtra	169	149
Orissa	424	358
Punjab	177	178
Rajasthan	501	445
Tamil Nadu	167	134
Uttar Pradesh	539	517
West Bengal	218	194

Note: Per 100000 Live Births
Source: Statistical Report, Registrar General of India, 2004

high maternal mortality, ASDRs should be normally high for female in the reproductive ages 15–49. But the situation may be true up to the age 24 years after which a contrasting picture is clearly noticed.

Mortality Risk

Mortality varies with age and sex prone to incidence of specific morbidity. Mortality risk for each sex could be estimated on the ASDRs calculated separately for males and females. Life tale function can also be used to estimate this risk. For example, nqx is one life table function which explains the probability of dying in a specified age interval. The World

Table 9
Gender Gap in Mortality Risk between Males and Females in India, 2001

	Male		*Female*		*Gender Gap in e^0_x*
Age Group	*nqx*	*ex*	*nqx*	*ex*	
<1	0.07093	60	0.07076	61.7	1.7
4-Jan	0.01943	63.5	0.02915	65.4	1.9
9-May	0.00849	60.8	0.01193	63.3	2.5
14-Oct	0.00645	56.2	0.00712	59.1	2.9
15-19	0.00987	51.6	0.01176	54.5	2.9
20-24	0.01302	47.1	0.01576	50.1	3
25-29	0.01591	42.7	0.01558	45.8	3.1
30-34	0.01882	38.3	0.0151	41.5	3.2
35-39	0.02571	34	0.01583	37.1	3.1
40-44	0.03212	29.8	0.02228	32.7	2.9
45-49	0.04649	25.8	0.03016	28.4	2.6
50-54	0.06628	21.9	0.04665	24.2	2.3
55-59	0.10514	18.3	0.0726	20.2	1.9
60-64	0.14421	15.1	0.1054	16.6	1.5
65-69	0.21119	12.2	0.17575	13.3	1.1
70-74	0.29375	9.8	0.26987	10.6	0.8
75-79	0.39902	7.9	0.34668	8.6	0.7
80-84	0.47854	6.5	0.44481	6.8	0.3
85-89	0.58562	5.1	0.56995	5.2	0.1
90-94	0.67599	3.9	0.67504	3.9	0
95-99	0.76122	2.8	0.76563	2.8	0
100+	1	2.1	1	2	0.1

Source: Estimated from the life table for India constructed by WHO, 2001.

Health Organizations constructed Life Tables for 191 countries. We made use of the tables constructed for India. Table 9 shows that *nqx* value explains the probability of dying per individual moving from one age to another age. Data show that this probability is slightly higher for female up to the age 24, after that males have high risk (probability). This is quite interesting observation. Irrespective of these probability differences, life expectancy for females is comparatively high in all the age groups.

Table 9 also explains the gender gap (ranging from 0.3 years to 3.2 year) in life expectancy. Of course, in the past Indian women had poor health condition which has been improving (close to condition for European Women) in consummation with females in developed countries. In the past, India was one among the few countries having high mortality rate for females compared to males. At present it has had low mortality rate as observed in European women. Obviously, Indian women used to consume less food and nutrition intake sanctifying her health for well being of family members. Under such circumstance, less mortality risk for females is quite interesting phenomena to be studied.

Cause of Death

At the national level, the Registrar General of India (RGI) is responsible for collection, collation and publication of cause of death statistics. At the state level, the Vital Statistics Division of the Directorate of Health deals with cause of death statistics. It is of vital importance to know the leading causes of deaths, as they are essential for prioritizing Public Health Initiatives and various National Health Programmes.

Medical Certification of cause of Death is an important tool of obtaining authentic & scientific information regarding causes of mortality. The Scheme is formulated by Office of the Registrar General; India is a big step towards the establishment of a system in the country for obtaining data on causes of death. The Scheme had undergone phase-wise implementation in the State, starting from medical college hospitals. In second phase, District hospitals, specialized hospitals were covered. The office of the Registrar General had given necessary administrative guidelines regarding coverage of MCCD Scheme in both urban & rural area. Attempts are being made to cover all private & govt. hospitals since 1998. A brief overview of the cause of death reporting systems in India is given below.

Medical Certification of Cause of Death

During the year 2000, the total number of 510580 medically certified deaths were registered in India under the civil registration system. The cause analysis revealed that about 73.33percent of the total medically certified deaths that has taken place in the year 2000 were under five major causes viz. Diseases of the circulatory system (I00-I99) (24.34%), Infectious and Parasitic Diseases (A00-B99) (15.72%), Symptoms, Signs and abnormal clinical & Laboratory finding not elsewhere classified (R00-R99) (14.21%), Injury, poisoning and certain other consequences of external causes (S00-T98) (11.28%), Certain conditions originating in the prenatal period (P00-P96) (7.79%) and the remaining 26.66 percent certified deaths were classified under the other causes. The MCCD data in terms of 19 major categories for the years 1998-2000 is presented in table 10 gender-wise

Tables 10 and 11 show that the distribution of medically certified causes of death by sex. The incidence of mortality is comparatively high among males. The major causes of death are 1.Infection, respiratory diseases, parasite diseases, 2.diseases of Circulatory System, 3.Cancer 4. Deaths by violence and 5 other causes and also for each cause, the incidence rate found to be high for males indicating better health situation for females.

Conclusions

In this study an attempt was made to analyse the gender difference or gap in mortality indicators of health. In general, gender gap in terms of socio-cultural, economic, demographic and environmental variables shows the most advantage position of men relative to women. But, in assessing health situation in terms of mortality indicators of health, women

Table 10
Distribution of Medically Certified Deaths by Causes and Age Group (Males)

Cause of Death & ICD 10	*Below 1 year*	*1-4 years*	*5-14 years*	*15-54 years*
Infectious and Parasitic Diseases	3468	1976	2032	26308
Neoplasms	103	142	271	3975
Diseases of the Blood and blood forming organs and certain disorder involving the immune mechanism	259	273	336	1642
Endocrine, Nutritional and Metabolic Diseases	238	142	83	2826
Mental and Behavioural Disorders	5	1	10	292
Diseases of Nervous System	1078	851	924	3859
Disease of eye and adnexa	2	3	2	18
Diseases of ear and mastoid process	1	3	5	11
Diseases of the circulatory system	840	337	658	26654
Diseases of the respiratory system	2904	1155	693	6866
Diseases of the digestive system	295	265	377	10063
Diseases of the skin and subcutaneous tissue	11	6	6	187
Diseases off Muscular skeletal system connective tissue	4	1	6	68
Diseases of the Genitourinary system	200	82	157	2503
Pregnancy, childbirth and Puerperioum	0	0	0	0
Certain conditions originating at prenatal period	24328	0	0	0
Congenital malformations, Deformations, & Chromosomal abnormalities	986	122	85	128
Symptoms, Signs and Abnormal Clinical & Laboratory finding not elsewhere classified	2258	851	1070	16585
Injury, Poisoning and Certain other Consequences of external causes	380	647	1539	24601
Total	37360	647	1539	126586

Table 11

Distribution of Medically Certified Deaths By Causes and Ag e group (Females)

Cause of Death & ICD 10	*Below 1 year*	*1-4 years*	*5-14 years*	*15-54 years*
Infectious and Parasitic Diseases	2157	1558	1767	12886
Neoplasms	82	66	137	3570
Diseases of the Blood and blood forming organs and certain disorder involving the immune mechanism	179	245	313	1891
Endocrine, Nutritional and Metabolic Diseases	235	143	95	1617
Mental and Behavioural Disorders	3	2	1	54
Diseases of Nervous System	676	651	669	2209
Disease of eye and adnexa	1	1	3	6
Diseases of ear and mastoid process	0	1	2	5
Diseases of the circulatory system	519	228	474	12425
Diseases of the respiratory system	2086	1028	561	3240
Diseases of the digestive system	167	140	283	2733
Diseases of the skin and subcutaneous tissue	14	6	6	117
Diseases off Mascular skeletal system connective tissue	5	1	2	62
Diseases of the Genitourinary system	104	58	1107	1211
Pregnancy, childbirth and Puerperioum	0	0	3	3891
Certain conditions originating at prenatal period	15456	0	0	0
Congenital malformations, Deformations, & Chromosomal abnormalities	552	81	31	134
Symptoms , Signs and abnormal clinical & Laboratory finding not elsewhere classified	1655	664	879	8579
Injury, Poisoning and certain other consequences of external causes	242	493	1223	17699
Total	24138	5366	6556	72629

are at advantage position. Actually the gender gap resulting from better position of women is really exceptional one. This study has clearly established gender gap in terms of mortality indicators which include Crude death rate, age specific death rate, standardized death rate, and expectation of life at birth, infant mortality rate, maternal mortality ratio, mortality risk, incidence of morbidity and mortality and cause of death by age and sex. Except infant mortality rate, females have better position in rest of the indictors. Therefore female infants are to be taken care of during pregnancy, delivery and post delivery period. Data show that sex ratio at birth is more favorable to male babies, under such condition how could mortality chance for females be more. This needs further exploration. Females have to face unfavorable circumstance (mortality risk) up to the age 24 years. After that males are put into similar circumstance. But the life expectancy of females is comparatively high in those specified age groups. This contrasting observation could be examined. Incidence of morbidity and mortality seems to be high for males. All aspects relating to health promotion in terms of food and nutrition intake (the amount and quantity of food intake), age at marriage, early pregnancy, unsafe motherhood, unsafe abortion, non use of contraceptives, frequent child births and high fertility, incidence of reproductive morbidity and mortality, treatment seeking behaviour, etc. Women used to forego their consumption for the growth and welfare of their children, husband and other family members. Gender difference is so obvious in utilizing health care services. Priority is given to promoting health of the family members, bearing the activities deteriorating health of women. Even under this condition, the data on mortality indicators and existence of gender gap indicate better health condition for women compared to men.

References

National Commission on Population, MOHFW (2007), *Report of Technical Group on Population Projections May 2006*. New Delhi: MOHFW.

Registrar General, India (1994), *Population Projections for India and States: 1996-2016*. New Delhi: Registrar General of India.

Registrar General, India (1995), *Sample Registration System, Occasional Paper No. 3*. New Delhi: Ministry of Home Affairs.

Registrar General, India (2004), *Statistical Report, 2003, India*. Delhi: Office of the Registrar General of India.

Registrar General, India (2008), *Sample Registration System Bulletin, October 2007*. New Delhi: Office of the Registrar General of India.

The Department of Health and Family Welfare (2006), *Family Welfare Year Book 2005*. New Delhi: Ministry of Health and Family Welfare.

The Department of Health and Family Welfare (2008), *Family Welfare Year Book, 2007*. New Delhi: Ministry of Health of Family Welfare.

United Nations (2008), ECAP Population Data Sheet. Bangkok: UN, The Emerging Social Issues Division.

World Health Organisation (2001), Life Table for 191 Countries. Switzerland: WHO.

15

Health at Old Ages in India: A Statistical Exposition of Its Socio-Cultural and Gender Dimensions

Sanjeev Bakshi, Prasanta Pathak

Introduction

Health is an indispensable integrant of Quality of Life (QOL). The concept has been defined as 'a state of complete physical, mental and social well being and not merely the absence of disease and infirmities' (WHO). The salience of sound health increases with age as it becomes pivotal to all the day to day activities. At the macro level as populations age the health at older ages becomes a matter of concern. The reasons for this concern are not difficult to discover especially in case of developing countries where the social security systems are under developed. Further, the public health systems are not well equipped to meet the health concerns of the **older Adults** (OA). Population ageing and health concerns blend together in the ageing experience of India. The OA constitutes about 7.28 per cent of the total population of India in 2001. This population of OA is heterogeneous with respect to socio-cultural, economic and health aspects.

Although, biological processes are responsible for the state of health nevertheless there are evidences to show the association between health and socio-cultural and economic factors (Gliksman et al, 1995; Smith et al., 1997; Chandola, 1998; Cambois et al., 2001; Adda et al., 2003; Zimmer et al., 2003; Kaneda et al., 2004; Baker et al., 2005; Ravito et al., 2005; Matthews et al., 2005; Matthews et al., 2006; Petrelli et al., 2006; Zimmer, 2006; Merkin et al., 2007). Even early childhood conditions have a lasting effect on the health at later life (Hayward et al., 2004). These factors can be viewed as exposures of various kinds an OA is subjected to during his/her lifetime. The health at older ages is the effect of these exposures. These exposures include economic status, occupation, marital status, number of children born during reproductive phase (for females) and education to name a few. Albeit, health is not a well defined concept and operational definition is needed for any quantitative analysis of health.

Health

One can broadly classify the components of health at older ages as morbidity, disability, self-rated health and mental health. At older ages the states of morbidity and disability are self evident. In any study on health it is most appropriate to study the prevalence of each disease and disability separately in a population. However, there are a large number of diseases that can affect the health status of an OA. Added to this is the association among various diseases (co-morbidities).

A simple measure of health status of an OA is the count of diseases and the count of disabilities. These two can serve as operational definitions of the corresponding components of the health of an OA. These definitions are based on the assumption that all the diseases considered in the study are equally severe. A count of c means a state of severity whatever these c diseases are. Further, we assume that all the diseases occur independently of each other. Thus, the difference in severity of the counts c and $c+1$ is same as the difference in severity of the counts $c+1$ and $c+2$.

Generation of a disease in an OA is a random event that takes place in response to various exposures. Thus, the count of diseases and disabilities are random variables that may or may not be associated. The distribution of these counts can be inferred and the corresponding parameters can be interpreted and estimated. Further, the effect of various exposures on these parameters can be estimated by applying appropriate models.

The present study peruses the following objectives:

1. To conceptualise the distribution of the count of diseases and disabilities
2. To investigate the association between diseases and disabilities
3. proposing model to investigate the effect of various socio-cultural and economic exposures on health

Source of Data

The 60th round of the National Sample Survey provides rich information on the health aspects like diseases, disabilities and health seeking behaviour of OA. It also provides rich details about the socio-cultural and economic aspects of the OA. The data provides information on 37 diseases and 5 disabilities. An OA is asked to list at most five diseases or disabilities in the decreasing order of severity. The following Tables 1 & 2 shows the frequency distribution of the count of diseases and disabilities.

Table 1
Frequency Distribution of the Count of Diseases in OA

Number of Diseases	*Frequency*	*Cumulative Frequency*
0	21317	73.249
1	6524	95.701
2	1084	99.427
3	151	99.944
4	15	99.994
5	2	100.000

Table 2
Frequency Distribution of the Count of Disabilities in OA

Number of Diseases	*Frequency*	*Cumulative Frequency*
0	24480	84.117
1	4181	98.482
2	394	99.836
3	41	99.976
4	7	100.000
5	0	100.000

From the tables it is evident that instances of suffering from more than 5 diseases/disabilities are rare and the data can be used to count the number of diseases for all practical purposes.

Distribution of Diseases and Disabilities

Letting D={D1, D2,....,Di,...} denote the set of all diseases possible in an OA where D_i denote the ith disease. There is a non-zero probabilityp_i that an OA suffers from the ith disease. This probability depends upon the socio-cultural and economic exposure of the OA. A random variable X_i is defined as follows:

$$P(X_i=1)=p_i \tag{1}$$

$$P(X_i=0)=1-p_i \tag{2}$$

Define
$$Y=\sum_i X_i \tag{3}$$

Then, Y denotes the count of diseases on an OA. Assuming independence of X_i s the moment generating function of Y is

$$M_Y(t)=\prod_i\left(1-p_i\left(1-e^t\right)\right) \tag{4}$$

The expression on the r.h.s can be expanded as follows,

$$1-\left(\sum_i p_i\right)\left(1-e^t\right)+\left(\sum_i\sum_{\substack{j\\i\neq j}} p_i p_j\right)\left(1-e^t\right)^2- \tag{5}$$

$$\left(\sum_i\sum_{\substack{j\\i\neq j\neq l}}\sum_l p_i p_j p_l\right)\left(1-e^t\right)^3+....+(-1)^k p_i p_j \cdots p_k$$

For low values of p_i's, the product terms in the above expression can be ignored. Thus, (4) can be approximately written as,

$$M_X(t) \approx 1 - \left(\sum_i p_i\right)\left(1 - e^t\right) \tag{6}$$

This resembles the m.g.f of a random variable having Poisson distribution with parameterl. Where, $\lambda = \sum_i p_i$. Hence, under the assumptions discussed earlier the distribution of the count of diseases/disabilities can be approximated as Poisson distribution (Agresti, 1996; Luke, 2004).

Association between Diseases and Disabilities

Since the variables number of diseases and the number of disabilities are ordinal, gamma can serve as a measure of association between diseases and disabilities. The values near to 0 depict weak association between the two variables and the values near +1 and -1 indicate strong positive and negative association respectively.

In what follows the variables that may influence the health of an OA are discussed.

Characteristics of the Individuals

Age

The natural process of ageing is inevitable and has a bearing on the health of an OA. This process coincides with the increasing age of an OA. Hence, age can be considered as a proxy to the natural process of ageing. The effect of age on health indicates the net effect of the process of ageing on health. Correct reporting of age is marred with high degree of digit preference error. Therefore, the present study includes age as a categorical variable with young-old (includes ages 60 to less than 69), old (includes ages 69 to less than 79) and old-old (includes ages 79 years and above) as categories. The category young-old can serve as a reference to compare the state of health in rest of the categories.

Marital Status

Risk of widowhood/widower hood looms large at older ages. In the Indian society remarriage/marriage at older ages is rare. Therefore, at older ages transition in marital status happens only from being married to being widow/widower. Therefore, the state of being widow/widower can be seen as the future transition state of married OA. Further, there may be OA who never got married, who are divorced or live life as a separated couple. But, this is a minority as the population of OA mostly comprise of married OA and widow/widower OA. In the present study the marital status of this minority shall be called 'others'. The other two categories of marital status are 'currently married' and 'widowed/widowers'. Widowhood/widowerhood may push an OA into ignorance and social neglect. This may affect his/her overall health. Therefore, in the present study the interest lies in comparing the effect of widowhood/widowerhood with the effect of being married on health.

It should be borne in mind that transition to widowhood and the on set of diseases in an OA does not coincide. It only means that widowhood/widowerhood may worsen the health condition. If health worsens, the extent of worsening of health has to be estimated from the statistical analysis that shall follow.

Level of Education

Health seeking behaviour of an OA is guided by his/her level of awareness regarding health. Awareness regarding health may be associated with the level of education. It is opined that more the level of education more is the regarding health. Therefore, the present study includes education as a categorical variable with three categories namely, 'illiterate', 'literate but below matriculation' and 'matriculation and above' in the increasing order of the level of education. The last category may be considered as a reference to compare the health status in rest of the categories.

Dependence

In the present study, dependence means economic dependence of an OA. Dependence can be categorised into four discrete states. When an OA is completely dependent on others for his day to day needs the state of dependence is called 'complete dependence. It may happen that an OA is partially dependent on others. This state of dependence is called 'partial dependence'. A state where no economic support is required by an OA is called 'non-dependence'. Such OA may have to support dependents like spouse, children or other relatives. Such a state is called 'non-dependence and supporting'. Finally, the OA who are not dependent and do not have dependents to support are said to be in a state of 'non-dependence and non-supporting'. Out of the four states of dependence it is the last one where an OA is least constrained. This state can serve as a reference for comparing the health in rest of the states.

Number of Children

Female's reproductive phase spans from the age of 15 years to the age of 49 years. During this span she may give birth to off springs. The effect of this biological process may have repercussions on health at older ages. The number of children indicates the extent to which a woman goes through such biological process. The effect of a unit increase in number of children on health needs investigation. Though the interpretation of the effect of number of children on the health of females is direct, similar interpretation is not sound in case of males.

Characteristics of the Households

Economic Condition of Households

Economic well being of a household is reflected in per capita monthly expenditure (PCME) of the household. The households are divided into five equal parts using quintiles for the PCME. These are called first, second, third, fourth and fifth quintiles. The first through fifth quintiles represent the positioning of economic strata in descending order. The lowest economic stratum Male shall be considered as reference for comparing the health status in rest of the strata. The quintiles are formed separately for rural and urban areas.

Classification of Households Based on Major Economic Activity

Net income of a household, during a reference period (past one year), may depend on a single economic activity or a host of economic activities. The activity that contributes the maximum to the net household income is called the major economic activity. This characteristic can be assumed to be more or less unvarying with time. For example, for a household reporting to be self-employed in agriculture in the reference period is likely to have remained so for the past also. The present study intends to compare the relative state of health of OA in households involved in different major economic activities. The broad groups for major economic activities, for rural and urban areas, are given in Table1.

Table 3
The Classification of Households Based on the Major Economic Activity in Rural and Urban Areas

Major Economic Activity	*Rural*	*Urban*
Type I	self-employed in non-agriculture	self-employed
Type II	agricultural labour	regular wage/salary earning
Type III	other labour	casual labour
Type IV	self-employed in agriculture	others
Type V	others	

The group 'others' can be set as a reference to compare the health status of the OA in rest of the categories.

Living Arrangements of OA (LA) and Size of Household

LA and size of the household determine indicate how OA live and how many members share the space. LA of the OA are of two types namely, alone and co-residence. Staying alone or with spouse only is called 'alone'; otherwise it is called 'co-residence'. In addition to LA the size of the household may have effect on the health of OA as increasing number of household members may mount pressure on the resources available for the OA.

Land Owned by the Household

Like PCME amount of land owned by a household is a measure of economic condition of the household. This may be more prominent in case of rural areas. The categories considered here are in increasing order of the amount of land starting from less than 0.005 hectares to more than 8 hectares. The last category can be taken as a reference category for comparing the health status in rest of the categories.

Socio-cultural Factors

Caste, religion and region constitute the socio-cultural factors. Social groups classifies as 'scheduled castes (SC)', 'scheduled tribes (ST)' and the rest of the population called 'others' constitute the three categories of caste. Due to socially disadvantageous position of SC and ST the study intends to compare the health status of OA belonging to these categories with respect to those belonging to the category 'others'. The religious categories considered in the present study are Christians, Muslims and the rest of the religious groups that serve as a reference. The country is divided into eight geographical regions namely north-eastern, eastern, northern I, northern II, western, peninsular, southern and south-western.

The Model

Form the preliminary analysis of the data it is evident that generally in a population the count of diseases adheres to a Poisson model. Whereas, the count of number of disabilities adhere to a model where over dispersion is taken into account. Hence, the study proposes Poisson model for diseases and Negative binomial model for disabilities. The models are described as follows:

$$\ln(\lambda_{diseases}) = \alpha + A_1 + A_2 + \ldots + A_n \quad \text{For diseases} \qquad (7)$$

$$\ln(\lambda_{disabiklities}) = \alpha + A_1 + A_2 + \ldots + A_n + \varepsilon \quad \text{, for disabilities} \ (8)$$

Where, e is distributes as a beta variable and A_1, A_2, ..., A_k are the effects of various socio-cultural and economic factors (Luke, 2004).

Findings and Analyses

Rates for Diseases

The rates are higher for old and old-old age groups when compared to young-old age group. For RURAL MALE the rates are higher (Table 4) by 1.198 and 1.250 times for old and old-old age groups respectively. The corresponding figures for RURAL FEMALE, URBAN MALE and URBAN FEMALE are 1.350 and 1.260, 1.322 and 1.182 and 1.236 and 1.094 (not significantly differing from young olds) respectively.

The marital status of an OA makes a significant difference in their health status. Consider the female populations. When compared to currently married females, the rates are higher for widowed ones by 1.311 and 1.186 times in RURAL FEMALE and URBAN FEMALE populations respectively. On the other hand the rates do not differ significantly between currently married females and category others that comprising of never married/divorced/separated females.

Education is found to be a significant (Table 4) factor in the model in case of rural populations only. For RURAL MALE the rates for the groups 'illiterate' and 'below matriculation' are lesser by 0.658 times and 0.868 times when compared to the reference group (above matriculation). But in case of RURAL FEMALE, the two groups mentioned above do not differ significantly from the reference group.

Dependence is not found to be a significant factor in the model for URBAN FEMALE. However, for RURAL FEMALE the females who are completely dependent have rate higher by 1.303 times when compared to the reference group (non-dependent non-supporting). In case of RURAL MALE the partially dependent and completely dependent males have rates higher by 1.477 and 2.132 times when compared to the reference group. The non-dependent and supporting URBAN MALE have rates lesser by 0.728 times when compared to the reference group. Further, economic well being of the household and health of OA are associated. Irrespective of the population, the rates are lower in all the higher economic strata when compared to the lowest economic strata.

OA and size of the household are not significant factor in the model except for the URBAN MALE. The rates for URBAN MALE who are living alone are 1.142 times more than those who are co-residing.

Possession of land is a significant factor in rural populations only. The effects do not show any monotonic trend. For RURAL MALE the households (Table 4) having land with ranges (0-0.005 ha), (0.005-0.01 ha), (2-3 ha), (3-4 ha) and (4-6 ha) differ from the reference (more than 8 ha). All these households show lesser rate of diseases when compared to the reference. Similarly the households having land with ranges (1-2 ha), (2-3 ha), (4-6 ha) and (6-8 ha) show lesser rate of diseases when compared to the reference.

The rates for scheduled tribes differ significantly from the other castes (reference) in all the populations. The rates are 0.851, 0.697, 0.619 and 0.703 times lesser in RURAL MALE, RURAL FEMALE, URBAN MALE and URBAN FEMALE respectively for scheduled tribes when compared to the reference.

The rate of diseases for OA belonging to religious groups namely Muslim and Christians differ significantly from the rest in case of rural populations only. When compared to the reference group, the rates are higher by 1.252 and 1.302 times in case of Christians and Muslims respectively for RURAL MALE. Similarly, for RURAL FEMALE the corresponding rates are 1.732 and 1.438 times higher in Christians and Muslims respectively.

Table 4
Results of Poisson Regression for the Count of Diseases for Rural Male, Rural Female, Urban Male and Urban Female Populations

	Rural Male			Rural Female			Urban Male			Urban Female		
Variables	*Effect b (p-value)*	*S.E*	*Exp (b)*	*Effect b (p-value)*	*S.E*	*Exp (b)*	*Effect b (p-value)*	*S.E*	*Exp (b)*	*Effect b (p-value)*	*S.E*	*Exp (b)*
Intercept	-1.275	0.2287		-1.377			-1.006			-0.866		
	(0.000)			(0.000)	0.3180		(0.001)	0.3164		(0.004)	0.2971	
Age Groups *(Young-old)*[R]												
Old-old	0.223	0.0675	1.250	0.233	0.0773	1.262	0.167	0.0753	1.182	0.090	0.0763	1.094
	(0.001)			(0.003)			(0.027)			(0.240)		
Old	0.181	0.0448	1.198	0.300	0.0468	1.350	0.279	0.0498	1.322	0.212	0.0490	1.236
	(0.000)			(0.000)			(0.000)			(0.000)		
Marital Status *(Currently Married)*[R]												
Others	-0.637	0.3190	0.529	0.217	0.2283	1.242	0.104	0.2382	1.110	0.219	0.2291	1.245
	(0.046)			(0.342)			(0.662)			(0.339)		
Widowed	-0.101	0.0524	0.904	0.271	0.0486	1.311	-0.256	0.0697	0.774	0.171	0.0512	1.186
	(0.054)			(0.000)			(0.000)			(0.001)		
Level of Education *(Matriculation and above)*[R]												
Illiterate	-0.418	0.0811	0.658	-0.309	0.2204	0.734	-0.055	0.0800	0.946	-0.086	0.0862	0.918
	(0.000)			(0.161)			(0.489)			(0.320)		
Below Matriculation	-0.145	0.0783	0.865	0.184	0.2218	1.202	0.029	0.0571	1.029	-0.005	0.0808	0.995
	(0.064)			(0.406)			(0.610)			(0.951)		
Dependence *(Not dependent /Not Supporting)*[R]												
Completely Dependent	0.757	0.1290	2.132	0.265	0.1158	1.303	-0.014	0.0989	0.986	0.048	0.0990	1.049
	(0.000)			(0.022)			(0.886)			(0.631)		
Partially Dependent	0.390	0.1338	1.477	0.141	0.1266	1.151	-0.089	0.1060	0.915	0.093	0.1174	1.097
	(0.004)			(0.266)			(0.339)			(0.427)		
Not Dependent / Supporting	0.136	0.1279	1.146	-0.107	0.1404	0.899	-0.317	0.0950	0.728	0.066	0.1180	1.068
	(0.287)			(0.445)			(0.001)			(0.577)		
No. of Children	0.028	0.0091	1.028	0.019	0.0065	1.019	0.048	0.124	1.049	0.033	0.0049	1.034
	(0.002)			(0.004)			(0.000)			(0.000)		

Contd.

	Rural Male			Rural Female			Urban Male			Urban Female		
Variables	*Effect b (p-value)*	*S.E*	*Exp (b)*	*Effect b (p-value)*	*S.E*	*Exp (b)*	*Effect b (p-value)*	*S.E*	*Exp (b)*	*Effect b (p-value)*	*S.E*	*Exp (b)*
Household Economic Condition *(Fifth)* [R]												
First	-0.345 (0.000)	0.0720	0.708	-0.494 (0.000)	0.0746	0.610	-0.652 (0.000)	0.0885	0.521	-0.532 (0.000)	0.0860	0.587
Second	-0.229 (0.001)	0.0659	0.795	-0.343 (0.000)	0.0691	0.710	-0.830 (0.000)	0.0822	0.436	-0.442 (0.000)	0.0758	0.656
Third	-0.164 (0.006)	0.0600	0.849	-0.273 (0.000)	0.0624	0.761	-0.573 (0.000)	0.0724	0.564	-0.336 (0.000)	0.0701	0.715
Fourth	-0.082 (0.165)	0.0591	0.921	-0.265 (0.000)	0.0635	0.767	-0.291 (0.000)	0.0684	0.748	-0.125 (0.081)	0.0719	0.882
Household Type *(Type V)* [R]												
Type I	0.101 (0.180)	0.0753	1.106	0.059 (0.423)	0.0734	1.061	-0.082 (0.264)	0.0736	0.921	0.016 (0.837)	0.0767	1.016
Type II	0.008 (0.912)	0.0759	1.008	-0.040 (0.595)	0.0755	0.961	0.083 (0.267)	0.0752	1.087	-0.034 (0.662)	0.0788	0.967
Type III	0.254 (0.003)	0.0868	1.289	0.145 (0.090)	0.0854	1.156	-0.321 (0.006)	0.1170	0.725	-0.029 (0.787)	0.1070	0.971
Type IV	0.055 (0.444)	0.0720	1.057	0.019 (0.792)	0.0734	1.019						
Living Arrangements (Co-residence) [R]												
Alone	0.003 (0.965)	0.0665	1.003	-0.004 (0.964)	0.0776	0.996	0.133 (0.093)	0.0789	1.142	-0.090 (0.336)	0.0935	0.914
Size of the Household	-0.003 (0.688)	0.0081	0.997	0.008 (0.390)	0.0091	1.008	0.037 (0.000)	0.0094	1.038	0.005 (0.570)	0.0093	1.005
Land Owned (Hectares) *(More than 8.0)* [R]												
Less than 0.005	-0.520 (0.004)	0.1805	0.595	-0.196 (0.312)	0.1940	0.822	0.316 (0.272)	0.2817	1.372	-0.034 (0.899)	0.2651	0.967
0.005 – 0.01	-0.361 (0.040)	0.1756	0.697	-0.310 (0.109)	0.1935	0.733	0.357 (0.212)	0.2862	1.429	-0.038 (0.886)	0.2649	0.963
0.02 – 0.20	-0.204 (0.238)	0.1728	0.815	-0.225 (0.238)	0.1908	0.799	0.265 (0.358)	0.2878	1.303	0.067 (0.800)	0.2661	1.069
0.21 – 0.40	-0.178 (0.299)	0.1711	0.837	-0.226 (0.232)	0.1890	0.798	0.364 (0.233)	0.3052	1.439	0.031 (0.914)	0.2827	1.031
0.41 – 1.00	-0.257 (0.118)	0.1640	0.773	-0.282 (0.121)	0.1819	0.754	0.074 (0.813)	0.3146	1.077	-0.224 (0.459)	0.3023	0.799
1.01 – 2.00	-0.163 (0.316)	0.1626	0.850	-0.396 (0.030)	0.1828	0.673	0.135 (0.674)	0.3199	1.145	-0.083 (0.783)	0.3013	0.920
2.01 – 3.00	-0.551 (0.002)	0.1767	0.576	-0.581 (0.004)	0.1999	0.559	-0.525 (0.229)	0.4364	0.592	-0.217 (0.537)	0.3513	0.805
3.01 – 4.00	-0.326 (0.076)	0.1838	0.722	-0.320 (0.125)	0.2084	0.726	0.213 (0.668)	0.4956	1.237	0.035 (0.922)	0.3560	1.036
4.01 – 6.0	-0.860 (0.000)	0.2182	0.423	-0.613 (0.007)	0.2294	0.542	0.382 (0.327)	0.3898	1.465	-0.078 (0.841)	0.3819	0.925
6.01 – 8.0	-0.218 (0.328)	0.2234	0.804	-0.664 (0.025)	0.2957	0.515	0.491 (0.298)	0.4719	1.634	-0.146 (0.795)	0.5642	0.864
Caste *(Other Castes)* [R]												
Scheduled Tribes	-0.161 (0.082)	0.0923	0.851	-0.361 (0.001)	0.1106	0.697	-0.479 (0.052)	0.2463	0.619	-0.353 (0.021)	0.1529	0.703
Scheduled Castes	-0.049 (0.386)	0.0568	0.952	0.054 (0.363)	0.0591	1.055	0.009 (0.913)	0.0794	1.009	0.000 (0.999)	0.0775	1.000
Religious Group *(Others)* [R]												
Christians	0.225 (0.053)	0.1164	1.252	0.549 (0.000)	0.1005	1.732	-0.165 (0.197)	0.1280	0.848	0.091 (0.397)	0.1080	1.095
Muslims	0.264 (0.000)	0.0659	1.302	0.363 (0.000)	0.0655	1.438	0.044 (0.553)	0.0739	1.045	0.032 (0.655)	0.0707	1.033

Contd.

	Rural Male			Rural Female			Urban Male			Urban Female		
Variables	Effect b (p-value)	S.E	Exp (b)	Effect b (p-value)	S.E	Exp (b)	Effect b (p-value)	S.E	Exp (b)	Effect b (p-value)	S.E	Exp (b)
Regions *(South Western)*[R]												
North Eastern	0.324 (0.007)	0.1194	1.383	0.526 (0.000)	0.1409	1.692	0.241 (0.258)	0.2128	1.273	-0.320 (0.011)	0.1256	0.726
Eastern	0.198 (0.004)	0.0683	1.219	0.471 (0.000)	0.0754	1.602	0.173 (0.014)	0.0701	1.189	-0.003 (0.969)	0.0799	0.997
Northern I	-0.023 (0.880)	0.1515	0.977	-0.133 (0.467)	0.1823	0.875	-0.151 (0.473)	0.2108	0.860	-0.636 (0.000)	0.1658	0.529
Northern II	0.188 (0.009)	0.0716	1.207	0.300 (0.000)	0.0772	1.350	-0.238 (0.002)	0.0750	0.788	-0.169 (0.026)	0.0757	0.845
Western	0.015 (0.861)	0.0849	1.015	-0.216 (0.030)	0.0994	0.806	-0.202 (0.018)	0.0856	0.817	-0.194 (0.030)	0.0891	0.824
Peninsular	0.170 (0.026)	0.0765	1.185	0.254 (0.002)	0.0824	1.289	-0.009 (0.912)	0.0777	0.991	0.078 (0.300)	0.0755	1.081
Southern	0.155 (0.051)	0.0797	1.168	0.147 (0.087)	0.0857	1.158	0.009 (0.903)	0.0740	1.009	-0.020 (0.788)	0.0750	0.980

Note: the p-value indicative of the test of the hypothesis that the effect is zero against the alternative that the effect is not zero

Rates for Disabilities

The rate of disabilities is higher in old and old-old age groups when compared to the reference (young-old age) group (Table 5). For example, in RURAL MALE the rate are higher by 1.418 and 2.303 times in old and old-old age groups respectively. The corresponding figures for RURAL FEMALE, URBAN MALE and URBAN FEMALE are 1.696 and 2.392, 1.573 and 1.939 and 1.528 and 2.010 respectively.

Widowhood/widowerhood is a comparatively disadvantageous state with respect to disabilities as the rates of disabilities (Table 5) are higher in this state when compared to married state. For RURAL MALE, the two states do not significantly differ with respect to the rate of disabilities. But the rates are higher in case of widows/widowers by 1.242, 1.487 and 1.283 times for RURAL FEMALE, URBAN MALE and URBAN FEMALE respectively.

In the model for RURAL MALE, RURAL FEMALE and URBAN FEMALE, the effects of the levels 'illiterate' and 'literate but below matriculation' are not found to be significantly different from the effect of the reference category 'matriculation and above'. However, in case of URBAN MALE the rates are higher by 1.288 times and 1.592 times higher respectively when compared to the reference category.

Prevalence of disabilities (Table 5) and economic dependency are associated. The rates for completely dependent OA are higher by 1.846, 1.351, 1.508 and 1.674 times in RURAL MALE, RURAL FEMALE, URBAN MALE and URBAN FEMALE respectively when compared to the reference group (non-dependent and non-supporting). Rest of the groups ate not found to be significantly differing from the reference group except in case of URBAN FEMALE. Here, the rates for partially dependent females are higher by 1.842 times higher than the reference group.

The association between the rate of disability and number of children is not significant in RURAL FEMALE; but in URBAN FEMALE the rates are reduced by 0.962 times with a unit increase in the number of children.

Table 5
Results of Poisson Regression for the Count of Disabilities for Rural Male, Rural Female, Urban Male and Urban Female Populations

	Rural Male			*Rural Female*			*Urban Male*			*Urban Female*		
Variables	*Effect b (p-value)*	*S.E*	*Exp (b)*	*Effect b (p-value)*	*S.E*	*Exp (b)*	*Effect b (p-value)*	*S.E*	*Exp (b)*	*Effect b (p-value)*	*S.E*	*Exp (b)*
Intercept	-1.601 (0.000)	0.3525		-1.616 (0.001)	0.5020		-4.415 (0.000)	1.0701		-2.097 (0.000)	0.5672	
Age Groups *(Young-Old)*[R]												
Old-old	0.834 (0.000)	0.0900	2.303	0.872 (0.000)	0.0950	2.392	0.662 (0.000)	0.1257	1.939	0.698 (0.000)	0.1120	2.010
Old	0.349 (0.000)	0.0666	1.418	0.528 (0.000)	0.0643	1.696	0.453 (0.000)	0.0947	1.573	0.424 (0.000)	0.0816	1.528
Marital Status *(Currently Married)*[R]												
Others	-0.904 (0.038)	0.4369	0.405	0.365 (0.210)	0.2916	1.441	0.432 (0.306)	0.4217	1.540	0.046 (0.915)	0.4279	1.047
Widowed	0.039 (0.598)	0.0733	1.040	0.217 (0.001)	0.0663	1.242	0.397 (0.000)	0.1054	1.487	0.249 (0.004)	0.0854	1.283
Level of Education *(Matriculation and above)*[R]												
Illiterate	-0.009 (0.952)	0.1399	0.991	0.432 (0.290)	0.4085	1.540	0.253 (0.083)	0.1461	1.288	0.119 (0.454)	0.1582	1.126
Below Matriculation	0.102 (0.460)	0.1382	1.107	0.219 (0.599)	0.4160	1.245	0.465 (0.000)	0.1141	1.592	0.114 (0.441)	0.1476	1.121
Dependence *(Not Dependent: Not Supporting)*[R]												
Completely Dependent	0.613 (0.000)	0.1551	1.846	0.301 (0.046)	0.1512	1.351	0.411 (0.049)	0.2088	1.508	0.515 (0.002)	0.1698	1.674
Partially Dependent	0.200 (0.224)	0.1645	1.221	0.111 (0.508)	0.1682	1.117	0.338 (0.127)	0.2216	1.402	0.611 (0.002)	0.1951	1.842
Not Dependent: Supporting	-0.227 (0.142)	0.1547	0.797	0.001 (0.997)	0.1800	1.001	0.078 (0.708)	0.2073	1.081	0.162 (0.429)	0.2051	1.176
No. of Children	-0.039 (0.009)	0.0150	0.962	0.015 (0.128)	0.0099	1.015	0.004 (0.866)	0.0230	1.004	-0.039 (0.037)	0.0189	0.962
Household Economic Condition *(Fifth)*[R]												
First	-0.273 (0.009)	0.1050	0.761	-0.077 (0.420)	0.0951	0.926	0.082 (0.629)	0.1695	1.085	-0.167 (0.223)	0.1368	0.846
Second	-0.004 (0.965)	0.0955	0.996	-0.249 (0.009)	0.0954	0.780	0.139 (0.379)	0.1584	1.149	-0.001 (0.992)	0.1269	0.999
Third	-0.057 (0.526)	0.0897	0.945	-0.093 (0.287)	0.0871	0.911	0.042 (0.785)	0.1536	1.043	-0.056 (0.643)	0.1207	0.946
Fourth	-0.175 (0.063)	0.0941	0.839	-0.239	0.0922	0.787	0.546 (0.000)	0.1461	1.726	-0.072 (0.589)	0.1326	0.931
Household Type (Type V)[R]												
Type I	0.001 (0.996)	0.1136	1.001	0.216 (0.043)	0.1070	1.241	-0.101 (0.463)	0.1374	0.904	0.201 (0.122)	0.1296	1.223
Type II	-0.062 (0.560)	0.1057	0.940	-0.008 (0.935)	0.1033	0.992	-0.140 (0.333)	0.1448	0.869	0.051 (0.705)	0.1352	1.052
Type III	0.321 (0.013)	0.1288	1.379	0.158 (0.212)	0.1269	1.171	0.208 (0.259)	0.1841	1.231	0.151 (0.363)	0.1659	1.163
Type IV	-0.122 (0.241)	0.1039	0.885	0.000 (0.998)	0.1034	1.000						
Living Arrangements (Co-residence)[R]												
Alone	0.220 (0.021)	0.0951	1.246	0.070 (0.502)	0.1044	1.073	0.361 (0.013)	0.1463	1.435	0.328 (0.023)	0.1447	1.388

Contd.

Variables	Rural Male			Rural Female			Urban Male			Urban Female		
	Effect b (p-value)	S.E	Exp (b)	Effect b (p-value)	S.E	Exp (b)	Effect b (p-value)	S.E	Exp (b)	Effect b (p-value)	S.E	Exp (b)
Size of the Household	-0.017 (0.171)	0.0122	0.983	-0.028 (0.026)	0.0125	0.972	0.010 (0.538)	0.0169	1.010	-0.020 (0.225)	0.0166	0.980
Land Owned (Hectares) *(More than 8.0)*[R]												
Less than 0.005	0.055 (0.853)	0.2943	1.057	-0.748 (0.003)	0.2484	0.473	1.432 (0.166)	1.0331	4.187	0.072 (0.886)	0.5050	1.075
0.005 – 0.01	0.038 (0.897)	0.2922	1.039	-0.682 (0.006)	0.2470	0.506	1.692 (0.101)	1.0321	5.430	-0.126 (0.803)	0.5046	0.882
0.02 – 0.20	-0.078 (0.791)	0.2933	0.925	-0.691 (0.005)	0.2458	0.501	1.796 (0.082)	1.0333	6.025	-0.127 (0.803)	0.5072	0.881
0.21 – 0.40	0.133 (0.647)	0.2819	1.142	-0.606 (0.012)	0.2417	0.546	1.435 (0.175)	1.0585	4.200	-0.104 (0.847)	0.5384	0.901
0.41 – 1.0	0.267 (0.336)	0.2779	1.306	-0.494 (0.032)	0.2299	0.610	1.414 (0.182)	1.0599	4.112	-1.051 (0.074)	0.5883	0.350
1.01 – 2.0	-0.008 (0.978)	0.2786	0.992	-0.465 (0.041)	0.2277	0.628	1.857 (0.077)	1.0517	6.404	-0.744 (0.209)	0.5925	0.475
2.01 – 3.0	0.578 (0.041)	0.2823	1.782	-0.346 (0.147)	0.2386	0.708	1.645 (0.130)	1.0862	5.181	-1.018 (0.192)	0.7796	0.361
3.01 – 4.0	0.507 (0.082)	0.2918	1.660	-0.499 (0.054)	0.2595	0.607	1.563 (0.221)	1.2768	4.773	0.265 (0.674)	0.6290	1.303
4.01 – 6.0	0.058 (0.858)	0.3214	1.160	-0.652 (0.019)	0.2785	0.521	-0.013 (0.993)	1.4555	0.987	-1.500 (0.089)	0.8822	0.223
6.01 – 8.0	-0.620 (0.159)	0.4404	0.538	-2.614 (0.000)	0.7483	0.073	0.659 (0.653)	1.4658	1.933	0.235 (0.783)	0.8538	1.265
Caste *(Other Castes)*[R]												
Scheduled Tribes	-0.281 (0.025)	0.1252	0.755	0.069 (0.531)	0.1100	1.071	-0.075 (0.825)	0.3383	0.928	-0.326 (0.282)	0.3029	0.722
Scheduled Castes	0.111 (0.163)	0.0799	1.117	0.076 (0.341)	0.0802	1.079	-0.032 (0.814)	0.1363	0.969	0.009 (0.940)	0.1183	1.009
Religious Group*(Other)*[R]												
Christian	0.550 (0.003)	0.1843	1.733	0.452 (0.010)	0.1751	1.571	0.270 (0.260)	0.2398	1.310	-0.054 (0.787)	0.2019	0.947
Muslim	0.257 (0.015)	0.1057	1.293	0.295 (0.003)	0.1009	1.343	0.113 (0.391)	0.1319	1.120	0.031 (0.784)	0.1115	1.031
Regions *(south western)*[R]												
North eastern	-0.786 (0.000)	0.2189	0.456	-0.222 (0.279)	0.2055	0.801	-0.884 (0.048)	0.4471	0.413	-0.412 (0.449)	0.5444	0.662
Eastern	-0.560 (0.000)	0.0914	0.571	-0.453 (0.000)	0.0911	0.636	-0.580 (0.000)	0.1325	0.560	-0.096 (0.429)	0.1208	0.908
Northern I	-0.357 (0.066)	0.1941	0.700	-0.758 (0.001)	0.2378	0.469	-1.114 (0.035)	0.5287	0.328	-0.951 (0.030)	0.4391	0.386
Northern II	-0.485 (0.000)	0.0955	0.616	-0.416 (0.000)	0.0900	0.660	-0.718 (0.000)	0.1332	0.488	-0.066 (0.548)	0.1091	0.936
Western	-0.851 (0.000)	0.1225	0.427	-0.947 (0.000)	0.1186	0.388	-0.594 (0.000)	0.1556	0.552	-0.467 (0.001)	0.1366	0.627
Peninsular	-0.319 (0.001)	0.0967	0.727	-0.499 (0.000)	0.0985	0.607	-0.201 (0.124)	0.1305	0.818	-0.344 (0.006)	0.1254	0.709
Southern	-0.958 (0.000)	0.1210	0.384	-0.700 (0.000)	0.1126	0.497	-1.240 (0.000)	0.1592	0.289	-0.575 (0.000)	0.1233	0.563

Note: the p-value indicative of the test of the hypothesis that the effect is zero against the alternative that the effect is not zero

The household economic conditions and rate of disabilities are found to be associated in the RURAL MALE, RURAL FEMALE and URBAN MALE populations. When compared to the lowest economic strata (reference group) the rates are lower by 0.780 and 0.787 times in second and fourth quintiles respectively for RURAL FEMALE. Similarly, for RURAL MALE the rates are lower by 0.761 times and 0.839 times in first and fourth quintiles respectively. However, in the fourth quintile, the rates are higher by 1.726 times in case of URBAN MALE.

The analysis shows that the variable 'household type' is significant in the model for rural populations only. For RURAL MALE, rates are higher by 1.379 times for households with major economic activity 'other labour' when compared to the reference. Whereas, for RURAL FEMALE the rate among the households that are self-employed in non-agriculture are higher by 1.070 times when compared to the reference.

Living arrangements have significant effect for RURAL MALE, URBAN MALE and URBAN FEMALE whereas size of the household has significant effect for RURAL FEMALE. Higher rates of disability are observed in living alone when compared to co-residence. The rates are higher by 1.246, 1.435 and 1.388 times in RURAL MALE, URBAN MALE and URBAN FEMALE respectively. On the other hand, for RURAL FEMALE with each unit of increase in size of the household the rate falls by 0.972 times.

Ownership of land by a household and rate of disability are associated but the nature of association differs from one population to another. In the case of RURAL FEMALE, when compared to the reference category the rates are found to be lesser in all the other categories. In case of RURAL MALE the rates are higher by 1.782 times and 1.660 times for categories (2.01–3.0 ha) and (3.01–4.0 ha) respectively. For URBAN MALE the rates are higher by 6.025 times and 6.404 times respectively for categories (0.02–0.20 ha) and (1.01–2.0 ha). For URBAN FEMALE, the rates are lower by 0.350 times and 0.223 times in categories (0.41–1.0 ha) and (4.01–6.0 ha) respectively.

Socio-cultural factors also have significant effects (Table 5) on the health of OA. Caste is a significant factor for RURAL MALE. For this population the schedules castes have rates lesser by 0.755 times than the other castes where as the scheduled tribes did not significantly differ from the other castes in this respect. On the other hand the effect of religion is significant for rural populations only. Rates among Christians and Muslims are higher then the others by 1.733 times and 1.293 times respectively for RURAL MALE. In case of RURAL FEMALE, the corresponding rates are higher by 1.571 times and 1.343 times respectively. Regional variations in rates also exist. The rates in all the regions are lower when compared to the reference (south western).

Discussion

Health care aspects of OA cannot be ignored in any planning of policies for the well being of OA. It comes out clearly from the study that the population of OA is not a homogeneous group with respect to health and its socio-cultural and economic associates. The old-old group is most vulnerable among the OA. It needs priority consideration in health policies. Widowhood in females is associated with bad health status. The reasons for this association may lie in the fall in the social status that accompanies widowhood. Similarly, economic dependency of OA is associated with lower health status. Further, household economic conditions play a significant role in health status of an OA. In a nut shell, lower the economic strata worse the health of OA. Health care needs to reach the economically disadvantaged households that have OA members. Further, co-residence has health benefits for OA. Therefore, public policies should encourage co-residence. Even regional variations in health status of OA exist. Region wise planning for health is needed.

References

Adda Jèrôme, Tarani Chandola and Michael Marmot (2003), "Socio-economic Status and Health: Causality and Pathways", *Journal of Econometrics* 112: 3-56.

Agresti, Alan (1996), *An Introduction to Categorical Data Analysis*. John Wiley & Sons, Inc.

Baker, Kristine R., Mary Beth Ofstedal, Zachary Zimmer, Zhe Tang and Yi-Li Chuang (2005), *Reciprocal Effects of Health and Economic Well-Being among Older Adults in Taiwan and Beijing*. Policy Research Division Working Paper ISSN: 1554-8538, Washington, D.C.: Population Council.

Cambois, Emmanuelle, Jean- Marie Robine and Mark D. Hayward, (2001), "Social Inequalities in Disability Free Life expectancy in the French Male Population, 1980-1991", *Demography* 38(4): 513-524.

Chandola, Tarani (1998), "Social Inequality in Coronary Heart Disease: A Companion of Occupational Classifications", *Social Science and Medicine* 47(4): 525-533.

Gliksman, M.D, R. Lazarus, A. Wilson and S.R. Leader (1995), Social Support, Marital Status and Living Arrangement Correlates of Cardiovascular Disease Risk Factors in the Elderly", *Social Science and Medicine* 40(6): 811-814.

Hayward, Mark. D. and Bridget K. Gorman (2004), "The long Arm of Childhood: The Influence of Early- Life Social Conditions on Men's Mortality", *Demography* 41(1): 87-107.

Kaneda Toshiko, Zachary Zimmer and Zhe Tang (2004), *Differentials in Life Expectancy and Active Life Expectancy by Socioeconomic Status among Older Adults in Beijing*. Policy Research Division Working Paper. Washington, D.C.: Population Council.

Luke, Douglas A. (2004), *Multilevel Modeling*. London: Sage Publications.

Matthews Ruth J., Levy K. Smith, Ruth M. Hamock., Carol Jagger and Nicola A. Spiers (2005), "Socio-Economic Factors Associated with the onset of Disability in Older Age: A Longitudinal Study of People Aged 75 Years and Over", *Social Science and Medicine* 61: 1567-1575.

Matthews, Ruth J., Carol Jogger, Ruth M. Harcock (2006), "Does Socio-Economic Advantage Lead to a Longer, Healthier Old Age?", *Social Science and Medicine* 62: 2489-2499.

Merkin, Sharon Stein, Ana V. Deiz Roux, Josef Coresh, Linda F. Fried, Sharon A. Jackson and Niel R. Powe (2007), "Individual and Neighbourhood Socio-Economic Status and Progressive

Chronic Kidney Disease in an Elderly Population: The Cardiovascular Health Study", *Social Science and Medicine* 65: 809-821.

Petrelli, Alessio, Roberto Gnavi, Chiara Marinnacci and Givseppe Costa (2006), "Socioeconomic Inequalities in Coronary Heart Disease in Italy: A Multilevel Population-Based study", *Social Science and Medicine* 63: 446-456.

Ravito, Nina, Eino Heikkinen and Shah Ebrahim (2005), "Socio-Economic Position and Its Relationship to Physical Capacity Among Elderly People Living in Jyvaskyla, Finland: Five and Ten-Year Follow-up Studies", *Social Science and Medicine* 60: 2405-2416.

Smith, James. P and Raynard Kington (1997), "Demographic and Economic Correlates of Health in Old Age", *Demography* 34(1): 159-170.

Zimmer, Zachary, Napaporn Chayovan, Hui-Sheng Lin and Josefina Natividad (2003), *How Indicators of Socioeconomic Status Relate to Physical Functioning of Older Adults in Three Asian Societies.* Policy Research Division Working Paper No. 172. Washington, D.C.: Population Council.

Zimmer Zachary (2006), *Poverty, Wealth Inequality, and Health among Older Adults in Rural Cambodia.* Policy Research Division Working Paper ISSN: 1554-8538, Washington D.C.: Population Council.

16

Changing Gender Disparity in Child Survival in India: Evidences from three National Family Health Surveys

Jagannath Behera

Introduction

The child mortality rate is commonly used more than any other measure as a general indicator of socioeconomic wellbeing and of general medical and public health conditions in a country. Despite of achieving a remarkable decline in the mortality level in world, as a result of improvement in socio-economic, demographic and family health care particularly mother and child health care factors as well as scientific and technological advancement in the medical field, the gender differential in child mortality still remained very high in many developing countries like India.

Rapid economic progress over the last two decades has significantly improved the health status of population in India. But gender disparity in child health status is remains a grate concern. Ensuring human rights of the population requires reduction and ultimate elimination of gender and socio-economic disparity in health. Strategies to promote economic progress may also help to improve overall efficiency of the women towards equal with men. But from the successive census results, female disadvantage is evident in India from the constantly declining juvenile sex ratio, lower literacy rate of females compared to males and lower participation of women than men in the work force. The juvenile sex ratio (females per 1000 males) declined from 976 in 1961 to 927 in 2001. The male literacy rate for 2001 was 76 percent compared with 54 percent for females. In the same year the work participation rates for males and females were 52 and 26 percent respectively.

Excessive female mortality in any country is one of the important factors for determining low sex ratio. Female and male children face alarmingly different rates of morbidity and mortality in India. The under-five mortality rate for girls (79 per 1000 live births) in 2005-2006 was substantially higher than for boys (70 per 1000 live births) (IIPS and Macro International, 2007). At birth, girl babies have an only marginally higher mortality rate (58 per 1000 live births) than boy babies (56 per 1000 live births). However, from age 1-4 years, the mortality rate for girls is 61 per cent higher than for boys, contributing to India's overall male-female population imbalance. The female to male sex ratio has declined substantially during the past decade, resulting in a substantial female deficit in the population.

A number of studies have found higher female mortality than males in many of the developing countries. Hill and Upchurch (1995) studied data from a large number of countries and compared their sex differentials in mortality. They concluded that girls in the developing countries have a higher risk of mortality than boys for a given level of mortality. Female disadvantage is maxima for girl ages 1-4 years, where care is more important than genetic factors in determining mortality risks. D' Souza and Chen (1980) found that in Matlab area of Bangladesh, females had 60 per cent higher risk of mortality than males after the neonatal period. Das Gupta (1987) in her study of rural Punjab found that excess female mortality is a part of family building strategy where girls are considered as burden and boys are resources. One study in north Indian states (Bhat and Sharma, 2006) shows that growth in incomes and education of women an equal status in society, have actually worked in a reverse direction in states like Punjab, Haryana and Himachal Pradesh. Discrimination against females is engineered even before birth through female foeticide. It seems that education and incomes, which were supposed to result in the emancipation of women, have actually increases, not lowered, the bias in favour of the male child. Since the interventions to encourage overall growth have been strengthened over the years, this study examines the effect of improved efficiency of socio-economic and health system on gender disparity in child mortality. Though in different socio-economic condition gender differential in child mortality occurs, here we will examine 'is there any changes occur over the study period'. The main objective of the study to know whether gender itself a determinant factor for child mortality and its trend from 1990's to 2001.

Data Source

The data sets used for this analysis are: first (1992-93), second (1998-99) and third (2005-06) round of National Family Health Surveys (NFHS). The unit of study is child. In the first NFHS 66449 children are acting as cases (sample) in the analysis. Likely 62528 and 57447 children are acting as cases in second and third NFHS, respectively.

Methodology

The individual data file of NFHS-1, NFHS-2 and NFHS-3 (IIPS, 1995; IIPS and ORC Macro, 2000; IIPS and Macro International, 2007) have used for the Bivariate and Logistic Regression analysis purpose. The logistic regression is used here because to know whether due to gender child are discriminated and it leads to child death. It shows after controlling all other factor what is the effect of one factor on child mortality. Data were extracted from birth file using SPSS (Statistical Package for Social Sciences) software and analysis also done through this software.

All respondent (mothers) in the national family health survey were asked to give a complete birth history, including sex, date of birth, survival status and age of the time of the survey or age at death for each live birth. For children who had died, age at death was recorded in days for children dying in the first month of life, in months for children dying after first month of life. This information was used to calculate the following direct estimates of child mortality rate. The number of child deaths within one to four year of age per 1000 live births within a specified period is called child mortality rate. The cohort mortality has been calculated from three National Family Health Surveys. The birth cohort within specific period chosen for calculating the mortality rates is given below. For NFHS-3, the survey period started from the November 2005 to August 2006 for all-India. For calculating child mortality rate the period taken 5 year cohort and it was five year before the survey (1997 to 2001). The period was calculated from the month of birth and date of survey. For calculating child mortality rates 60 months has been deducted from the starting date of survey, after five year cohort has taken to calculate mortality rates. The live births in this period completely exposed to die within one to four year at the time of survey. The same procedure has applied for NFHS-2 and NFHS-3.

Variables Used

The dependant variable is child survival (1 to 4 years), and it is dichotomous (two categories), if child is died it is coded as 1 otherwise zero for logistic regression. The independent variables are sex of child, place of residence, standard of living of household, caste, education of mother, religion, child's birth order, source of drinking water, and toilet facility of household.

Results and Discussion

In the first part of the study the bivariate result is analyzed and in the second part result of logistic regression is analyzed. The bivariate result shows the gross effect of individual socio-economic and demographic factor, where as logistic regression shows net effect of these factors. The female children are more risk of dying than male children in both rural and urban area shown in Table 1.

Table 1
The gender disparity of child mortality (Relative Risk: Female/Male mortality) by background characteristics in India

Background Variables	*NFHS-1*	*NFHS-2*	*NFHS-3*
Place of Residence			
Urban	1.35	1.27	1.36
Rural	1.34	1.34	1.35
Religion			
Hindu	1.38	1.52	1.44
Muslim	1.30	0.92	1.50
Others (Non Hindu/Muslim)	1.18	0.69	0.82
Education of Mother			
Illiterate	1.40	1.29	1.43
Primary	1.21	1.44	1.27
Secondary	1.00	1.38	0.88
Higher	0.67	2.00	0.75
Caste/Tribe			
Others(non SC/ST)	1.46	1.24	1.46
SC	1.23	1.89	1.53
ST	1.14	0.98	0.93
Standard of Living			
Low	1.54	1.33	1.48
Medium	1.33	1.38	1.21
High	1.38	0.90	1.29
Birth Order of Child			
1st Order Child	1.13	1.05	1.00
2nd & 3rd Order Child	1.37	1.38	1.43
4th & above Order Child	1.47	1.39	1.37
Overall average disparity	*1.32*	*1.31*	*1.29*

Source: Calculated from individual data file of NFHS 1, NFHS-2, NFHS-3

Gender disparity in child mortality is same for both the rural and urban area and over the study periods (NFHS-1, NFHS-2 and NFHS-3) there has no change. The female are disadvantage groups and gender disparity in child mortality is increasing for children belonging to Hindu and Muslim religion over the study period but for children belonging to other (Non Hindu/Muslim) religion it is declining. The female children are more risk of dying than male children for the children of illiterate and primary educated mother; and over the study period the disparity has not substantially changed. But the disparity declined for children of secondary and higher educated mother and female are the advantage groups. It shows that increasing mother's education have an effect on reducing gender disparity in child mortality.

It is shows that gender disparity in child mortality is approximately same over the study period and female are disadvantage groups for childıen belonging to other (Non SC/ST) caste. The gender disparity in child mortality is increasing over the study period and female are disadvantage groups for children belonging to scheduled caste but is reverse for children belonging to scheduled tribe. The disparity in child mortality for all categories of standard of living has not changed substantially and it is high for children belonging to low standard of living household. The gender disparity in child mortality increasing with birth order of child and female are the disadvantage group and over the study period disparity has not changed substantially.

In Table 2, it is shown that in the first National Family Health Survey female child are more likely (odds is 1.496) to risk of dying in childhood period (1 to 4 years) compared to male child after controlling all other factors constant. In the second National Family Health Survey female child are also more likely (odds is 1.329) to risk of dying than male child. In the third National Family Health Survey female child are also more likely (odds is 1.332) to risk of dying than male child after keeping all other variable constant. Though the gender disparity is high in all three national family health surveys but over the period it marginally declined. The gender disparity in child survival has not substantially changed over the study period (NFHS-1, NFHS-2 and NFHS-3). Here one can predict our policies to reduce gender discrimination not much effective to reduce child mortality.

Child mortality disparities according to place of residence are not significant in three National Family Health Surveys. Those mother who are having higher education their child are very less (odds is 0.160) likely to risk of dying compared to child of illiterate mother. Mother's level of education has strong negative relationship with the child mortality and throughout the study period it has constant level of relationship. Standard of living of household also has strong negative relationship with child mortality. Throughout the study period the disparity in child mortality according to standard of living of household has not substantially changed. In NFHS-1 children belonging to scheduled caste are more likely to risk of dying compared to children of other (non SC/ST) caste. But in NFHS-2 and NFHS-3 the children

Table2
Results of Logistic Regression Analysis of Child Mortality on Socio-economic, Demographic and Sanitation Variables, India, NFHS - 1, 2 and 3

Explanatory Variables	*Odds Ratios*		
	NFHS-1	*NFHS-2*	*NFHS-3*
Sex of Child - Male ®			
Female	1.496***	1.329***	1.332***
Place of Residence - Urban ®			
Rural	1.178	1.014	1.038
Maternal Education - Illiterate ®			
Primary	0.743***	0.678***	0.792**
Secondary	0.516***	0.359***	0.484***
Higher	0.160*	0.168***	0.369***
Standard of Living - Low ®			
Medium	0.623***	0.704***	0.782***
High	0.460***	0.515***	0.477***
Ethnicity - Others (Non SC/ST)®			
SC	1.317***	1.218***	1.161*
ST	1.007	1.552***	1.426***
Religion - Hindu®			
Muslim	0.897	0.891	0.908
Non Hindu/Muslim	0.731**	0.936	1.016
Birth order of Child - First child®			
2nd & 3rd Child	1.226**	1.321***	1.246**
4th & above Child	1.274**	1.529***	1.834***
Drinking water Source - Safe water®			
Unsafe Water	0.984	0.981	1.000
Toilet Facility - With toilet®			
Without Toilet	0.959	1.376***	1.201**
Constant	-3.485	-3.813	-4.116
-2 Log likelihood	7875.38	15426.59	9608.44
Nagelkerke R^2	0.034	0.055	0.053
N	26977	61199	52352

Note: ***P < 0.01; **P < 0.05; *P < 0.1
® : indicates reference category

belonging to scheduled tribe are more likely to risk of dying compared to children of other (non SC/ST) caste after controlling all other factors. The net child mortality differential by religious groups is not significant over the study period.

The birth order of children has positive relationship with child mortality. The fourth and above order children are more likely to dying than the preceding birth order and over the study period it is increasing. After controlling all other factors constant, child mortality disparity by source of drinking water is not significant over the study period. The children of households with toilet facility are less risk of dying compared to children of households without toilet facility in NFHS-2 and NFHS-3.

Conclusions

The results of the study show that gender disparity in child mortality marginally declined. Still female children are discriminated and facing more risk of dying in childhood period despite of biologically stronger than male children. Achieving gender equality is an important aim of the public policy in a welfare country like India. But it has been found that both in micro and macro level disparities exist in India. Child survival and overall health of Indians has improved over the past sixty years. But not all Indians are benefiting equally from advances in health sector. The disparities in health status among male and female children still not decline as expected.

From the study it is found that, disparity in child mortality between male and female children not narrowed down substantially over the study period in India. In this context it can be said that probably the advanced socio-economic and reproductive and child health programme has not been effective to reduce the gender disparity in child survival in India. It is generally believed that strong son preference exists in India. The mother who has a son gets more respect than the mother who has daughter in the family. So the mother as well as family members discriminate female children particularly in feeding practices and care, which leads to higher child mortality among female children than male children. Reducing gender inequality would have a catalytic effect on cutting child mortality. So we need some more meticulous policy for reducing gender disparity in child survival. One of the important finding of this paper shows that with increasing level of mother's education the gender disparity in child mortality decline. So our public policy should aim at increasing the level of women's education but not simply literacy of women, which will helpful for reducing gender disparity in child survival in the long run. If our health as well as public policy focuses on changes in attitude of family members towards reducing gender discrimination, it will helpful to decline female child mortality.

References

Bhat, R. L and Sharma, Namita (2006), "Missing Girls: Evidences from some north Indian states", *Indian Journal of Gender Studies* 13: 351-374.

Bongaarts, John (1987), "Does Family Planning Reduce Infant Mortality Rates?", *Population and Development Review* 13(2): 323-334.

Das Gupta, Monica (1987), "Selective Discrimination against Female Children in Rural Punjab, India", *Population and Development Review* 13(1): 77-100.

D'Souza, Stan and Lincoln C. Chen (1980), "Sex Differentials in Mortality in Rural Bangladesh", *Population and Development Review* 6(2): 257-270.

Hill, Kenneth and Upchurch, M. (1995), "Gender Differences in Child Health: Evidences from the Demographic and Health Surveys", *Population and Development Review* 21(1): 127-151.

International Institute for Population Science (IIPS) and Macro International (2007), *National Family Health Survey (NFHS-3), 2005-06, India.* Mumbai: IIPS.

International Institute for Population Science (IIPS) and ORC Macro (2000), *National Family Health Survey (NFHS-2), 1998-99, India.* Mumbai: IIPS.

International Institute for Population Science (IIPS) (1995), *National Family Health Survey (NFHS-1), 1992-93, India.* Mumbai: IIPS.

SECTION – 5

Policies and Health Programs to reduce Vulnerability

17

National Rural Health Mission (2005-2012): An Overview of the Salient Features

H.C. Srivastava

Introduction

The National Rural Health Mission was launched by the Honorable Prime Minister on 12th April 2005, to provide accessible, affordable and accountable quality health services even to the poorest households in the remotest rural regions. The difficult areas with unsatisfactory health indicators were classified as special focus States to ensure greatest attention where needed. The thrust of the Mission was on establishing a fully functional, community owned, decentralized health delivery system with inter sectoral convergence at all levels, to ensure simultaneous action on a wide range of determinants of health like water, sanitation, education, nutrition, social and gender equality. Institutional integration within the fragmented health sector was expected to provide a focus on outcomes, measured against Indian Public Health Standards for all health facilities. From narrowly defined schemes, the NRHM was shifting the focus to a functional health system at all levels, from the village to the district.

The mission adopted a synergistic approach by relating health to determinants of good health viz. nutrition, sanitation, hygiene and safe drinking water. The plan of action of NRHM includes increasing public expenditure on health, reducing regional imbalance in health infrastructure, pooling resources, integration of organisational structures, and optimisation of health manpower, decentralisation and district management of health programmes. In addition it emphasises community participation and ownership of assets, induction of management and financial personnel into district health system, and operationalising Community Health Centres into functional hospitals meeting Indian Public Health Standards in each block of the country. NRHM (2005-2012) seeks to provide effective healthcare to rural population throughout the country with special focus on 18 states, which have weak public health indicators and/or weak infrastructure.

Some of the goals of NRHM include reduction in Infant Mortality Rate and Maternal Mortality Ratio, prevention and control of communicable and non-communicable diseases, population stabilisation gender and demographic balance, mainstream AYUSH and promotion of healthy life style among the people. To achieve these goals the Government has formulated several strategies, amongst them some important are to train and enhance the capacity of *Panchayati Raj* Institutions (PRIs) to own, control and manage public health services, promote access to improved healthcare at household level through the female health activist (ASHA), developing capacities for preventive health care at all levels and promotion of public private partnerships for achieving public health goals. .

The Vision of NRHM

The Mission document seeks to provide effective healthcare to rural population throughout the country with special focus on 18 states, which have weak public health indicators and/ or weak infrastructure, namely, Arunachal Pradesh, Assam, Bihar, Chhattisgarh, Himachal Pradesh, Jharkhand, Jammu & Kashmir, Manipur, Mizoram, Meghalaya, Madhya Pradesh,

Nagaland, Orissa, Rajasthan, Sikkim, Tripura, Uttaranchal and Uttar Pradesh.

Also, it aims to undertake architectural correction of the health system to enable it to effectively handle increased allocations as promised under the National Common Minimum Programme of the Government and promote policies that strengthen public health management and service delivery in the country. Further, the Mission considered provision of a female health activist in each village; a village health plan prepared through a local team headed by the Health & Sanitation Committee of the Panchayat; strengthening of the rural hospital for effective curative care and made measurable and accountable to the community through Indian Public Health Standards (IPHS), as its key components.

It aims at effective integration of health concerns with determinants of health like sanitation and hygiene, nutrition, and safe drinking water through a District Plan for Health. Also it seeks to revitalize local health traditions and mainstream AYUSH into the public health system.

The NRHM emphasizes decentralization of programmes for district management of health and therefore seeks to address the inter-State and inter-district disparities, especially among the aforementioned 18 high focus States, including unmet needs for public health infrastructure. Besides, it tries to improve access of rural people, especially poor women and children, to equitable, affordable, accountable and effective primary healthcare.

Goals of NRHM

1. Reduction in Infant Mortality Rate (IMR) and Maternal Mortality Ratio (MMR).
2. Universal access to public health services such as Women's health, child health, water, sanitation & hygiene, immunization, and Nutrition.
3. Prevention and control of communicable and non-communicable diseases, including locally endemic diseases.

4. Access to integrated comprehensive primary healthcare.
5. Population stabilization, gender and demographic balance.
6. Revitalize local health traditions and mainstream AYUSH.
7. Promotion of healthy life styles.

Strategies Adopted for NRHM

Several strategies are adopted for achieving the goals of NRHM. However, these strategies can be divided into two broad groups namely, core strategies and supplementary strategies. Some of the strategies are described in the following lines:

Core Strategies of NRHM

1. Train and enhance capacity of *Panchayati Raj* Institutions (PRIs) to own, control and manage public health services.
2. Promote access to improved healthcare at household level through the female health activist (ASHA).
3. Health Plan for each village through Village Health Committee of the Panchayat.
4. Strengthening sub-centre through an untied fund to enable local planning and action and more Multi Purpose Workers (MPWs).
5. Strengthening existing PHCs and CHCs, and provision of 30-50 bedded CHC per lakh
6. Population for improved curative care to a normative standard (Indian Public Health Standards defining personnel, equipment and management standards).
7. Preparation and Implementation of an inter-sectoral District Health Plan prepared by the District Health Mission, including drinking water, sanitation & hygiene and nutrition.
8. Technical Support to National, State and District Health Missions, for Public Health Management.
9. Strengthening capacities for data collection, assessment and review for evidence based planning, monitoring and supervision.

10. Developing capacities for preventive health care at all levels for promoting healthy life styles, reduction in consumption of tobacco and alcohol etc.

Supplementary Strategies

1. Regulation of Private Sector including the informal rural practitioners to ensure availability of quality service to citizens at reasonable cost.
2. Promotion of Public Private Partnerships for achieving public health goals.
3. Mainstreaming AYUSH–revitalizing local health traditions.
4. Reorienting medical education to support rural health issues including regulation of Medical care and Medical Ethics.
5. Effective and viable risk pooling and social health insurance to provide health security to the poor by ensuring accessible, affordable, accountable and good quality hospital care.

Plan of Action

To fulfill the goals of the NRHM the policy of the Government has suggested a wide range of components. Altogether there are eleven components but important features of some amongst them are described below;

Accredited Social Health Activist (ASHA)

(a) Every village/large habitat will have a female ASHA - chosen by and accountable to the *panchayat*- to act as the interface between the community and the public health system. States should choose State specific models.
(b) ASHA would act as a bridge between the ANM and the village and be accountable to the *Panchayat.*
(c) She will be trained on pedagogy of public health developed and mentored through a Standing Mentoring Group at National level incorporating best practices and

implemented through active involvement of community health resource organizations.

(d) She will be promoted allover the country with special emphasis on the 18 high focus states. The government of India will bear the cost of training, incentives and medical kits. The remaining components will be funded under Financial Envelope given to the states under the programme.

(e) She will be given a Drug Kit containing generic AYUSH and allopathic formulations for common ailments. The drug kit would be replenished from time to time.

(f) Training for ASHA would require partnership with NGOs/ICDS Training Centres and State Health Institutes.

Strengthening Sub-Centers (SC)

(a) Each sub-centre will have an Untied Fund for local action @ Rs. 10,000 per annum. This Fund will be deposited in a joint Bank Account of the ANM & *Sarpanch* and operated by the ANM, in consultation with the Village Health Committee.

(b) Regularize the supply of essential drugs to the Sub-centres; both allopathic and AYUSH.

Strengthening Primary Health Centers (PHC)

(a) Mission aims at strengthening PHC for quality preventive, promotive, curative, supervisory and Outreach health care services through;

(b) Adequate and regular supply of essential quality drugs and equipment (including Supply of Auto Disabled Syringes for immunization) to PHCs.

(c) Provision of 24 hour service in at least 50% PHCs by addressing shortage of doctors, especially in high focus States, through mainstreaming AYUSH manpower.

(d) Observance of standard treatment guidelines and protocols.

Strengthening Community Health Centers (CHCs) for First Referral Care

(a) Operationalising 3222 existing Community Health Centers (30-50 beds) as 24 Hour First Referral Units, including posting of anesthetists.

(b) Promotion of Stakeholder Committees *(Rogi Kalyan Samitis)* for hospital management.

(c) Developing standards of services and costs in hospital care.

District Health Plan

(a) District Health Plan would be an amalgamation of field responses through Village Health Plans, State and National priorities for Health, Water Supply, Sanitation and Nutrition.

(b) Health Plans would form the core unit of action proposed in areas like water supply, sanitation, hygiene and nutrition. Implementing Departments would integrate into District Health Mission for monitoring.

(c) District becomes core unit of planning, budgeting and implementation.

(d) All vertical Health and Family Welfare Programmes at District and State level merge into one common 'District Health Mission" at district level and the state Health Mission at the state level.

Converging Sanitation and Hygiene under NRHM

(a) Total Sanitation Campaign (TSC) is presently implemented in 350 districts, and is proposed to cover all districts in 10th Plan.

(b) Components of TSC include IEC activities, rural sanitary marts, individual household toilets, women sanitary complex, and School Sanitation Programme.

(c) The District Health Mission would therefore guide activities of sanitation at district level, and promote joint IEC for public health, sanitation and hygiene, through

Village Health & Sanitation Committee, and promote household toilets and School Sanitation Programme. ASHA would be incentivised for promoting household toilets by the Mission.

Strengthening Disease Control Programmes

(a) National Disease Control Programmes for Malaria, TB, Kala Azar, Filarial, Blindness and Iodine Deficiency and Integrated Disease Surveillance Programme shall be integrated under the Mission, for improved programme delivery.

(b) New Initiatives would be launched for control of Non Communicable Diseases.

(c) Disease surveillance system at village level would be strengthened.

(d) Supply of generic drugs (both AYUSH & Allopathic) for common ailments at village, SC, PHC/CHC level.

Public-Private Partnership for Public Health Goals including Regulation of Private sector

(a) Since almost 75% of health services are being currently provided by the private sector, there is a need to refine regulation.

(b) Regulation to be transparent and accountable.

(c) Need to develop guidelines for Public-Private Partnership (PPP) in health sector. Identifying areas of partnership, which are need based, thematic and geographic.

Health Financing Mechanisms

(a) Progressively the District Health Missions to move towards paying hospitals for services by way of reimbursement, on the principle of "money follows the patient."

(b) Standardization of services - outpatient, in-patient, laboratory, surgical interventions- and costs will be done periodically by a committee of experts in each state.

(c) A National Expert Group to monitor these standards and give suitable advice and guidance on protocols and cost comparisons.

Reorienting Health / Medical Education to Support Rural Health Issues

(a) While district and tertiary hospitals are necessarily located in urban centres, they form an integral part of the referral care chain serving the needs of the rural people.

(b) Medical and Para-medical education facilities need to be created in states, based on need assessment.

Institutional Mechanisms of NRHM

Village Health and Sanitation Samiti

Village Health and Sanitation *Samiti* to be established and performed at village level, consisting of *Panchayat* Representative/s, ANM/MPW, *Anganwadi* worker, teacher, ASHA, community health volunteers.

Rogi Kalyan Samiti

Rogi Kalyan Samiti (or equivalent) to be constituted for community management of public hospitals.

District Health Mission

District Health Mission, under the leadership of *Zila Parishad* with District Health Head as Convener and all relevant departments, NGOs, private professionals etc represented on it.

State Health Mission

State Health Mission, Chaired by Chief Minister and co-chaired by Health Minister and with the State Health Secretary as Convener- representation of related departments, NGOs, private professionals etc.

Empowered Programme Committee

Empowered Programme Committee chaired by Secretary HFW, to be the Executive Body of the Mission.

Role of Panchayati Raj Institutions in NRHM

1. States to indicate in their Memorandum of Understandings (MoUs) the commitment for devolution of funds, functionaries and programmes for health, to PRIs.
2. The District Health Mission (DHM) to be led by the *Zilla Parishad*. The DHM will control, guide and manage all public health institutions in the district, Sub-centres, PHCs and CHCs.
3. ASHAs would be selected by and be accountable to the Village *Panchayat*.
4. The Village Health Committee of the Panchayat would prepare the Village Health Plan, and promote intersectoral integration.
5. PRI involvement in *Rogi Kalyan Samitis* for good hospital management.
6. Provision of training to members of PRIs.
7. Making available health related databases to all stakeholders, including Panchayats at all levels.

Role of Non Governmental Organizations (NGOs) in NRHM

1. NGOs should be Included in institutional arrangement at National, State and District levels, including Standing Mentoring Group for ASHA.
2. Provision of Training, BCC and Technical Support for ASHAs/DHM.
3. Work as Health Resource Organizations.
4. Provide Service delivery for identified population groups on select themes.
5. Looking after monitoring, evaluation and social audit.

Mainstreaming Ayush

1. The Mission seeks to revitalize local health traditions and mainstream AYUSH infrastructure, including manpower, and drugs, to strengthen the public health system at all levels.

2. AYUSH medications shall be included in the Drug Kit provided at village levels to ASHA.
3. Single doctor PHCs shall be upgraded to two doctor PHCs by mainstreaming AYUSH practitioner at that level.

Expected Outcomes

National Level

1. Infant Mortality Rate reduced to 30/1000 live births.
2. Maternal Mortality Ratio reduced to 100/100,000.
3. Total Fertility Rate reduced to 2.1.
4. Malaria Mortality Reduction Rate -50%upto 2010, additional105 by 2012.
5. Upgrading Community health centers to Indian public health standards.
6. Increase utilization of First referral units from less than 205 to 755.

Community Level

1. Availability of trained community level worker at village level, with a drug kit for generic ailments.
2. Health Day at *Anganwadi* level on a fixed day/month for provision of immunization, ante/post natal checkups and services related to mother and child healthcare, including nutrition.
3. Availability of generic drugs for common ailments at Sub-centre and hospital level
4. Good hospital care through assured availability of doctors, drugs and quality services at PHC/CHC level.
5. Improved access to Universal Immunization through induction of Auto Disabled Syringes, alternate vaccine delivery and improved mobilization services under the programme.
6. Improved facilities for institutional delivery through provision of referral, transport, escort and improved

hospital care subsidized under the Janani Suraksha Yojana (JSY) for the Below Poverty Line families.

The Progress so far

The NRHM is only two and half years old and already there are some very significant gains in the health sector, in partnership with States. Illustrative evidence from States of the programme so far is presented in the following lines;

Areas of Improvement

Out Patient Cases

Reports from different States indicate significant improvement in health care service as well as health care seeking behaviour amongst the population. For example, in Bihar, the average number of patients visiting a Primary Health Centre every month has gone up from 39 in January 2006 to 3015 in August 2006. In Punjab, with the Alternate Health Delivery involving service providers under PRIs at 1310 Subsidiary Health Centers, out patient cases have gone up by 290 percent between June to October 2006. Further,39.6 percent improvement in cataract operations performed, 11.8 percent increase in new TB cases detected, and 25.1 percent increase in students examined under the School Health Programme has been reported. In Gujarat, so far out Patient cases have gone up from 33.6 lakhs per year to more than 24.92 lakhs per year.

Institutional Deliveries

Institutional deliveries have also been found increased significantly because of demand side financing under the scheme of Janani Suraksha Yojana (JSY). The number of JSY has increased from six lakhs to 21 lakhs. In 50 Blocks of *Madhya Pradesh* under the Dhanwantari Yojana, institutional deliveries recorded more than 100% increase (From 26% to 53%) in 1152 PHCs. In Orissa, figures from three CHCs in Malkangiri and Koraput districts also shows an increase in institutional delivery from 88 to 149, 59 to 120 and 97 to 169 respectively over a corresponding time period. In Haryana, with the innovative delivery hut scheme, the institutional deliveries went up from 28 percent in 2004-05 to 43.6 percent in 2005-06.

Availability of Medicines

States have put in place effective systems of procurements of drugs. NRHM has advocated decentralized procurement in line with the successful Tamil Nadu Medical Supplies Corporation (TNMSC). Funds for procurement under NRHM were released to States. Even a state like Bihar, where procurement was ineffective, very efficient and effective drug procurement arrangement has put in place. States of Uttar Pradesh and Jharkhand revised the per capita allocation for drugs, which lead to better availability of drugs at health facilities. A few North Eastern States like Assam are also procuring drugs from the TNMSC.

Immunization

Efforts have been made to ensure improvement in immunization coverage by promoting alternate vaccine delivery, providing incentives for immunization sessions, conducting catch up rounds like Jharkhand, and ensuring proper maintenance of the cold chain. Recent evaluation of UNICEF shows improvements in child immunization in States like Uttar Pradesh, Bihar and Jharkhand. With popularization of the Monthly Health Days at *Aanganwadi* Centers routine immunization has got a further stimulus.

Monthly Health Days

More than 10 lakh Monthly health Days have been organized at *Aanganwadi* Centers, facilitating ANC / PNC, immunization, availability of basic drugs, etc. Evidence of successful Monthly Health Days in the presence of ANMs/ AWWs are being reported from all the States, including States like Tripura, Orissa, *Madhya Pradesh,* Rajasthan, Chhatisgarh, etc. Orissa uses the Monthly Health Days in the malaria affected areas. With Village Health and Sanitation Committees being set up in every village, public health measures will be the focus of these Monthly Health Days.

Resident Community workers / functional Sub Centers

More than 4.35 lakh ASHAs, Community Workers, Maintainers, Link Workers have been selected and are at various stages of selection. They are playing a key role in community mobilization, immunization and other health services, JSY, public health measures, advocacy, nutrition and health education and improving health seeking behaviour of households.

By engagement of contractual ANMs wherever required and by provision of Rs. 10,000 annual untied grant, nearly all 1,46,026 Sub Health Centers have been made functional Sub-centres. Sub-centres may judiciously use the united funds as per need, buying B.P. Equipment, weighing machine, repairing the examination table, cleaning the Sub-centre, etc. Early evidence suggests that deliveries have started taking place in a few Sub-centers because of the untied grants. A second ANM is already in place in 7699 Sub-centers.

PHCs with 2 Additional Nurses

2230 PHCs have been made available in all time with a provision of two additional Nurses. Out of these 2230 PHCs, 600 have been made in Tamil Nadu itself.

Community Pressure for Services from CHCs/Sub-District/ District Hospital

Demand side financing under JSY and ASHAs/ Community Workers are putting pressure on services from CHCs/Sub-District and District Hospitals in all the States. The community pressure is putting pressure on the Health Facility to improve its performance. Rupees twenty lakhs have been provided to all the 3346 CHCs as first installment to move towards Indian Public Health Standards. 1554 CHCs have carried out Facility Surveys to plan for the gaps as per IPHS. Facility Surveys of CHCs are available on this Ministry's web site. Rs. 50,000 Annual Maintenance Grant and Rs. 25000 as untied grant for PHCs have been sanctioned for each of the 23236 PHCs, to be used under the supervision of the RKS. Works have been completed in some facilities and is under way in a large number of them. It has taken a little time as Facility Surveys had to be completed as a pre requisite.

Rogi Kalyan Samitis (RKSs)

More than 8000 *Rogi Kalyan Samitis*/Hospital Development Committees have been set up in the country. Nearly all District/ Sub District Hospitals and CHCs have opened their own Bank Accounts. PHCs are also in the process of doing so. Rs. 5 lakhs has been provided for District Hospital RKSs and Rs. One lakh has been allotted for Sub District/ CHC/ PHCs. They are also expected to make the functioning of the Hospitals more accountable, transparent and need based.

Improved Outreach through Mobile Medical Units (MMUs)

States have already started more than 224 Mobile Medical Units from their own sources /NRHM. NRHM has approved MMUs for 314 districts and most of these units are expected to be operationalised in the current financial year. NGOs are involved in such arrangements in many States. Gujarat, Andhra Pradesh, West Bengal, Orissa have set up effective systems for mobile units to improve outreach of services in remote areas.

Partnerships with Non Governmental Providers

Useful partnerships with Non Governmental providers have been attempted in every State. Reputed NGOs like VHAI and Karuna Trust have taken the responsibility of running PHCs in remote locations of Arunachal Pradesh. Non Governmental specialists are being paid on a per case basis for work done in the Government Hospitals. Under the Chiranjeevi Scheme in the 5 tribal districts of Gujarat, institutional delivery of Below Poverty Line women is taking place in nursing homes of private gynecologists at government's cost. NGOs are playing a very important role in facilitating ASHAs and community workers and in their capacity building efforts in every State. 1825 Non-Governmental providers have been accredited under the Janani Suraksha Yojana.

Capacity Building Initiatives

More than 1200 Programme Management, Finance Management and Data Management professionals have joined the system at State and District levels. More are joining as Block Public Health Managers in a few States. The introduction of these skills has improved programme management, monitoring and evaluation, financial reporting and record keeping. The National, the North Eastern Regional and State Resource Centres are further strengthening this process.

Decentralized Planning and Appraisal of District Health Action Plans

The process of decentralized planning has been initiated across the country with planning village upwards. Each and every district of *Madhya Pradesh* and Chhatisgarh has completed the District Planning process. The other States are also at an advanced stage of district planning. A grant of Rupees ten lakhs was provided to every district for decentralised planning. Nearly all the 606 districts are expected to complete this process by March 2007. These District Health Action Plans have been prepared through a consultative process involving communities and health functionaries at each level. Chhattisgarh has undertaken the innovative exercise of developing a human development index for each Panchayat and for awarding Panchayats on the basis of their Human Development ranking.

Effective Monitoring and Evaluation

NRHM has set up effective systems of monitoring and evaluation. A detailed Management Information System (MIS) that provides disaggregated information about performance with respect to vulnerable groups like SCs and STs, has been operationalised. An effective Financial Management Reporting System has become functional with quarterly, activity wise reports from States. A pilot initiative on community monitoring is being initiated in partnership with NGOs. The Institute of Public Auditors of India has started field work in five States (Bihar, Assam, UP, Tamil Nadu and Kerala). Assessment of ASHA programme in *Madhya Pradesh*, Rajasthan, Orissa, UP, Bihar is under way with the support of UNFPA/ UNICEF. A system of independent assessment of performance of States by institutions of excellence is in the process of finalization. An intensive field based joint review mechanism is in place for the RCH–II that covers core areas of NRHM as well. Three such reviews have already been conducted.

The Way Ahead

As is evident from the progress, a lot has been achieved in the last two years in partnership with States. This is a sector that requires simultaneous action on many fronts. The institutional platform of Village Health and Sanitation Committees, the *Rogi Kalyan Samitis* and the *Panchayati Raj* Institution committees at various levels is providing a rare opportunity for convergent action on all determinants of health. An army of locally resident Accredited Social health Activists with strong referral links with the strengthened health system will put even greater pressure on the public sector health system to delivery quality services. Along with need based and transparent partnerships with non governmental providers for public health goals, the strengthened system will have positive consequences for all interventions, whether they are for family welfare, disease surveillance, National Health Programmes, etc. The innovative engagement of human resource as per need and the arrangements for incentives at each level will help craft a new and innovative system of public health delivery. The experience of the last two years gives us the confidence that we are on the right track and that we need to deepen institutional reforms and effective decentralization through a concerted effort at capacity building.

The setting up of a National Health System Resource Centre is a step in that direction. States are also in the process of setting up their resource Centers. The North Eastern Regional Resource Centre is already playing a critical role in developing need based programmes in the eight North Eastern States.

Reference

Ministry of Health and Family Welfare, Government of India (2006), *National Rural Health Mission (2005-2012), Mission Document,* Available from http//mohfw.nic.in/NRHM/

18

Vulnerability of Kolkata Slum Population in Financial Management of Health Problems

Prasanta Pathak

Introduction

Kolkata, like other major metropolitan districts in India, has a significant percentage of its population residing in the slum areas. The percentage has increased from 22 in 1961 to nearly 33 in 2001. Though the relative incidence of migrants in the Kolkata metropolitan district, measured in terms of ratio per centum of total population, shows a declining trend (Chakraborty, 1990) from 1971, increasing slum population is a matter of serious concern for the policy makers, the planners and the plan implementers. The growth rate among the slum dwellers was always more as compared to that in the other residential areas. Lack of education as well as their demand for more potential earning members in the family made them avoiding the family planning methods (Roy, 1978).

Limited success out of the efforts to clear the slum areas and rehabilitate the slum dwellers at places outside the city in previous five year plans, made the planners concentrate their attention more on the scheme of Environmental Improvement of Urban Slums from the Fifth Five year plan onward. The scheme was subsequently brought under the Minimum Needs Programme (Roy, 1994). Starting with the Sixth Five Year Plan, vigorous efforts have been put for a sustainable development of the urban slums. It is now well-understood that improvement of the state of living of the slum dwellers is essential for improving the state of living of all urban residents.

It was CMDA which took a major initiative to improve the city life. Its report on health and socio-economic status of the city dwellers with specific information on the slum dwellers was a major contribution which was found useful for subsequent planning (CMDA, 1983). Though the report contained a big quantum of useful information, the ample scope of in-depth data analysis remained unutilized. The study by the Child-in-Need Institute (CINI)-ASHA (CINI-ASHA, 1999) attempted to develop a self-sustainable model for cost-effective provision of quality primary health care to the slum population. It found out the prevalent common illnesses and the quality of available treatment procedures. It tried to develop a standard management protocol for the prevalent common illnesses for monitoring the quality of care, explored different insurance options and planned an insurance coverage for the slum population based on their need, expenditure pattern and willingness to participate in a health care scheme. Though the study had good quantity of useful information, including the standard management protocol, inadequacy of the sample size did not allow the study purposes to get served fully.

A Number of studies have been done on the socio-economic profile of the households in the Kolkata metropolitan area (Sen, 1960; Roy and Bandyopadhyay, 1976; Roy and Chaudhuri, 1976; CMDA, 1983; Jagannathan and Halder, 1988; Chakraborty and Halder, 1991). But, the two studies mentioned above have only been found significant in relating health with socio-economic status. Here we present a part of the findings of a micro-level pilot study done on five selected slum areas in Kolkata (Pathak, 2002). Variation in seeking health care by the household members in different categories of economic activity and in different slabs of economic condition, measured in terms of reported monthly income and per capita monthly consumption expense, and the expenditures incurred on health care by the same categorized household members have been already reported in Pathak (2006). Here our focus is on the most vulnerable groups in the slum population who need special attention in any intervention aimed at improving the living condition of the slum population. It has been assumed that under the existing poor economic status of the slum population, priced health care products and/or services are sought only when these are absolutely necessary. The validity of the assumption may be verified through another study where probing questions on reasons behind not seeking health care outside in spite of suffering from some health problems may be investigated.

Objectives of the Study

1. To know the relation between the total expenditure incurred for having medical treatment and per capita monthly consumption expenditure (PCMCE) in a household,
2. To find out various expense head wise mean percentage of total expenditure for availing different types of health care for children, mothers and adult males and females,
3. To understand the importance of different sources of financing the household expenditure on managing health problems, and
4. To find out the vulnerability of the households to fall in debt trap.

Methodology of the Study

The state of economic well-being has been measured by reported monthly income of a household and by estimated per capita monthly consumption expense. Given the variables, on which information are to be collected to achieve the objectives, and the information that are already available on the Kolkata slums through different past studies and other secondary sources, finding out an appropriate sample size has been a difficult task. Available information was either too old or not useful to serve the purpose in the context of the slum population. The study, thus, is an exploratory one. Based on available information, it has been known that the cases of hospitalization are rarer than the cases of sickness. Additionally, it has been felt that the percentages of such cases in different age groups and economic groups might be less than 10. In such a situation, Haldane's (1945) inverse sampling method becomes very useful. As per this method, 102 cases of, say, hospitalization is to be identified to estimate the proportion of hospitalized cases in a population with coefficient of variation less than 10 per cent. Again, the assumption of Normality on a statistic estimating a very small Binomial proportion like 0.5 holds true at 95 per cent confidence level and with 5.5 per cent error provided the sample size is 1,400 (Selvin, 1991). Thirdly, under given time and budget constraints and based on both the plan of data collection and the plan of doing tabular analysis, it has been thought that to have at least 5 cases of hospitalization or sickness per cell in a multivariate table with maximum 200 cells there should be at least 1000 cases in its totality.

Taking into account the aspects of non-sampling error and design effect, ultimately a sample of 1,500 households with each sampled unit having one or both of the following stated characteristics has been found suitable for this study. For best possible representation of the Kolkata slums under the given budget and time constraints, Ward 13 in the northern Kolkata, Ward 33 in the eastern Kolkata, Ward 29 in the central Kolkata, Ward 69 in the southern Kolkata and Ward 134 in the western Kolkata have been chosen in consultation with the appropriate authorities in the Kolkata Municipal Corporation as the study areas. From each of the chosen slum areas, about 300 sample households with either or both of the following characteristics have been chosen for detailed data collection.

Characteristic 1 : One or more household members hospitalized once or more than once in a period of 365 days prior to the date of data collection.

Characteristic 2 : One or more household members fallen sick once or more than once in a period of 30 days prior to the date of data collection.

The sample households with one or both of the above mentioned characteristics have been identified by visiting sequentially one after another household in each area in the period February 13, 2002 to March 27, 2002, and noting down on a House Listing Schedule few basic information about the broad age structure of the household members and the events of falling sick in the last 30 days and/or getting hospitalized in the last 365 days, experienced by them. The households with the above stated characteristics have been chosen for collection of detailed information on a structured Household Schedule.

Results and Discussion

Health Care Providers

Health service providers play an important role in giving proper guidance to the patients and their immediate relatives. Expenditure incurred in availing health services also depends on the providers' guidance. Thus, before going in depth to the financial aspects of availing health services, it will be worth seeing the distribution of various types of health service providers who are consulted to solve various health problems. It is seen from Table 1 that private allopathic doctors were consulted in majority of the pre-hospitalization cases (about 63%). These doctors were also consulted maximum for post-delivery complications (about 54%), childhood sickness (about 48%) and sickness among adult persons (about 58%). Except the cases of consultation for female reproductive health problems, the demand for consulting the private and the government allopathic doctors had been there in at least 82

Table 1

Chosen Health Service Providers for Solving Various Types of Health Problems

	Percentage of Times Consulted for Treatment						
Health Provider	*Female Reproductive Health Problems*	*Pregnancy Complications*	*Post-delivery Complications*	*Pre-Hospitalization Health Problems*	*Post-Hospitalization Health Problems*	*Sickness of Children Aged 12 Years and Less*	*Sickness of Adults Aged 13 Years and More*
(1)	*(2)*	*(3)*	*(4)*	*(5)*	*(6)*	*(7)*	*(8)*
Private Allopathic Doctor	27.9	40.1	54.5	63.4	48.0	48.5	57.6
Government Allopathic Doctor	24.4	47.5	45.5	27.2	48.0	34.9	25.7
Private Homeopathic Doctor	11.6	1.5	0.0	1.6	1.1	7.8	6.2
Government Health Worker/Compounder	1.2	2.2	0.0	1.6	0.6	2.8	3.5
Private Health Worker/Compounder	2.3	0.0	0.0	0.6	0.0	1.8	0.5
Other Qualified Private Doctor	4.7	1.5	0.0	2.2	0.6	1.2	1.4
Treatment at Home with Medicine without Consulting Any Medical Person	4.7	0.0	0.0	0.0	0.6	0.4	1.2
Private Pharmacist/Chemist	2.3	0.7	0.0	1.6	0.6	0.2	0.9
Other Qualified Government Doctor	2.3	2.9	0.0	0.6	0.0	0.6	0.8
Government Homeopathic Doctor	1.2	2.2	0.0	0.3	0.0	1.0	1.4
Quack/Faith Healer	0.0	0.7	0.0	0.3	0.0	0.2	0.5
Others (including treatment at home without use of medicines	0.0	0.7	0.0	0.3	0.5	0.6	0.3
None	17.4	0.0	0.0	0.3	0.0	0.0	0.0
Total Consultation Number (Per Cent)	86 (100.0)	137 (100.0)	22 (100.0)	320 (100.0)	177 (100.0)	499 (100.0)	778 (100.0)

per cent cases. For female reproductive health problems, the private and the government allopathic doctors were consulted in about 52 per cent cases. No medical help was sought in about 17 per cent cases and private homeopathic doctors were consulted in about 12 per cent cases. There were about 5 per cent cases where help was sought from qualified non-allopathic and non-homeopathic doctors. Another 5 per cent cases of female reproductive health problems were treated at home with medicines without consulting any medical person. Services of the private homeopathic doctors were also demanded in significant per cent of cases of sickness among the children and the adult persons. They were consulted in about 8 per cent and 6 per cent cases, respectively.

Expenditure Features by Various Types of Seeking Health Care in Different Categories of PCMCE

Broad types of health care sought by the sampled households in different PCMCE categories with varying age profiles of health seeking persons and varying expenses for treatment, incurred directly or indirectly, have been presented in Table 2. While about 5 per cent households on the whole reported occurrences of female reproductive health problems, the per centages were lower for the households belonging to the highest and the lowest PCMCE categories (about 2 per cent and 4 per cent respectively). As a whole, about 2 per cent females faced reproductive health problems, but the per centages were nearly unity for those belonging to the lowest and the highest PCMCE categories. The median age of all the females who faced reproductive health problems was about 31 years. This had been higher and about 35 years for the females in the lowest PCMCE category. The minimum age of these females had also been higher and it was about 28 years. Overall median total expenditure incurred for treatment of female reproductive health problems had been nearly Rs. 365. The expenditure range had been Rs. 5 to Rs. 20,210. The median and the mean expenditures corresponding to various PCMCE categories indicate that the expenditure on treatment increases with the increase in the level of PCMCE.

Table 2

Distribution of Households, Household Members, Age-Sex Characteristics of Cases and Expense Features for Cases by Various Types of Seeking Health Care in Different Categories of Per Capita Monthly Consumption Expenses

Type of Seeking Health Care and Per Capita Monthly Consumption Expense (in Rs)	% of Households (with Cases)	Household Members: Male (%)	Household Members: Female (%)	Household Members: Overall (%)	Percentage of Cases: M	Percentage of Cases: F	Percentage of Cases: T
(1)	(2)	(3)	(4)	(5)	(6)	(7)	(8)
A. Reproductive Health Problems Among Females							
1 - 300	12.7 (3.7)	687 (50.1)	683 (49.9)	1370 (100)	–	1.0	–
300 - 500	35.7 (6.3)	1621 (51.2)	1548 (48.8)	3169 (100)	–	2.3	–
500 - 700	28.9 (5.5)	1173 (51.7)	1094 (48.3)	2267 (100)	–	2.3	–
700 - 900	13.9 (5.3)	460 (51.1)	440 (48.9)	900 (100)	–	2.7	–
≥ 900	8.8 (2.3)	295 (55.7)	235 (44.3)	530 (100)	–	1.3	–
Total (%)	1502100.0 (5.3)	4236 (51.4)	4000(48.6)	8236 (100)	–	2.1	–
B. Other Health Problems Among Adults							
1 - 300	12.7 (34.0)	687 (50.1)	683 (49.9)	1370 (100)	3.2	7.5	5.3
300 - 500	35.7 (34.0)	1621 (51.2)	1548 (48.8)	3169 (100)	5.4	7.9	6.6
500 - 700	28.9 (39.6)	1173 (51.7)	1094 (48.3)	2267 (100)	8.1	11.1	9.5
700 - 900	13.9 (42.6)	460 (51.1)	440 (48.9)	900 (100)	10.2	12.5	11.3
≥ 900	8.8 (39.4)	295 (55.7)	235 (44.3)	530 (100)	9.2	13.2	10.9
Total (%)	1502100.0 (37.3)	4236 (51.4)	4000 (48.6)	8236 (100)	6.6	9.5	8.0

Contd.

C. Health Problems Among Children							
1 - 300	12.7 (16.8)	678 (50.1)	683 (49.9)	1370 (100)	2.5	2.8	2.6
300 - 500	35.7 (27.4)	1621 (51.2)	1548 (48.8)	3169 (100)	5.9	4.6	5.2
500 - 700	28.9 (29.0)	1173 (51.7)	1094 (48.3)	2267 (100)	6.3	6.8	6.5
700 - 900	13.9 (20.6)	460 (51.1)	400 (48.9)	900 (100)	5.0	5.2	5.1
≥ 900	8.8 (12.9)	295 (55.7)	235 (44.3)	530 (100)	3.7	3.4	3.6
Total (%)	1502100.0 (24.3)	4236(51.4)	4000(48.6)	8236(100)	5.2	4.9	5.0
D. Pre-hospitalization Care							
1 - 300	12.7 (13.1)	687 (50.1)	683 (49.9)	1370 (100)	1.2	2.5	1.8
300 - 500	35.7 (17.5)	1621 (51.2)	1548 (48.8)	3169 (100)	3.1	2.8	3.0
500 - 700	28.9 (17.3)	1173 (51.7)	1094 (48.3)	2267 (100)	3.8	2.9	3.4
700 - 900	13.9 (24.4)	460 (51.1)	400 (48.9)	900 (100)	5.2	6.6	5.9
≥ 900	8.8 (30.3)	295 (55.7)	235 (44.3)	530 (100)	7.1	8.9	7.9
Total (%)	1502100.0 (19.0)	423651.4)	4000(48.6)	8236(100.0)	3.5	3.6	3.5
E. Care in Hospital							
1 - 300	12.7 (20.9)	687 (50.1)	683 (49.9)	1370 (100)	1.9	4.4	3.1
300 - 500	35.7 (28.2)	1621 (51.2)	1548 (48.8)	3169 (100)	5.1	4.9	5.0
500 - 700	28.9 (31.1)	1173 (51.7)	1094 (48.3)	2267 (100)	6.3	5.9	6.1
700 - 900	13.9 (38.8)	460 (51.1)	440 (48.9)	900 (100)	7.6	11.4	9.4
≥ 900	8.8 (45.5)	295 (55.7)	235 (44.3)	530 (100)	12.2	12.8	12.5
Total (%)	1502100.0 (31.2)	4236(51.4)	4000(48.6)	8236(100.0)	5.7	6.3	6.0
F. Post-hospitalization Care							
1 - 300	12.7 (5.2)	687 (50.1)	683 (49.9)	1370 (100)	0.3	1.2	0.7
300 - 500	35.7 (6.5)	1621 (51.2)	1548 (48.8)	3169 (100)	1.3	0.9	1.1
500 - 700	28.9 (10.8)	1173 (51.7)	1094 (48.3)	2267 (100)	2.0	2.2	2.1
700 - 900	13.9 (20.6)	460 (51.1)	440(48.9)	900 (100)	4.3	5.5	4.9
≥ 900	8.8 (23.5)	295 (55.7)	235(44.3)	530 (100)	6.8	6.0	6.4
Total	1502100.0 (11.1)	4236(51.4)	4000 (48.6)	8236(100)	2.0	2.1	2.1

Contd...

	Age of Member (in years)					Expense (Direct + Indirect) Incurred (in Rs.)				
	Min.	Max.	Median	Mean	CV	Min.	Max.	Median	Mean*	CV*
	(9)	(10)	(11)	(12)	(13)	(14)	(15)	(16)	(17)	(18)
A.	28	62	35.0	45.0	26.9	20	1250	213.0	424.0	118.2
	14	70	30.0	33.8	37.0	20	1500	325.0	453.9	93.6
	13	60	28.0	33.5	41.8	5	20210	550.0	1594.0	270.5
	15	83	24.0	35.8	61.5	20	4500	515.5	1116.8	116.5
	20	28	20.0	24.7	13.8	4460	4460	4460.0	4460.0	0.0
	13	83	31.0	34.6	43.4	5	20210	365.0	986.8	259.7
B.	13	70	35.0	37.7	43.2	5	4140	222.5	408.6	148.0
	13	80	34.0	35.8	47.2	1	4360	290.0	571.6	132.2
	13	84	35.0	37.3	46.9	1	9470	322.0	681.7	172.7
	13	80	35.0	37.5	44.5	1	9700	375.0	672.5	172.0
	13	70	39.0	36.2	41.2	1	5750	570.0	938.3	129.8
	13	84	35.0	36.8	45.9	1	9700	315.0	638.6	159.1
C.	1	12	3.0	4.0	80.0	2	2000	115.5	273.0	144.0
	1	12	5.3	5.6	60.7	1	5300	180.0	338.6	156.6
	1	12	5.0	5.3	60.4	1	3400	160.0	314.0	137.2
	1	11	6.0	6.4	51.6	1	3145	255.0	453.3	134.2
	1	11	6.0	6.0	55.0	18	8100	200.0	878.6	221.9
	1	12	5.0	5.4	63.0	1	8100	190.0	361.8	180.1

Contd.

	(9)	(10)	(11)	(12)	(13)	(14)	(15)	(16)	(17)	(18)
D.	2	70	25.0	27.4	71.9	40	4650	570.0	853.0	113.4
	1	80	32.0	34.6	56.4	30	4500	515.0	792.5	107.8
	1	85	33.0	35.1	65.8	10	16434	492.5	1171.7	195.4
	2	74	39.0	38.0	54.5	40	6000	550.0	1060.7	110.7
	1	95	35.0	36.5	61.6	70	15610	960.0	2006.8	139.8
	1	95	34.0	35.0	60.9	10	16434	608.0	1121.8	160.4
E.	1	70	22.5	26.9	76.6	13	12000	532.5	1400.1	153.8
	1	80	32.0	34.7	61.4	20	14351	812.0	1714.2	131.1
	1	85	30.0	32.7	69.1	25	120000	1380.0	3438.3	307.3
	2	75	37.5	36.6	58.2	70	27600	2197.5	4410.8	123.8
	1	95	34.0	35.0	58.9	210	50000	4265.0	8265.2	127.8
	1	95	32.0	33.8	64.2	13	120000	1450.0	3515.7	217.4
F.	1	45	15.5	18.3	84.2	10	560	241.0	223.4	78.7
	1	72	25.0	35.5	63.7	50	2950	245.0	435.6	131.0
	1	70	25.0	28.5	70.9	26	5600	290.0	744.8	155.9
	2	74	39.0	37.9	54.4	30	5300	555.0	1105.6	113.8
	2	65	35.0	33.1	52.3	130	9000	600.0	1530.5	135.8
	1	74	32.5	32.6	63.2	10	9000	372.5	901.9	152.1

* **Excluding** *the cases with zero expenditure.*

Other health problems among adult males and females were found in about 37 per cent households. The per centages were lower for the households with PCMCE below Rs. 500 and higher for those with PCMCE Rs. 500 and above. The per centages of adult males in different PCMCE categories, who sought care for their health problems, were generally having an increasing trend with increasing PCMCE level. The same had been noticed for the adult females. Additionally, the per centages for the females in different PCMCE categories were in general higher than those for the males. The overall per centage had been about 8.0. The age profile of the adult males and the adult females who sought care for their health problems, however, had been more or less same for all the PCMCE categories. The total expense incurred for having treatment, inclusive of both direct and indirect expenses, had its median and mean estimates increasing with increasing PCMCE. The overall median total expenditure incurred for treatment of these health problems had been Rs. 315.

As far as children's health problems are concerned, the table shows that there were nearly 24 per cent households that sought care for childhood sickness. The percentages were higher for the households with PCMCE between Rs. 300 and Rs. 700. The percentages of male children in different PCMCE categories who sought health care were generally similar to those estimated for the female children. The overall percentage had been 5.0. The overall mean and the median ages of the sick children were about 5.4 and 5.0 years, respectively. It is seen here also that the median and the mean total expenses incurred for having treatment increase with increasing PCMCE. The overall median total expense had been Rs. 190.

The per centages of households with cases of pre-hospitalization care were found increasing with increasing PCMCE level. The overall per centage had been 19.0. The percentages of cases among the males were somewhat higher than that among the females for the households with PCMCE below Rs. 700, but it had been otherwise for the remaining households. The median and the mean ages of the persons who had undergone pre-hospitalization care were remarkably low in the lowest PCMCE category (about 25 and 27 years, respectively). The median total expense incurred for having pre-hospitalization care had been Rs. 608.

The percentages of households with cases of hospitalization also showed an increasing trend with increasing PCMCE level, but these were generally higher than the corresponding percentages of pre-hospitalization care. The former had been in the range of 20 to 46 and the latter in the range of 13 to 30. The overall percentage had been about 31. The percentages of cases among the males were similar to those among the females for all the PCMCE categories except the lowest one and the one corresponding to the PCMCE category Rs. 700 to Rs. 900. There were not much variation in the age profile of persons from one PCMCE category to another except that the hospitalised cases in the lowest PCMCE category were generally more young than the other cases. Both the median and the mean total expenses incurred to have hospital care show an increasing trend with increasing PCMCE. The overall median total expense had been Rs. 1450.

Post-hospitalization care had been had by only about 11 per cent of all considered households. The percentages were only about 5 and 6 for the persons in the two lowest PCMCE categories and these again showed an increasing trend with increasing PCMCE level. The percentages of cases among the males and that among the females were more or less same and it was about 2. Increasing median and mean total expenses for having post-hospitalization care with increasing PCMCE level is noted here also with the overall median total expense about Rs. 372.

Distribution of Cases by Different Categories of Incurred Expenditures for Various Types of Health Care

Varying level of expenditure for availing various types of health care has been detailed in Table 3. Out of 82 cases of seeking reproductive heath care for females (nearly 3 per cent of the total 3,050 of cases of seeking various types of health care), nearly 21 per cent had treatment at no cost. About 24 per cent cases had treatment by spending some amount below

Table 3
Percentage Distribution of Cases by Different Categories of Incurred Expenditures for Various Types of Health Care and Few Summary Statistics

Types of Seeking Health Care	Total Cases (row % /col. %)	Percentage of Cases with Expenditure Incurred (in Rs.) 0	1-200	200-400	400-600	600-800
(1)	(2)	(3)	(4)	(5)	(6)	(7)
A. Treatment of Reproductive Health Problems of females	82(100.0/2.7)	20.7	24.4	17.1	6.1	8.5
Overall (A)	82(100.0/2.7)	17(20.7)	20(24.4)	14(17.1)	5(6.1)	7(8.5)
B. Pregnancy and Child Birth						
1. Pregnancy Complications	131(100.0/4.3)	0.8	12.2	21.4	18.3	13.0
2. Pre – Natal Care	454(100.0/14.9)	24.2	11.5	20.7	22.0	3.1
3. Natal care (including abortion)	335(100.0/11.0)	7.5	15.8	29.0	14.6	6.3
4. Post-natal Care	22(100.0/0.7)	0.0	18.2	40.9	9.1	9.1
Overall (B) 942(100.0/30.8)	136(14.4)	125(13.3)	228(24.2)	175(18.6)	54(5.7)	
C. Hospitalization						
1. Prior to hospitalization	291(100.0/9.5)	0.3	17.9	18.6	12.4	1.7
2. In hospital	491(100.0/16.1)	2.6	7.1	13.0	9.2	6.3
3. Post-hospitalization	170(100.0/5.6)	2.4	21.8	27.6	10.0	9.4
Overall (C) 952(100.0/31.2)	18(1.9)	124(13.0)	165(17.3)	98(10.3)	78(8.2)	
D. Childhood Illnesses						
1. Male	220(100.0/7.2)	1.8	47.7	27.7	9.1	4.5
2. Female	195(100.0/6.4)	1.0	51.3	21.5	9.7	5.1
Overall (D)	415(100.0/13.6)	6(1.4)	205(49.4)	103(24.8)	39(9.4)	20(4.8)
E. Other Health Problems						
1. Adult Male	279(100.0/9.1)	0.7	33.7	20.4	13.3	8.6
2. Adult Female	380(100.0/12.4)	2.1	35.0	20.5	11.1	12.4
Overall (E) 659(100.0/21.6)	10(1.5)	227(34.4)	135(20.5)	79(12.0)	71(10.8)	

Contd.

	800-1000	1000-1500	1500-2000	2000-3000	3000-4000	4000-5000	^{3} 5000	Median	Mean*	C.V.*
	(8)	(9)	(10)	(11)	(12)	(13)	(14)	(15)	(16)	(17)
	(2.4)	(12.2)	2.4	2.4	0.0	2.4	1.2	365.0	986.8	259.7
Overall A	2(2.4)	10(12.2)	2(2.4)	2(2.4)	0(0.0)	2(2.4)	1(1.2)	365.0	986.8	259.7
	6.1	13.0	9.2	3.1	0.8	0.8	1.5	565.0	868.0	112.1
	1.1	9.3	5.1	0.9	1.1	0.7	0.4	420.0	659.3	121.2
	3.9	11.3	3.6	4.5	0.6	0.3	2.7	400.0	810.4	149.7
	0.0	13.6	4.5	0.0	0.0	0.0	4.5	345.0	697.4	157.1
Overall B	26(2.8)	100(10.6)	48(5.1)	23(2.4)	8(0.8)	5(0.5)	14(1.5)	420.0	752.2	135.0
	7.6	13.1	6.2	4.8	3.8	2.7	2.1	608.0	1121.8	160.4
	4.5	9.2	8.4	9.6	6.5	4.7	18.9	1450.0	3515.7	217.4
	7.1	5.9	4.7	4.1	2.4	2.4	2.4	372.5	901.9	152.1
Overall C	56(5.9)	93(9.8)	67(7.0)	68(7.1)	47(4.9)	35(3.7)	103(10.8)	800.0	2307.8	248.0
	3.2	2.3	1.4	0.5	0.9	0.5	0.5	200.0	373.3	198.1
	3.6	4.6	1.5	1.0	0.0	0.0	0.5	170.0	348.8	153.6
Overall D	14(3.4)	14(3.4)	6(1.4)	3(0.7)	2(0.5)	1(0.2)	2(0.5)	190.0	361.8	180.1
	6.8	6.5	3.2	3.2	1.4	1.8	0.4	325.0	639.5	148.2
	3.4	6.8	1.6	3.4	1.6	1.1	1.1	315.0	638.0	166.8
	32(4.9)	44(6.7)	15(2.3)	22(3.3)	10(1.5)	9(1.4)	8(0.8)	315.0	638.6	159.1
Overall E	131(4.3)	261(8.5)	138(4.5)	118(3.9)	67(2.2)	52(1.7)	125(4.1)	420.0	1182.2	293.4

* Excluding the cases with zero expenditure

Rs. 200. An amount between Rs. 200 and Rs. 400 had been spent in about 17 per cent cases. There were about 12 per cent cases for which the spent amount had been between Rs. 1,000 and Rs. 1,500. Nearly 8 per cent cases had undergone treatment at a cost between Rs. 600 and Rs. 800. The median and the mean expenditures were Rs. 365 and Rs. 987 respectively.

About 31 per cent of the total considered cases had been concerning pregnancy and childbirth. Among these, about 4 per cent were concerning pregnancy complication, 15 per cent were concerning pre-natal care, 11 per cent concerning natal care (including care for abortion) and 1 per cent concerning post-natal care. In about 65 per cent cases of pregnancy complication, the expenditure incurred had been below Rs. 800 and in another 28 per cent cases, the range had been from Rs. 800 to Rs. 2,000. The median and the mean expenditure were Rs. 565 and Rs. 868, respectively.

Nearly 24 per cent cases had availed pre-natal care free of cost and 54 per cent cases had pre-natal care by spending less than Rs. 600. The median and the mean expenditures on pre-natal care had been about Rs. 420 and Rs. 659, respectively. Natal care (including abortion) was availed free of cost by about 8 per cent women. For about 59 per cent cases of natal care the range of expenditure had been below Rs. 600 and for 11 per cent cases, it had been in the range of Rs. 1,000 to Rs. 1,500. The median expense was found to be Rs. 400 and the mean was nearly Rs. 810. In about 59 per cent cases of post-natal care, the expenditure had been below Rs. 400 and in another 32 per cent cases, the spent amount had been Rs. 400 to Rs. 1,500. The median and the mean expenses were Rs. 345 and Rs. 697, respectively.

The cases of hosptialisation were about 31 per cent of the total considered cases of seeking various types of health care. Among these cases, about 10 per cent had availed pre-hospitalization care, 16 per cent had hospitalization care and about 6 per cent had post-hospitalization care. While pre-hospitalization care was had in about 59 per cent cases of hospitalization, post-hospitalization care was had in only about 35 per cent cases. The expenditure had been below Rs.

600 in about 49 per cent cases of pre-hospitalization care and it had been between Rs. 600 and Rs. 2,000 in about 27 per cent cases. The median and the mean expenses on pre-hospitalization care were Rs. 608 and Rs. 1,122, respectively. Nearly 19 per cent cases of hospitalization were such that the expenditure incurred had been Rs. 5,000 and above. In about 40 per cent cases, the expense had been below Rs. 1,000 and in another 38 per cent cases the expense range had been from Rs. 1,000 to Rs. 5,000. The median and the mean expenses had been Rs. 1,450 and Rs. 3,516, respectively. The expense on post-hospitalization care had been below Rs. 1,000 in about 76 per cent cases of post-hospitalization care. The median and the mean expenditures had been Rs. 372 and Rs. 902, respectively.

There were about 14 per cent cases of childhood sickness and a little above half of them were among the male children. Irrespective of the sex of the considered children, the expenditure incurred in more than 80 per cent cases had been below Rs. 600. In the cases of the male children, the median and the mean expenses were Rs. 200 and Rs. 373, respectively and in the cases of the female children, these were Rs. 170 and Rs. 349, respectively.

The cases of other health problems among adult males and females were about 21 per cent of the total considered cases. Among these, 9 per cent cases were found among the males and about 12 per cent cases were found among the females. The expenditure on dealing with the health problems was below Rs. 800 for about 76 per cent males and about 79 per cent females. The median and the mean expenses were Rs. 325 and Rs. 640 for the male cases, and Rs. 315 and Rs. 638 for the female cases.

Per centage of Total Expenditure Incurred Under Different Expense Heads to Avail Various Types of Health Care

Table 4 gives the mean per centages of total expenditure incurred under various heads while availing different types of health care. It gives simultaneously the coefficients of variation. Clearly, the mean per centage of the total expense

Table 4
Various Expense Head wise Mean Percentage of Total Expenditure Incurred Under Various Heads for Availing Different Types of Health Care and Coefficient of Variation

Type of Health Care	Percentage of Total Expenditure Incurred Under								
	Direct Payment to Hospital, etc.	Consul-tation Fee		Medicines		Blood Test and /or Transfusion		X-ray/ECG/ EEG/Scan/ Sonography etc	
	Mean*	CV*	Mean*	CV*	Mean*	CV*	Mean*	CV*	Mean*
(1)	(2)	(3)	(4)	(5)	(6)	(7)	(8)	(9)	(10)
A) Reproductive Health Care for Females	—	—	25.1	93.2	61.6	41.6	—	—	29.5
B) Managing Pregnancy Complication	—	—	19.4	88.7	56.3	42.3	21.7	80.2	33.4
C) Managing Delivery	16.7	107.2	—	—	67.7	40.0	20.7	101.9	21.8
D) Managing Post-Delivery Complication	—	—	16.7	68.9	78.4	30.5	31.8	55.3	10.0
E) Pre-hospitalisation Care	—	—	18.8	98.4	58.9	40.1	19.9	105.0	27.0
F) Care in Hospital	5.9	144.1	20.6	120.9	57.7	49.2	10.6	114.2	13.8
G) Post-hospitalisation Care	—	—	17.6	89.2	84.7	25.6	15.5	92.9	32.5
H) Managing Sickness of Children	—	—	24.4	71.7	73.2	28.8	20.2	81.2	27.7
I) Managing Other Health Problems of Adults	—	—	20.4	80.4	69.3	34.5	17.8	78.1	26.7

Contd.

Other Diagnostic Tests		Purchase of Personal Medical Appliances		Transport/ Communication		Escorts Board & Lodging Charges		Attendant Charges			Other	
CV*	Mean*	CV*	Mean*	CV*	Mean*	CV*	Mean*	CV*	Mean*	CV*	Mean*	CV*
(11)	(12)	(13)	(14)	(15)	(16)	(17)	(18)	(19)	(20)	(21)	(22)	(23)
53.9	20.7	50.7	11.9	63.9	13.7	139.4	—	—	—	—	10.4	
62.9	19.3	70.5	15.6	76.9	11.8	77.1	—	—	—	—	13.2	125.0
56.0	17.5	88.6	—	—	—	—	—	—	—	—	16.7	107.2
0.0	55.0	81.8	19.5	64.1	11.4	55.3	—	—	—	—	27.0	0.0
73.0	14.7	66.7	12.4	75.8	10.1	109.9	—	—	—	—	11.3	147.8
98.6	9.0	103.3	11.9	118.5	12.3	152.0	12.2	123.0	18.0	122.2	5.9	144.1
73.5	16.3	62.6	4.0	0.0	11.4	93.9	—	—	—	—	25.3	96.4
79.1	20.3	60.6	16.8	63.1	18.4	171.2	—	—	—	—	15.9	120.1
80.9	18.0	78.3	22.5	104.0	13.7	159.1	—	—	—	—	15.0	172.0

* Excluding zero expense.

which was spent on medicines had been, in general, the highest for each type of health care. It had been in the range of about 56 per cent to about 85 per cent with the former corresponding to managing the pregnancy complications and the latter corresponding to the post-hospitalization care. The mean percentage of expenditures on X-ray/ECG/EEG/Scan/ Sonography, etc. had been, in general, the second highest with all per centages falling between 22 and 33 except the cases of post-delivery complications with the mean per centage about 10 and the cases of having care in hospital with the mean per centage about 14.

The third important head had been the consultation fee, on which about 16 to 25 per cent of the total expenditure was spent. The next two important heads had been the blood tests and/or transfusion and other diagnostic tests. Except the hospitalization cases and the cases of post-delivery complications, the mean per centages had been in the range of 15 to 22 for the former and in the range of 14 to 21 for the latter. The mean per centages were about 11 and 9 respectively for the hospitalization cases and were about 32 and 55 for the cases with post-delivery complications.

The mean per centage of expense on purchase of personal medical appliances had been 4, the minimum, corresponding to post-hospitalization care. For other types of health care, the mean per centages had been in the range of about 12 to 22. As far as the expenses on transport/ communications were concerned, the mean per centages had been in the range of 10 to 18.

The mean per centage of direct payment to hospitals, nursing homes, etc. had been nearly 17 in the cases of managing delivery, and it was higher than 6 as far as the mean per centage of direct such payment in the cases of availing care from hospitals, nursing homes, etc. for other purposes are concerned. For the latter cases, the mean per centages of expenses on attendant charges and escorts' board and lodging charges had been about 18 and 12, respectively.

The Sources of Finance for Meeting Expenditures on Various Types of Health Care

As shown in Table 5, the money earmarked for monthly spending had been the most important source of finance for managing almost all the considered health problems except the ones, managed through hospitalization. Generally, 42 to 65 per cent cases of managing various health problems were financed through making use of the money, earmarked by households for monthly spending. Majority of the cases of childhood sickness had undergone treatment with this sort of financing. Management of health problems among the adults was the next most important category which got financed the same way in about 59 per cent cases. The third in this series was post-hospitalization care, about 50 per cent cases of which were also managed by making use of the money, meant for monthly spending. Pre-hospitalization care had been the fourth broad category with nearly 49 per cent cases managed financially the same way.

Loan had been the next most important source of finance and its use had been maximum for the cases of hospitalization. Nearly 53 per cent cases of hospitalization were managed financially by making use of loan. The money earmarked for monthly spending was utilised in about 38 per cent cases of hospitalization. Loan had been an important source of financing for post-hospitalization care also. Nearly 41 per cent cases of post-hospitalization care were managed financially by borrowing money. The third and the fourth broad categories of managing health care with significant dependence on loan as a source of finance had been pre-hospitalization care (with about 36% cases) and care for other health problems among the adults (with about 33% cases).

For managing the cases of delivery and abortion, savings had been an important source of finance, next to the money earmarked for monthly spending and the loan. About 24 per cent delivery and abortion cases were financially managed by making use of the savings. Use of savings as the third most important source of finance had also been noted in about

Table 5

Distribution of Cases by Sources of Finance for Expenditures Incurred on Various Types of Seeking Health Care

Type of Seeking Health Care	No. of Cases with Zero Expense (row% /col.%)	*Sources of Finance for Other Cases (row% / col.%)* Money earmarked for monthly spending	Saving	Reimbursement by Employer	Reimbursement by Other Agencies
(1)	(2)	(3)	(4)	(5)	(6)
1. Reproductive Health Care for Female	18(22.0/26.1)	(42.7/2.6)	(7.3/1.4)	(4.9/4.5)	(0.0/0.0)
2. Care for Pregnancy Complications	1(0.8/1.4)	(42.0/4.1)	(11.5/3.6)	(4.6/6.7)	(1.5/9.1)
3. Care During Delivery / Abortion	26(7.8/37.7)	(46.9/11.8)	(24.2/19.4)	(0.0/0.0)	(0.0/0.0)
4. Post - delivery Care	0(0.0/0.0)	(50.0/0.8)	(0.0/0.0)	(9.1/2.2)	(0.0/0.0)
5. Pre - hospitalization Care					
a) Male	0(0.0/0.0)	(52.7/5.9)	(16.2/5.7)	(2.0/3.4)	(1.4/9.1)
b) Female	1(0.7/1.4)	(44.8/4.8)	(21.7/7.4)	(2.8/4.5)	(0.0/0.0)
c) Persons	1(0.3/1.4)	(48.8/10.7)	(18.9/13.2)	(2.4/7.9)	(0.7/9.1)
6. Care Through Hospitalization					
a) Male	2(0.8/2.9)	(38.3/6.9)	(14.2/8.1)	(5.0/13.5)	(2.1/22.7)
b) Female	6(2.4/8.7)	(37.5/7.1)	(22.3/13.4)	(3.6/10.1)	(2.0/22.7)
c) Persons	8(1.6/11.6)	(37.9/14.0)	(18.3/21.5)	(4.3/23.6)	(2.0/45.5)
7. Post-hospitalization Care					
a) Male	0(0.0/0.0)	(47.7/3.1)	(10.5/2.2)	(1.2/1.1)	(1.2/4.5)
b) Female	2(2.4/2.9)	(52.4/3.3)	(16.7/3.3)	(4.8/4.5)	(0.0/0.0)
c) Persons	2(1.2/2.9)	(50.0/6.4)	(13.5/5.5)	(2.9/5.6)	(0.6/4.5)
8. Care for Sick Children					
a) Male	3(1.4/4.3)	(63.2/10.5)	(16.8/8.9)	(5.0/12.4)	(0.5/4.5)
b) Female	1(0.5/1.4)	(66.7/9.8)	(16.9/7.9)	(4.1/9.0)	(1.5/13.6)
c) All	4(1.0/5.8)	(64.8/20.2)	(16.9/16.7)	(4.6/21.3)	(1.0/18.2)
9. Care for Other Health Problems of Adults					
a) Male	2(0.7/2.9)	(59.1/12.4)	(13.6/9.1)	(5.0/15.7)	(0.4/4.5)
b) Female	6(1.6/8.7)	(58.2/16.6)	(10.5/9.6)	(2.9/12.4)	(0.5/9.1)
c) All	8(1.2/11.6)	(58.6/29.0)	(11.8/18.7)	(3.8/28.1)	(0.5/13.6)
Total	69(2.7/100.0)	1329(51.1/100.0)	418(16..1/100..0)	89(3.4/100.0)	22(0.8/100.0)

Contd.

Loan	*Help/Gift/ Donation*	*Selling of Household Goods/ Ornaments/ Physical Assets*	*Selling of Cattle/ Animals*	*Mortgaging Ornaments/ Durable Goods/ Physical Assets*	*Total Cases (row % col. %)*
(7)	*(8)*	*(9)*	*(10)*	*(11)*	*(12)*
(23.2/2.0)	(4.9/1.7)	(2.4/2.9)	(0.0/0.0)	(0.0/0.0)	82(100.0/3.2)
(35.1/4.9)	(9.2/5.2)	(9.2/17.6)	(0.0/0.0)	(3.8/9.3)	131(100.0/5.0)
(33.7/12.2)	(10.1/14.7)	(0.6/2.9)	(0.0/0.0)	(1.5/9.3)	335(100.0/12.9)
(22.7/0.5)	(13.6/1.3)	(0.0/0.0)	(0.0/0.0)	(9.1/3.7)	22(100.0/0.8)
(39.9/6.3)	(9.5/6.1)	(2.7/5.9)	(0.0/0.0)	(2.0/5.6)	148(100.0/5.7)
(32.2/4.9)	(14.0/8.7)	(6.3/13.2)	(0.0/0.0)	(2.8/7.4)	143(100.0/5.5)
(36.1/11.3)	(11.7/14.7)	(4.5/19.1)	(0.0/0.0)	(2.4/13.0)	291(100.0/11.2)
(52.9/13.7)	(15.0/15.6/)	(2.9/10.3)	(0.0/0.0)	(3.3/14.8)	240(100.0/9.2)
(53.0/14.3)	(17.5/19.0)	(3.6/13.2)	(0.4/50.0)	(1.6/7.4)	251(100.0/9.6)
(53.0/28.0)	(16.3/34.6)	(3.3/23.5)	(0.2/50.0)	(2.4/22.2)	491(100.0/18.9)
(48.8/4.5)	(5.8/2.2)	(4.7/5.9)	(0.0/0.0)	(5.8/9.3)	86(100.0/3.3)
(33.3/3.0)	(13.1/4.8)	(0.0/0.0)	(0.0/0.0)	(1.2/1.9)	84(100.0/3.2)
(41.2/7.5)	(9.4/6.9)	(2.4/5.9)	(0.0/0.0)	(3.5/11.1)	170(100.0/6.5)
(23.2/5.5)	(3.2/3.0)	(1.8/5.9)	(0.0/0.0)	(1.4/5.6)	220(100.0/8.5)
(22.6/4.7)	(0.00.0)	(1.0/2.9)	(0.0/0.0)	(1.0/3.7)	195(100.0/7.5)
(22.9/10.2)	(1.7/3.0)	(1.4/8.8)	(0.0/0.0)	(1.2/9.3)	415(100.0/15.9)
(28.7/8.6)	(5.7/6.9)	(2.5/10.3)	(0.4/50.0)	(1.8/9.3)	279(100.0/10.7)
(35.5/14.5)	(6.6/10.8)	(1.6/8.8)	(0.0/0.0)	(1.8/13.0)	380(100.0/14.6)
(32.6/23.1)	(6.2/17.7)	(2.0/19.1)	(0.2/50.0)	(1.8/22.2)	659(100.0/25.3)
930(35.7/100.0)	231(8.9/100.0)	68(2.6/100.0)	2(0.1/100.0)	54(2.1/100.0)	2602(100.0/100.0)

17 to 19 per cent cases of pre-hospitalization care, care through hospitalization and care for the sick children.

Out of 1329 cases where the money earmarked for monthly spending had been used as a source of finance, the categories of care which received maximum attention of the households had been in decreasing order of importance (1) care for other health problems among the adults (about 29% cases), (2) care for the sick children (about 20% cases), (3) care through hospitalization (about 14% cases), (4) care during delivery/ abortion (about 12% cases) and (5) pre-hospitalization care (about 11% cases). In about 930 cases of utilising loan, maximum attention had been on (1) care through hospitalization (about 28% cases), (2) care for other health problems among the adults (about 23% cases), (3) care during delivery / abortion (about 12% cases), (4) pre-hospitalization care (about 11% cases), (5) care for the sick children (about 10% cases). In about 418 cases of utilisation of savings as a source of finance, maximum attention of the households had been on (1) care through hospitalization (about 22% cases), (2) care during delivery / abortion (in about 19% cases), (3) care for other health problems among the adults (about 19% cases), (4) care for the sick children (about 17% cases) and (5) pre-hospitalization care (about 13% cases).

Sources of Finance for Different Slabs of Expenditures Incurred to Avail Various Types of Health Care

Table 6 tries to show how the sources of finance vary with changing level of incurred expenses on availing different types of health care. Almost for all types of health care, majority of the cases in the lowest expense category had been using the money earmarked for monthly spending and/or savings as the finance source to meet the expenses on treatment. The per centages of such cases were in the range of 68 to 82 for all types of health care except managing non-institutional delivery and care in hospital. For these exceptional types of health care, nearly one-third of the cases had utilised loan as a source of finance. For other types of care, loan had been utilised as a source of finance by about 13 to 22 per cent cases in the

Table 6

Sources of Finance Corresponding to Different Slabs of Expenditure Incurred to Avail Various Types of Health Care

Type of Health Care	Total Number of Cases(%)	Cases with Zero Expense(%)	Expense Slabs (in Rs.)	Percentage of Other Cases with Sources of Finance: Money earmarked for monthly spending and/ or savings	Reimbu-rsement by employer or other agency	Loan	Help/gift/ donation	Selling/ mortgaging household goods/ ornaments/ physical assets/ cattle	Total Use of Various Sources (%)
(1)	(2)	(3)	(4)	(5)	(6)	(7)	(8)	(9)	(10)
A) Reproductive Health Care for Females	82(100.0)	17(25.0)	1 - 300	81.5	0.0	14.8	3.7	0.0	27 (39.7)
			300 - 600	57.1	0.0	28.6	7.1	7.1	14 (20.6)
			600 - 900	55.6	11.1	22.2	11.1	0.0	9 (13.2)
			≥ 900	22.2	16.7	50.0	5.6	5.6	18 (26.5)
B) Managing Pregnancy Complication	131(100.0)	1(0.7)	1 - 300	71.0	6.5	12.9	6.5	3.2	31 (20.9)
			300 - 600	31.7	2.4	41.5	9.8	14.6	41 (27.7)
			600 - 900	44.4	11.1	25.9	11.1	7.4	27 (18.2)
			≥ 900	38.8	4.1	36.7	6.1	14.3	49 (33.1)
C. 1) Managing Delivery (Institutional)	284(100.0)	22(7.1)	1 - 300	74.4	0.0	17.9	5.1	2.6	78 (25.1)
			300 - 600	63.3	0.0	26.7	8.9	1.1	90 (28.9)
			600 - 900	57.9	0.0	34.2	5.3	2.6	38 (12.2)
			≥ 900	44.8	0.0	40.0	13.3	1.9	105 (33.8)
C. 2) Managing Delivery (Non-institutional)	51(100.0)	51(3.7)	1 - 300	54.1	0.0	32.4	13.5	0.0	37 (69.8)
			300 - 600	45.5	0.0	54.5	0.0	0.0	11 (20.8)
			600 - 900	25.0	0.0	50.0	25.0	0.0	4 (7.5)
			≥ 900	100.0	0.0	0.0	0.0	0.0	1 (1.9)

Contd.

D) Managing Post-delivery Complications	22(100.0)	0(0.0)	1 - 300	72.7	0.0	18.2	9.1	0.0	11 (47.8)
			300 - 600	60.0	0.0	20.0	0.0	20.0	5 (21.7)
			600 - 900	0.0	0.0	100.0	0.0	0.0	2 (8.7)
			≥ 900	0.0	40.0	0.0	40.0	20.0	5 (21.7)
E) Pre-hospitalisation Care	291(100.0)	1(0.3)	1 - 300	67.8	2.2	20.0	8.9	1.1	90 (25.9)
			300 - 600	62.9	0.0	24.3	7.1	5.7	70 (20.2)
			600 - 900	48.1	5.8	34.6	5.8	5.8	52 (15.0)
			≥ 900	37.8	3.0	38.5	13.3	7.4	135 (38.9)
F) Care in Hospital	491(100.0)	13(2.1)	1 - 300	51.7	3.4	31.5	11.2	2.2	89 (14.1)
			300 - 600	48.7	2.6	29.5	15.4	3.8	78 (12.4)
			600 - 900	55.8	3.8	30.8	9.6	0.0	52 (8.3)
			≥ 900	30.5	4.9	47.1	12.9	4.6	410(65.2)
G) Post-hospitalisation Care	170(100.0)	4(2.0)	1 - 300	68.1	2.8	22.2	6.9	0.0	72 (35.6)
			300 - 600	52.4	0.0	42.9	2.4	2.4	42 (20.8)
			600 - 900	43.3	3.3	26.7	16.7	10.0	30 (14.9)
			≥ 900	32.8	3.4	48.3	8.6	6.9	58 (28.7)
H) Managing Sickness of Children	415(100.0)	6(1.4)	1 - 300	78.0	5.0	15.2	1.4	0.4	282 (64.2)
			300 - 600	65.1	4.8	26.5	2.4	1.2	83 (18.9)
			600 - 900	39.5	10.5	42.1	2.6	5.3	38 (8.7)
			≥ 900	44.4	2.8	36.1	0.0	16.7	36 (8.2)
I) Managing Other Health Problems of Adults	659(100.0)	10(1.4)	1 - 300	73.0	3.4	15.5	6.8	1.2	322 (43.8)
			300 - 600	49.4	4.8	37.5	4.8	3.6	168 (22.8)
			600 - 900	58.6	2.7	32.4	2.7	3.6	111 (15.1)
			≥ 900	32.6	4.4	48.9	5.9	8.1	135 (18.3)

lowest expense category. Help/gift/donation, etc. had been used as the sources of finance in 5 per cent or more cases only when the types of care were (1) managing pregnancy complication (6.5%), (2) managing institutional delivery (5.1%), (3) managing non-institutional delivery (13.5%), (4) managing post-delivery complications (9.1%), (5) pre-hospitalization care (8.9%), (6) care in hospital (11.2%), (7) post-hospitalization care (6.9%) and (8) managing other health problems among the adults (6.8%).

It is noteworthy that there had been a general trend to depend less on the money earmarked for monthly spending and/or savings as the expense incurred in a case increased. Leaving aside the per centages, calculated based on inadequate number of sampled cases, the trend generally holds for others. For example, the per centages of cases who had utilised the money earmarked for monthly spending and/or savings for treatment of female reproductive health problems were about 82, 57, 56 and 22 corresponding to the expense categories of less than Rs. 300, Rs. 300 - 600, Rs. 600–900 and Rs. 900 and above respectively. Similar examples are there in the cases of managing institutional deliveries, non-institutional deliveries, pre-hospitalization care, post-hospitalization care, sickness of children and other adult health problems.

While the table shows that increase in treatment expense makes the cases depend less on the money earmarked for monthly spending and/or savings, it also shows that with decreasing dependence on the money earmarked for monthly spending and/or savings, the cases tend to depend more and more on loan. Leaving aside the per centages that are less reliable due to inadequacy of number of sampled cases and excepting the cases of managing pregnancy complications, the last stated dependency is generally quite evident from the per centages presented in the table. For example, with decreasing utilisation of the money earmarked for monthly spending and/or savings, as indicated by the per centages 82, 57, 56 and 22 corresponding to the expense levels of Rs. 1–300, Rs. 300–600, Rs. 600–900 and Rs. 900 and above, respectively, the per centages of cases of female reproductive health problems where loan got used as a source of finance were about 15, 29, 22 and 50, respectively. Similar association could be noticed for other types of health care also.

With increasing treatment expense, decreasing dependence on money earmarked for monthly spending and/ or savings also make more and more patients explore getting money in the form of help, gift, donation, etc. Though the association is not that clearly pronounced as could be seen from the relevant per centages given in the table, but with larger sample size, the association might get more pronounced. Selling of household goods/ornaments/physical assets/cattle, etc. as a source of finance was least found for the cases with treatment expense less than Rs. 300. Also, this source was least used for institutional and non-institutional deliveries, irrespective of the level of expense. For other types of health care, this source got used without having any clear association directly or indirectly with the level of expense. However at times, a good per centages of cases were dependent on this source. Notable were some cases of pregnancy complications, female reproductive health problems, pre- and post-hospitalization care, childhood sickness and other adult health problems.

Cases of reimbursement by employer or other agency were not there among the cases of institutional or non-institutional deliveries and the cases of post delivery complications. Such cases were there among the cases of female reproductive health problems when the treatment expense was Rs. 600 and above. Among other types of health care, good number of such cases had been found for managing pregnancy complications and managing childhood sickness. Excluding the per centages based on small samples, the maximum per centages of such cases among all types of health care had been about 17.

Vulnerability

It has been shown by Pathak (2002) that the percentage of monthly consumption expense spent on health care by a slum household having PCMCE not exceeding Rs.1,500 has the median ranging from 3per cent to 6per cent and the mean ranging between 5per cent to 14per cent. The percentage of households with PCMCE above Rs.1, 500 has been only 1.3. While average household size on the whole in the slum areas has been found in between 5 and 6, the percentage of households with size below 6 has been 58 and the percentage with size between 6 and 12 has been about 41. Thus, if a household with size either 4 or 5 encounters one of the said types of health problems for a family member and spends Rs.300, the minimum PCMCE which the household should have so as to spend the amount earmarked for its monthly spending on health, on managing the new health problem will have to be either Rs.1, 875 or Rs.1, 500. This is based on the assumption that 4per cent of the total monthly consumption expense is spent on an average on health. If the household size is between 6 and 12, the PCMCE in a similar circumstance is needed to be between Rs.625 and Rs.1250. It has been found out that the percentage of households with PCMCE Rs.600 and above is only 35.7 per cent or nearly 36 per cent.

Thus, about 64 per cent households are not capable of managing the stated types of health problems by simply utilizing what is normally earmarked for spending on health out of the total monthly consumption expense. In other words, the households with PCMCE below Rs.600 are highly vulnerable to fall in debt traps as going for loan is their second preferred source of finance for managing health problems. The seventh column of Table 6 gives an idea in general for each type of health problem, how the vulnerability increases with increasing expense on the health problems. Given this vulnerability pattern and the percentages of households with and without cases of sickness and/or hospitalization, as shown in Table 2 by different classes of PCMCE, one could estimate how many households might fall in debt traps at any point of time.

Conclusions

It is clear from the above findings that the better the economic status as measured by the level of PCMCE the greater the tendency of the households to spend more on health care. The percentage of households with health problems among adults except female reproductive health problems has been the maximum (about 37%). This is followed by the percentage of households with cases of hospitalization, which have been about 31. The other types of health problems with decreasing order of corresponding percentages are health problems among children (about 24%), pre-hospitalization care (about 19%), post-hospitalization care (about 11%) and female reproductive health problems (about 5%). In decreasing order of median expenses, incurred for managing the said types of health problems, the most expensive are the cases of hospitalization with median expense Rs.1, 450. Other problems in the series are pre-hospitalization care (Rs.608), post-hospitalization care (Rs.372), female reproductive health problems (Rs.365), other health problems among adults (Rs.315) and child health problems (Rs.190).

The input that costs maximum in the management of various health problems are the medicines. The second most expensive input has been various diagnostic tests such as X-ray, ECG, EEG, Scan, Sonography, etc. The third most expensive input has been consultation with doctors. These doctors have been mostly the government and the private allopathic doctors. The fourth and the fifth expensive input are blood test and/or transfusion and other diagnostic tests. Remaining important input in decreasing order of incurred expenses on it are personal medical appliances, transport/ communications, direct and indirect payment to hospitals, nursing homes, etc.

The money earmarked for monthly spending by a household has been the most important source of finance for managing almost all types of health problems except the ones managed through hospitalization. Loan has been the second most important source of finance and it has been utilized maximum in the cases of hospitalization (about 53%). This source has also been used significantly for the cases of post-hospitalization care, pre-hospitalization care, reproductive health care for females (inclusive of reproductive health problems and management of pregnancy and delivery) and other health problems among adults. Savings has been the third most important source of finance and it has been used maximum in the cases of delivery and abortion (about 24% cases).

Majority of the households have been found vulnerable to fall in debt traps as most of them have PCMCE below Rs.1, 500 and the percentages of households with cases requiring high financing for proper management of the health problems are rather high.

References

Calcutta Metropolitan Development Authority (CMDA) (1983), Report on *"Health and Socio-Economic Survey in Calcutta Metropolitan Area"*. Calcutta: CMDA.

Chakraborty, S.C. (1990), "The Growth of Calcutta in the Twentieth Century", In: Chaudhuri Sukanta, (ed.), *Calcutta the Living City: The Present and the Future, Vol. II.* Calcutta: Oxford University Press, pp. 1-14.

Chakraborty, A.M., and Halder, A. (1991), *Slum Dwellers of Calcutta: Socio-economic Profile–1989-90.* Calcutta: CMDA.

Child-in-Need Institute (CINI)–ASHA (1999), *A Study to Evolve Alternative Models of Service Delivery in the Urban Slums,* Calcutta: CINI-ASHA.

Haldane, J.B.S. (1945), "On a Method of Estimating Frequencies", *Biometrika* 33:222-225.

Jagannathan, N.V. and Halder, A. (1988), *Pavement Dwellers of Calcutta-1987: A Socio-economic Study.* Calcutta: CMDA.

Pathak, Prasanta (2002), *Health Problems in Kolkata Slums and Means of Its Financial Management at Household Level: A Project Report,* Kolkata: Indian Statistical Institute.

Pathak, Prasanta (2006), "Hospitalization and Health Care Seeking Pattern among Slum Dwellers of Kolkata, India", In: Arvind

Pandey, (ed.) *Bio-statistical Aspects of Health and Population*. New Delhi: Hindustan Publishing Corporation, pp. 204-218.

Roy, D.K. (1978), "*Environmental Improvement of Calcutta Slums - A Mid-term Appraisa*", Calcutta: CMDA.

Roy, J., nd Bandyopadhyay, S. (1976), *Calcutta, 1976: A Socio-economic Survey of Households with Municipal Address-Tables with Notes*. Calcutta: Indian Statistical Institute.

Roy, J., and Chaudhuri, A. (1976), *Calcutta, 1976: A Socio-economic Survey of Pavement Dwellers-Tables with Notes*. Calcutta: Indian Statistical Institute.

Roy, Bardhan, Maitreyi (1994), *Calcutta Slums: Public Policy in Retrospect*. Calcutta: Minerva Associates (Publications) Pvt. Ltd.

Selvin, Steve (1991), "*Statistical Analysis of Epidemiological Data*" New York: Oxford University Press, p. 14.

Sen, S.N. (1960), *The City of Calcutta: A Socio-economic Survey, 1954-55 to 1957-58*. Calcutta: Bookland Private Ltd.

19

The IMNCI Approach towards Realising the MDG Goal: A Community Study in Madhya Pradesh

Disha Tewari

Introduction

Various health intervention programs are implemented with the support of the government, civil societies and international organizations to reduce infant and child mortality and to improve the health indicators in India. But the socio-cultural web is complex and needs to be explored before introducing any kind of health intervention within a specific community, as the success of these programs rest on the acceptance by community for which they are implemented. Thus a holistic understanding of socio-economic and cultural beliefs is required to understand the contributions and achievements of various health programs toward curtailing infant deaths. The Integrated Management of Neonatal and Childhood Illness (IMNCI) approach was started by the state Government of Madhya Pradesh in 2005 with the UNICEF support to reduce the neonatal deaths in various districts as an initiative. This research work is based on the integrated management programme on child illness in the socio-economic context of unequal power relations where the villagers are dependent on the medical health providers to get relevant information for their children.

Social Context in Health

The existing literature available on infant mortality discusses the perspective of demography and policy-oriented maternal and child health. Both these perspectives interpret high rates of death and disease characteristic in young life as inevitable consequences of largely impersonal ecological, climactic or demographic conditions in the developing world. Both these approaches, however, obscure the role of economic relations in the social production of morbidity and mortality (Schepher-Hughes, 1984; Kidanemariam and Gallagher, 1992). Elling (1981) in his attempt to place the public health system of medicines in societies emphasized the role of political economy in health. He demonstrated that the mix of modern and traditional elements, their degree of integration, and availability has some kind of social control and seems to be related to resource levels and is economy driven. Morgan (1987) opined that no one perspective is widely incorporated into the corpus of socio-medical literature, and can explain the diversity in health literature. He studied three separate theoretical perspectives of political economy of health namely: orthodox Marxist approaches, cultural critiques of medicine, and dependency theories. He argued that the Marxists see health status and the organisation of health-care as direct results of the capitalist socio-economic formation. By insisting that health should be analyzed within the context of capitalism, the Marxists draw attention to the interplay between social class formation and the power of the postindustrial nation-state (Morgan, 1987). Furthermore, cultural critiques question the value of medical services and argued that biomedicine is detrimental to individual health and to standards of social equality as it supports and replicates the status quo by keeping women and minorities subordinate. In this aspect the cultural critiques are similar to the orthodox Marxist approach as both analyse individuals within the context of unequal power relations based on gender, race and socio-economic status .However, the dependency theory popularly known as the "world system theory" has referred to a "generic sense of global dependency and interpretation, dominated by the capitalist relations of production" (Morgan, 1987).

Andes (1992) further placed emphasis on the "community contexts" and argued that characteristics of a community play an important role in infant and child mortality. According to her, societies under transition due to modernization pressures face confusion about the available services and care for childbearing and argued that the existence of services does not necessarily insure the use of services. The composition of social classes affects the child mortality, thus the poorest members of a community who may be the largest proportion of a population may not have access to the facilities. This result in some groups being more vulnerable than the others In addition, Jain and Visaria (1988) demonstrated that to understand the implementation of various programs to reduce infant mortality at the macro level, the "community" becomes important in mortality studies.

Social scientists are always debating the issue of the nature/culture dichotomy to explore ideas about gender. This concept of dichotomy is further effective in understanding how the members of the community transcends this dichotomy in to their treatment seeking behavior, and choose the best form of medical service available at the time of emergency or any ailment. Their responses and reactions change with their experiences with sickness and its' cures in biomedicine. According to Richards (1969), there exists a third kind of behavior; "presumed behavior" that links the ideal-real dichotomy. The influence varies with factors such as communication and access to information about real behavior. Pelto and Pelto (1997) further re-emphasised the model of belief systems by stating that all people, whether they are trained in biomedicine or are rural villagers, have cultural belief systems about the causes of sickness and possible remedial measures.

Thus the socio-economic context, unequal power relations and the presumed behavior including the beliefs prevalent in the society, are the factors influencing peoples' perceptions about the available health-care services for their children.

Policy Interventions and the Millennium Development Goals and IMNCI

To improve the basic reproductive and child health, health-care services are integrated in India at the primary health centers in the rural areas through the Auxiliary Nurse Midwife (ANM) at the peripheral level. They are given an additional training and required to be a counselor, educator, service provider and a person who can arrange transportation in emergency to the nearest hospitals, coordinate with other programs. However, the health-care programs prior to the implementation of IMNCI approach could not address the key concerns of neonates in India. More specifically, "the rule of two-thirds" states that two-thirds of India's Under 5 Mortality Rate is due to IMR, while two-thirds of IMR is due to NMR, and two-thirds of NMR occur within the first week of neonatal life. To address this concern, UNICEF (2007a) along with the Government of India took an initiative to improve the health conditions of infants and children less than five years of age. For this purpose, the Government of India acknowledged Integrated Management of Childhood Illness (IMCI), a global strategy encompassing a range of interventions to prevent and manage under-five childhood illnesses. In order to address neonatal health in India, the IMCI approach was adapted to Integrated Management of Neonatal and Childhood Illness (IMNCI). The IMNCI approach was launched in 2003, a strategy that supported the NRHM policy framework and the RCH program in India as one of the prime interventions to realize MDG goal 4 (WHO India, 2007).

Objectives

This paper examines the community's responses by specifically addressing the issue of neonatal, infant and child deaths in one of the largest states of India: Madhya Pradesh, and discusses the role of the Integrated Management of Neonatal and Childhood Illness (IMNCI) approach in combating neonatal deaths in the Shivpuri district. Further an attempt is made to understand how IMNCI reaches rural families in the Shivpuri District by trying to situate IMNCI in the cultural and economic context of nurturing newborns and explore the problems faced by the service providers in convincing the community members to seek medical help when an infant is born. Finally, it discusses the concerns and fears of the community people who are not able to access the health-care facility.

Data and Methodology

Madhya Pradesh is one of the highest populated states, with over 48 districts. Large interstate disparities of Infant Mortality Rate and under five mortality rate (U5MR) exist within India, posing differing degrees of complexity that IMNCI must combat. The health situation in MP is still very poor compared to other adjoining states. The other critical indicator that many infants die in the first year of their birth due to poor nutrition that their mothers received during pregnancy and inadequate immunization from tetanus, lack of hemoglobin, poor sanitation and health conditions (MPHDR, 2007). Most of the deaths occur in infancy due to water borne and respiratory diseases. These deaths indicate poverty, poor levels of awareness, an unclean environment, the poor state of the health delivery system, and the lack of post natal care. Shivpuri district of Madhya Pradesh has an IMR of 98 per 1000 live births, one of the highest in the state. Shivpuri has many distal factors such as geographically remote areas, low socio-economic status, and high illiteracy rates, in addition to the lack of health facilities that greatly contribute to its poor health indicators. IMNCI was piloted in the Shivpuri district, in Madhya Pradesh throughout 2005 and 2006; community workers have been gradually trained to begin IMNCI in Madhya Pradesh.

An emphasis has been placed on linking the information from diverse sources and attention is given to the development of more coherent and comprehensive multidisciplinary explanations to understand the processes leading to high infant mortality in the Shivpuri district. Using a medical anthropology perspective, the cultural beliefs with respect to peoples' social behavior towards infant and child mortality is understood. By applying both these perspectives, a systematic data is produced, thus linking cultural beliefs, knowledge production and biomedicine. However, there is a difference in how the public-health professionals conceptualize knowledge production and beliefs. They view *knowledge* production and *beliefs* as contrasting terms and define *knowledge* as the information that is "scientific," in contrast *beliefs* is used to connote "traditional ideas or folk models" (Pelto and Pelto, 1997). In the anthropological lexicon, *beliefs* and *knowledge* are not contrastive terms. For the purpose of this paper, the terms are used synonymously and the belief systems of the people are supported by the empirical data produced as a result of a survey conducted in the eight villages of the Shivpuri district.

For this research, the use of mixed method approach offered at least three advantages to the study. First the fieldwork enabled this research to obtain the empirical data on the knowledge received from the ANM or AWW and the referrals made by them, in addition to getting the qualitative data from the mothers interviewed. The quantitative data was gathered by the mothers using a questionnaire in the local language of the people. Second, the qualitative data was also gathered both from the mothers and the service providers (AWWs, ANMs, ASHAs, LHWs and unregistered medical providers). Third, the interpretation from both the qualitative and the quantitative data in analysis enabled this research to relate the perceptions of the people of the community, health-care providers to the IMNCI approach and the ways in which IMNCI could be improved to curtail infant and child mortality.

Results

For the purpose of analysis, the findings section is divided into two parts, in first part, responses from the health-care providers are discussed while in the second the experiences and narratives of the mothers of the infants and children are discussed separately. This would keep the two kinds of interviews separate for understanding the responses and challenges from the perspective of the health-care providers and mothers to the IMNCI.

Anganwadi Workers (AWW) the Crucial Players in IMNCI

According to UNICEF, almost fifty percent of newborn deaths occur during the first seven days after birth in India (UNICEF, 2007b). Emphasis is placed on AWWs as frontline workers as they are acquainted with the community they are residing in. An eight day training program is designed for the AWWs that incorporates an integrated and multidisciplinary learning approach while focusing on problem based learning, video presentations, and fieldwork. In addition, half of the training is dedicated to focusing on the management of young infants (0-2 months). Specifically, the training aims to increase the skill set of the individual community health worker so that she is able to instill prevention practices, counsel family members and identify, classify, treat (only a few cases) and refer sick children to the health-care center.

As of June 2007, 68 batches have received basic IMNCI training in the Shivpuri district. This has enabled 1,624 individuals to become familiar with the IMNCI strategy and placed them ready to perform in their given localities. Table 1 indicates the number and position of those who have undergone IMNCI training.

A trained AWW quoted "with the help of booklets we can classify and identify the illnesses of children which help to reduce the national IMR." Every AWW interviewed found the training beneficial and reported utilizing the skills which they have learned. Another AWW trained in IMNCI pointed out that after obtaining the training, she is able to refer sick children, "if I see a malnourished child on my way, I ask them whether you give him any treatment, if they say no, I refer him immediately. 'Go to Karera, or Shivpuri.' If she goes and get the treatment I feel very nice to know the fact that this child got admitted." Such quotes from the community health-care providers reiterate the importance of breastfeeding as a crucial step towards saving infants and children under five years of age. Another benefit rendered to the community is possible only through the trained AWWs who can identify sick children and send them to the nearby health center.

Table 1
Training Completed in Shivpuri District Since June 2007

Position	*Number Trained*
AWWs	1038
ANMs	247
Direct Supervisors	264
Medical Officers	62
Other (Government officials, trainers, NGO Reps.)	72
Total	1683

Source: Quarterly Report UNICEF, June 2007

Integral to successful implementation of IMNCI is the responsibility of the AWW to serve as a community resource for families of children under five when the child is ill. The goal of the AWW serving as the initial contact is to provide children with preliminary treatment, gauge the gravity of the condition, and refer the child to the government sector when the condition exceeds their training. Figure 1 illustrates the percentage of referrals being made by AWWs to the interviewed mothers since the IMNCI implementation. As shown in the figure 1, 17.3 percent (19 out of 110) of mothers have received a referral for their sick child when needed.

Before IMNCI implementation, no referrals were taking place as AWWs lacked this skill set of identifying any danger signs. Furthermore, it is important to note that not every child seen by the AWW requires a referral.

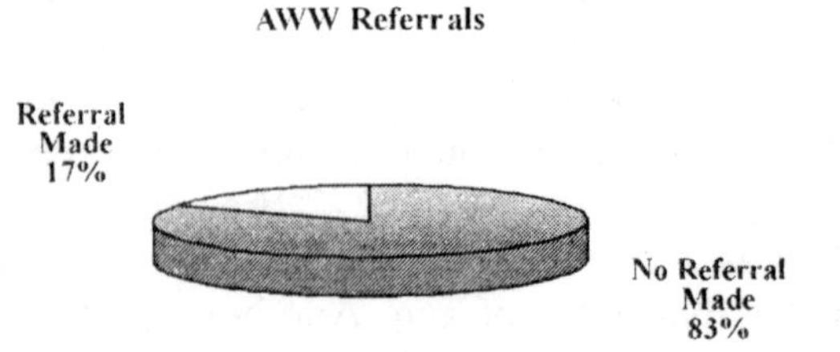

Source: Survey conducted in 2007; N=110

Fig. 1: Percentage of referrals being made by AWWs in the Study Area

Thus, the percentage of referrals made represents a positive change, and demonstrates the ability of an AWW to refer infants and children. It was observed that many AWWs who were interviewed could list and explain how to diagnose all danger signs directly from memory while others knew exactly what material to refer to quickly identify the danger signs. However, operating the weighing scale and completing the IMNCI forms still proved problematic for some AWWs, but it was quite apparent that a differential retention of IMNCI knowledge existed among them.

Another observation is that there is still a need for the full coverage of IMNCI. Out of the mothers surveyed with children under two years of age (with a gradual rollout of IMNCI beginning in 2005, only mothers with children under two years of age were quantified), eighty percent (46 out of 57) have never been seen by an AWW or ANM within their child's first week of life. It is important to note that with the government's initiatives such as Janani Suraksha Yojana to promoting the institutional deliveries and soliciting the mother to remain in the hospital for three days following labor, the responsibility of the AWW may only be to perform two home visits as opposed to three (MOHFW, 2006). However, only twelve percent (eight out of 57) of mothers surveyed received one visit, and five percent (three out of 57) received two.

An additional responsibility of the AWWs is also to inspire mothers regarding proper breastfeeding, hygiene, and early recognition of danger signs. This prevention based approach aims to instill proper knowledge to mothers and mitigate the severity of health maladies as they arise. Figure 2 depicts that 24 percent of the mothers surveyed (24 out of 99) reported being counseled regarding breastfeeding while 17.6 percent (12 out of 99) of mothers reported receiving more than one type of health promotion practice. However, 69 percent (68 out of 99) of mothers reported that they did not receive any kind of information from AWWs or ANMs.

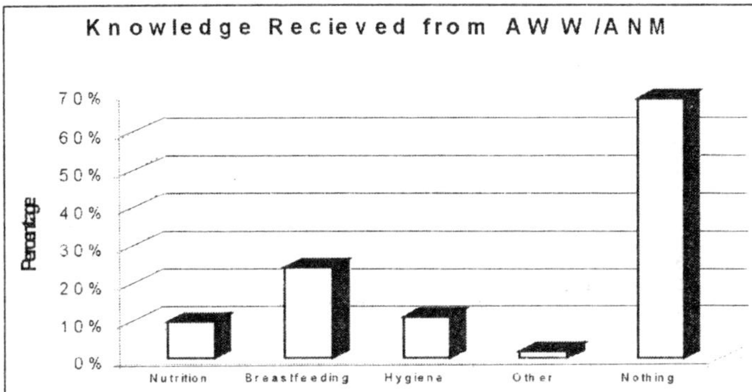

Source: Survey conducted in 2007; n=110

Fig. 2: Knowledge Imparted to Mothers by AWWs or ANMs

The skewed figures of the visits by the ANMs and AWWs and the knowledge imparted do not mean that IMNCI is unable to create an impact in the community. Since the socio-economic context is complex, issues surrounding the IMNCI implementation are explored to clarify the persisting situation. While the issues of economics and access often affect many members in the villages, decisions to seek the medical care of quacks (untrained medical practitioners), social norms and previous distrust in the government health-care services were some of the larger concerns that the AWWs were combating. An AWW from a village "Kota Naka" quoted "they do not believe in the government hospitals and they do not believe in medicines at the government hospitals. People think that private doctors give good medicines, because the government provides medicines for free. They think that free medicines do not work." However, in cases where families had positive experiences and beneficial outcomes, the credibility of the

AWWs has increased along with the trust in the medical health-care system. Although with each negative encounter, trust is lost in the government health-care system. A quote from an AWW at "Bhadarwas village" revealed that one girl died after she was given polio drops. This could have happened because she might be suffering from some other ailment, but since she died after having the vaccine; her parents blamed this AWW for killing their daughter. Such instances at times do pose a hindrance in convincing people about the efficacy of biomedicine from the government hospital to protect infants and young children.

Despite of all the aforementioned influences operating within the rural health-care system, AWWs are still finding ways to persevere and make changes which are saving lives of children in the Shivpuri district. The next part of this section brings out the issues from the community's perspective and presents how IMNCI is perceived by the community members.

IMNCI from the Community's Perspective

This part first discusses the importance of breastfeeding in an infant's life by exploring mothers' experiences with their infants. This provides an insight to their responses to breastfeeding, and these responses are informed by the diverse social, emotional and practical concerns (Marshall et al., 2007).

Importance of breastfeeding to infants

During the fieldwork and the interviews, it was observed that mothers were encouraged by the ANMs and AWWs to breastfeed their newborns at least for 6 months regularly and were advised not to wean children before the age of two years. It was noticed that the value attached to breastfeeding was synonymous with being a "good mother" and the benefits of breastfeeding, which is very popular in the medical discourse were constantly delivered by the health-care providers. However, the infant feeding practices and the beliefs vary across the cultures and the socio-economic context (Marshall et al., 2007). Until the IMNCI approach was actually introduced in the Shivpuri district, most of the mothers did not know the best position of breastfeeding a child due to which most of the infants were unable to receive full nourishment from the mother in the initial period of their lives. The next paragraph deals with the problems and crisis of infant's life and discusses the nuances in the first year of life.

What are the crises that an infant suffers in the first year of his / her life?

The faith in the efficacy of biomedicine is challenged very often, especially when an infant or a child falls sick and does not get timely help from the health-care provider. In many cases, the mothers were adamant against taking the child to the hospital, even though the ANM/ AWW constantly advised them to do so. One such case was encountered during the fieldwork where the mother was not willing to seek medical help, but on the request of the AWW, she finally sought medical help. The same mother initially lost her first son who had similar symptoms and admitted that "In case of that child, I wasn't able to pay much attention; I took him to the private doctor. He also had chest in-drawling and wheezing. The neighboring health worker came, but I could not take him to the hospital because it was evening. In the morning I took him, the baby died that day." After seeing the positive results, she instantly sought medical help as and when her child has some kind of sickness symptoms "I just go to the hospital and see the doctor...earlier I didn't have that much information I used to rub Vicks (a cold balm) on the baby. I did not have enough information. Now because of this madam, we have enough information. The baby is doing well he is able to feed properly. He is excreting and breathing well". While in the other case, a mother lost her 15 days old child due to tetanus. According to her, the AWW did not pay much attention towards the community and was busy doing chores at her home. This mother's second child was absolutely fine and did not have any symptoms of ailment.

When such compelling narratives of incompliance and indifference were presented in front of the AWWs, where they were pointed by the members of the community for not fulfilling their duties properly, they defended their stance by answering that many people say that they will not take their child anywhere. "We hardly care whether the child dies or survives." Such a belief pose a hindrance to the smooth working of the AWWs thus making harder for the AWWS to convince the parents of the ailing child and take him to the medical center. One AWW reported an incidence where she tried hard to convince the parents to take their sick daughter to the medical doctor. When with continuous coaxing the AWW did not succeed in convincing them, she stood against them and took the sick girl to the doctor. She said: "I will come along and I forcefully took her there. Now her daughter is doing well. Most of the people do not go, very few people go". This implies that it is very hard o convince people to take their ailing child to a medical doctor for treatment.

People who are less educated and have less understanding say that the government doctors give less effective medicines. A mother quoted that "the child had chest in drawing and wheezing for two days. I took him to the doctor to get an injection, but he did not get any relief". Lack of education and/or not getting quick relief creates a dilemma and restrains many people from seeking health-care from the qualified doctors and health practitioners. Furthermore, many people believed that the government medicines were not so good and were less effective.

Another perception of the community was revealed by an unlicensed health practitioner. An interview with him revealed that his treatment was cheaper than the government hospitals and thus he is very popular within the community. He said, "here they get the treatment for 20 rupees, there (the government hospital) they get treatment for 50 rupees. So why would they go there?" Furthermore, he added his opinion that "either they do not get good treatment in the hospital or they either come in the evening or after 12. If they come in the evening or after 12, they [the doctors] charge their fees." This implied that there was a fixed time during the day when the medical doctors were available within the health facility for free; however, in the evening if anybody visited the hospital, the doctors charged the consultation fee. After enquiring further into this matter, it was found out that the OPD ward of the hospital was opened during the first half of the day and in the evening and night only for the emergency cases. This question of not accessing the hospital facility was put up in front of the parents and they admitted that it was difficult for them to commute and reach the dispensary or the hospital as there was no transportation available. Moreover, they had to finish their daily chores before they could go to see the doctor or the health provider. In such cases, they rather preferred the private facility. One mother committed, "I go to the private facility, if I don't get any results then I go there [government hospital]". Thus, it was inferred in the end that private practitioners were favorite within the community because they charge less and were available any time of the day or night. Once that treatment failed, people resort to the government hospitals and mostly in critical situations implying that they wait to take a sick child to the hospitals and seek treatment from an unlicensed health practitioner until the child is extremely ill before taking the child for treatment in the hospital. It is thus very important to look at the belief system of the community members to reflect on their responses and perceptions toward the government health-care facilities.

Fears and Beliefs of the community members towards the government health facility

By further exploring into the matter of not accessing the health facilities, people from the rural areas who did not go very often into the town or the city expressed their concern of getting lost in the market area. One mother stated that "...if we go to the government hospital nobody asks where you are coming from. No body even recognizes us. If some worker assists us and tells us, then only we will be able to go there."

One AWW reported the fear people had for seeking the medical help in a nearby town or a city and how she dealt with those fears. According to her:

We [people] will forget the way in the market. We are not even sure whether somebody will admit us or not. So I say, I am coming with you. I admit them and at times I stay for one night and come back in the morning.

So she took initiatives in assisting people to the heath-care center as a result of which she was unavailable in the village to attend the cases of any ailment. After talking to the community members, financial constraint also came up as a major factor of deterring people to go to the health facilities. "We do not have money to pay for the traveling. We are poor people. What do we do, should we treat this child or feed the other children?" The issue of identity also came up as an important factor hindering people from seeking medical help. One mother reported that "If I go to the government hospital, no on asks me my name or where I have come from. Only if someone takes me, then only I will go." Thus the complexity of the socio-economic context needs more attention and an in depth research to unwind the processes and to make IMNCI a success in the Shivpuri district.

Discussion and Conclusion

The effectiveness and full implementation of IMNCI is contingent upon the continued support and coordination between the Government of India, health providers and members of the community. IMNCI is making significant strides towards improving neonatal and childhood health in rural Shivpuri but still has much ground to cover. Still the functioning of IMNCI is obstructed by many unforeseeable factors from reaching its maximum potential. As suggested by Andes (1992) "community contexts" are very important characteristics and play an important role to determine infant and child mortality. The existence of services does not necessarily translate into its utilization. As recorded during the fieldwork, most of the people who were aware of the nearest available health facility did not want to go either because they did not have money for transportation or could not take time off from their daily chores to take the child to the health-care center. Such impediments are quite common in a situation where both the parents have to strive hard to earn their daily wages. Furthermore, the social behavior towards use and disuse of biomedicine can not be neglected. Most of the members in the community were taking their children to the private, untrained, unlicensed health practitioner whose treatments are inexpensive compared to visiting a qualified government doctor. This practice was continued until they were cured by him, but in emergency situations most of the people contacted the nearby health center or the government hospital. This behavior also demonstrates the ideal/real dichotomy that persists within the community. The ideal system promoted by the service providers is through using biomedicine by seeking help from the trained personnel, but in real practice people are seeking help from untrained personnel without questioning his or her credibility. Furthermore, this also points towards the presumed behavior quoted by Richards (1969) where people tend to follow specific behavior of other members within the community followed, such as seeking medical-care from an unlicensed practitioner, questioning the credibility of the qualified doctors and the hospitals.

Thus to conclude it was observed that successful attempts were made to actively involve the community through the recruitment of the Anganwadi Workers (AWW) for providing nutritional supplements to young children, educating mothers and providing assistance in the maternal and child health services. However, there was lack of dissemination of information, and mothers were still unaware of whether their child needed prompt care or not. In certain cases, the service provider was not present to assist the mother and take the ailing child to the health center. Information dissemination to the rural community needs to be improved so that people are aware and can access IMNCI services. The lack of information in the community presents one of the largest barriers to successful IMNCI program implementation. Hence the successful implementation of communication strategy will provide essential information, and will create awareness among the community members of the villages regarding the responsibilities of the ANMs and AWWs and the services currently being offered in their area. Furthermore, knowledge of such services will enable villagers to seek the assistance and support of AWWs which will ensure the complete access to information and will check the infant and under five mortality rates.

Acknowledgements

The fieldwork for the paper was facilitated by UNICEF. Special Thanks to Genessa, Martin and Rachel for their support during the fieldwork.

References

Andes, N. (1992), "Child Survival in Community Contexts", *Central Issues in Anthropology* 10: 16-22.

Elling, R.H. (1981), "Political Economy, Cultural Hegemony, and Mixes of Traditional and Modern Medicine", *Social Science and Medicine* 15A: 89-99.

Jain, A.K., and Visaria, P., (1988), "Infant Mortality in India: An Overview", In: A. K. Jain and P. Visaria, (eds.), *Infant Mortality in India: Differentials and Determinants*. New Delhi: Sage Publicaitons, pp. 23-64.

Kidanemariam, A. and Gallagher, E.B. (1992), "Theoretical Perspectives for Explaining Infant Mortality in the Third World", *Central Issues in Anthropology* 10: 8-15.

Madhya Pradesh Human Development Report (2007), http://www.dif. Madhya Pradesh.gov.in/MADHYA PRADESHHDR 2007.htm accessed on July 10, 2007.

Marshall, J.L., Godfrey, M. and Renfrew, M. J. (2007), "Being a 'Good Mother': Managing Breastfeeding and Merging Identities", *Social Science and Medicine* 65: 2147-2159.

Ministry of Health and Family Welfare (2006), *Janani Suraksha Yojana: Guidelines for Implementation*. New Delhi: Dept. of Family Welfare.

Morgan, L.M. (1987), "Dependency Theory in the Political Economy of Health: An Anthropological Critique", *Medical Anthropology Quarterly (New Series)* 1(2): 131-154.

Pelto, P.J. and Pelto, G.H. (1997), "Studying Knowledge, Culture, and Behavior in Applied Medical Anthropology, *Medical Anthropology Quarterly* 11(2): 147-163.

Richards, C.E. (1969), "Presumed Behavior: Modification of the Ideal-Real Dichotomy", *American Anthropologist (New Series)* 71(6): 1115-1117.

Scheper-Hughes, N. (1987), *"The Cultural Politics of Child Survival"*, In: Schepher-Hughes, (ed.), *Child Survival*. Dordrecht: Reidel, pp. 1-29.

UNICEF (2007a), *Integrated Management of Neonatal and Childhood Illness (IMNCI) Making Change Possible for India's Newborns: A Working Paper*. New Delhi: UNICEF.

UNICEF (2007b), *Integrated Management of Childhood and Neonatal Illnesses*. "Making Change Possible for India's Newborns", http://www.unicef.org/india/health_369.htm accessed on July 25, 2007.

WHO India, (2007), Chapter-II *Goal 4: Reduce Child Mortality in Millennium Development Goals and Health-India,* 12-17. http://www.whoindia.org/LinkFiles/MDG_Chapter-02.pdf accessed on July 29: 2005.

20

Influence of Education on Health in India

Rekha Gupta

Introduction

Education and health are two basic objectives of development; they are important means as well as an end in themselves. Health is central to well-being, while education is essential for a life to be capable of making authentic choice and living a quality life, both are fundamental in the broader notion of expanded human capabilities that lie at the heart of all the development of nations. At the same time education plays a key role in the ability of a developing country to absorb modern technology and to develop the capacity for self-sustaining growth and development. Moreover, health is a prerequisite for increases in productivity, while achievement in education largely relies on adequate health as well. Thus, both health and education can also be seen as vital components of growth or development of economies (Sen and Dreze, 1995). Education and health are treated together because of their inherent relationship. The connections between health and education include similar analytical treatment, because both are the means of human capital (Schultz, 1961), important basic needs (Streeten, 1977), important indicator of human development index (UNDP, 1990), and important factor in the process of expanding the capabilities of people (Sen, 1999).

Education plays an important role in improving health. Greater education capital improves the return to investments in health, because many health programs rely on basic skills often learned at school, including personal hygiene and sanitation. Education is also needed for the formation and training of health personnel. The relationship between education and health has been studied widely by economists, sociologists and health researchers. Many of the researchers have found significant and positive relationship between education and health improvements. With the use of time lag and semi-log regression equation Tilak (2005) has find that the effect of secondary and higher education on infant mortality is confined to rural areas, but in case of urban areas, the regression coefficients are not statistically significant (at 10% level) and also in case of life expectancy, another important measure of health conditions, also, the effect of secondary and higher education is significant in rural areas, but not in urban areas, though in all cases, the sign of the regression coefficient is positive but not statistically significant.

Ethiopia Demographic and Health Survey (2005) also find that the relationship between education, fertility, and health is well documented. Educated women have fewer children, are more likely to use family planning, and receive better health care. Women's education also influences the health of her children. The children of an educated mother has higher chances of living long and healthy life than to a children of an uneducated mother, moreover they are less likely to face nutritional deficits, and more likely to receive appropriate care when sick. Such as with the help of multilevel discrete-time hazard model estimated with data from the National Family Health Survey II, Kravdal (2004) find that the average education of women in a census enumeration area has a strong impact on child mortality, in addition to the effect of the mother's own education. Kennedy (2002) has examined the strength of the empirical relationship between education and health for Australia and Canada with three important explanations of the education and health relationship: technical efficiency, allocative efficiency and time preference explanations and he find that education is indeed related to health and to a very similar extent in both countries.

Adriana et al. (2002) examined one of the mechanisms by which education may impact health outcomes. They investigated whether education is correlated with adoption of newer prescription drugs. If more educated people are more likely to adopt newer drugs, due to more information or better ability to learn, and those newer drugs improve health, then this may be one mechanism by which education leads to better health. They find that education is correlated with the purchase of drugs that are more recently approved, after controlling for the medical condition, individual income and health insurance status. The impact of education is generally felt only for chronic conditions, where prescriptions are bought regularly for the same condition. This suggests that the more educated are better able to learn from experience.

As the World Bank (1980a; 1980b) has argued, fulfillment of any one of the basic needs (nutrition, safe drinking water, health, shelter and education) can be beneficial to the fulfillment of each of the others and, conversely, lack of any one has adverse effect on the satisfaction of other basic needs. However, education was accorded a higher place among the several basic needs: education forms a critically important factor in the basic needs framework, as it is fundamental to the satisfaction of all basic needs (Noor, 1980). The interrelation between educations on health resulting in human development (Noor, 1980) is given in the following frame work (figure1)

It has been explained in the figure 1 that education influences basic human needs such as food, shelter, water and health. Increase in these basic needs leads to higher production, reduces fertility and increases longevity which influences human development. Further there is a feed back mechanism influencing education.

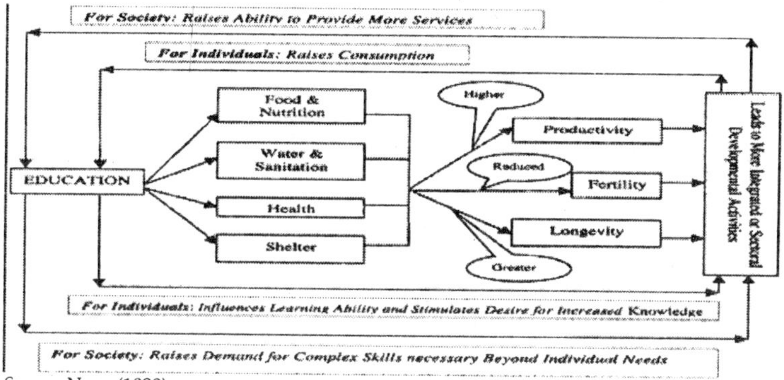

Source: Noor (1980)

Fig. 1: Framework of Basic Needs of Education

Keeping the aforesaid framework mechanism in view, in this paper, an attempt is made to understand the influence of education on health and social outcomes.

Objectives

1. To find out do education has any significant role in health outcomes in India?
2. Do variation in educational level affects health outcomes?
3. Do women's educations have more contribution in health improvement?

Data and Methodology

Data of the variables has been taken from secondary sources; they are UGC annual report, Selected Educational Statistics, Annual Report of Health Information of India. In this study ten years time series data has taken. The data of health indicators has taken from Annual Report of Health Information of India from year 1995 to 2004. The data of enrolment in higher education has taken from UGC annual report from year 1990-1991 to 1999-2000 (because of time lag of five years). The data of enrolment in secondary education has taken from Selected Educational Statistics from year 1990-1991 to 1999-2000 (because of time lag of five years). The data of enrolment in primary education has taken from Selected Educational Statistics from year 1987-1998 to 1996-1997 (because of time lag of eight years).Data used for the present study is given in the Appendix-1.

It is assumed that improving the education of a population will improve their health outcomes. The relationship between education and health has been studied widely by economists, sociologists and health researchers. Whilst there is general acceptance of a positive relationship between education and health, explanations of this relationship are still much debated. The demographic and health surveys conducted in more than 90 countries have consistently shown a positive relationship between education and improved health, lower fertility and lower infant mortality. But many questions remain: At what level of education among women and men does an improvement in health become noticeable? Is women's education play more significant role in improving health?

Variables Considered for Analysis

The term education also has a broad sense. There is using enrolment in different level of education as indicator of education such as Enrolment in Primary Education (PE), Enrolment in Secondary Education (SE), and Enrolment in Higher Education (HE) in the study. Enrolment in education has not immediately effect on health indicators. So the study used the variables of enrolment in different level of education with time lag. The average year of completing higher and secondary education is five year and eight year of primary education. So here we have taken five year lag for higher and secondary education and eight year time lag for primary education.

The concept of health improvement or outcomes has very large ambit. The question is which indicators of health to be used that would be the good representative of health outcomes. Considering above mention facts this study has taken the basic health indicators such as Birth Rate (BR), Death Rate (DR), Infant Mortality Rate (IMR), Total Fertility Rate (TFR) and Expectation of Life (EoL) as representative of Health indicators (SRS, 2007).

For the analysis of the role of education on health indicators, simple regression analysis has been used in the study.

The Regression Equations are given as follows:

$Y_{i1}=\beta_i + \beta_i X_{i1} + \mu_i$ (1)

$Y_{i2}=\beta_i + \beta_i X_{i1} + \mu_i$ (2)

$Y_{i3}=\beta_i + \beta_i X_{i1} + \mu_i$ (3)

$Y_{i4}=\beta_i + \beta_i X_{i1} + \mu_i$ (4)

$Y_{i5}=\beta_i + \beta_i X_{i1} + \mu_i$ (5)

$Y_{i1}=\beta_i + \beta_i X_{i2} + \mu_i$ (6)

$Y_{i2}=\beta_i + \beta_i X_{i2} + \mu_i$ (7)

$Y_{i3}=\beta_i + \beta_i X_{i2} + \mu_i$ (8)

$Y_{i4}=\beta_i + \beta_i X_{i2} + \mu_i$ (9)

$Y_{i5}=\beta_i + \beta_i X_{i2} + \mu_i$ (10)

$Y_{i1}=\beta_i + \beta_i X_{i3} + \mu_i$ (11)

$Y_{i2}=\beta_i + \beta_i X_{i3} + \mu_i$ (12)

$Y_{i3}=\beta_i + \beta_i X_{i3} + \mu_i$ (13)

$Y_{i4}=\beta_i + \beta_i X_{i3} + \mu_i$ (14)

$Y_{i5}=\beta_i + \beta_i X_{i3} + \mu_i$ (15)

Where,

i- year/s.

- Y_{i1} is Birth Rate,
- Y_{i2} is Death Rate,
- Y_{i3} is IMR,
- Y_{i4} is TFR,
- Y_{i5} is Expectation of Life, and
- β_i is regression coefficient in each equation,
- X_{i1} is Enrolment in Primary Education with time lag of eight years,
- X_{i2} is Enrolment in Secondary Education with time lag of five years,
- X_{i3} is Enrolment in Higher Education with time lag of five years,
- μ_i is error term in each equation.

Analysis is carried out by using the data at different points of time (i) at all India level and by sex wise to show the disparities in education by sex. Regression analysis results are given in the Table 1 and 2.

Results

The regression equations from 1 to 5 gives the influence of Primary education on health indicators, equation 6-10 shows influence of Secondary education on health indicators followed by equation 11-15 shows influence of Higher education on health indicators in India

Table 1
Influence of Different Levels of Education and Health Indicators in India

	Health Indicators				
Level of Education	*Birth Rate*	*Death Rate*	*IMR*	*TFR*	*EoL*
Constant Enrolment in Primary Education (PE)					
R^2	.917	.774	.782	.842	.929
Adjusted R^2	.907	.746	.755	.822	.920
Beta	-.958	-.880	-.884	-.917	.964
T	-9.403	-5.235	-5.356	-6.518	10.256
Sig.	.000	.001	.001	.000	.000
Constant Enrolment in Secondary Education (SE)					
R^2	.932	.889	.926	.918	.970
Adjusted R^2	.924	.875	.917	.907	.966
Beta	-.966	-.943	-.962	-.958	.985
T	-10.511	-7.997	-10.024	-9.449	16.027
Sig.	.000	.000	.000	.000	.000
Constant Enrolment in Higher Education (HE)					
R^2	.960	.936	.962	.932	.988
Adjusted R^2	.954	.928	.957	.923	.986
Beta	-.980	-.967	-.981	-.965	.994
T	-13.770	-10.784	-14.142	-10.442	25.249
Sig.	.000	.000	.000	.000	.000

The analysis shows (Table 1) that there is 96 percent contribution of primary education on birth rate while it reduces death rate by 88 percent, 89 percent in IMR, 91 Percent in TFR, and 96 percent in expectation of life. The enrolment in primary education is significantly negatively related to birth rate, death rate, IMR, and TFR and significantly positively related to expectation of life. It means that increase in enrolment in primary education wills indirectly influences reeducation in birth rate, death rate, IMR, and TFR and will increase the expectation of life.

In the case of enrolment in secondary education (Table 1) there is around 97 percent contribution of secondary education on birth rate whereas around 94 percent in death rate, 96 percent in IMR, 95Percent in TFR, and 98 percent in expectation of life. The enrolment in Secondary education is significantly negatively related to birth rate, death rate, IMR, and TFR and significantly positively related to expectation of life. It means as well as enrolment in secondary education will indirectly affects in reducing, birth rate, death rate, IMR, and TFR will increase in expectation of life.

In the case of enrolment in higher education (Table 1) there is around 97 percent contribution of higher education in birth rate whereas around 94 percent in death rate, 96 percent in IMR, 95 Percent in TFR, and 98 percent in expectation of life. The enrolment in higher education is highly significantly negatively related to birth rate, death rate, IMR, and TFR and significantly positively related to expectation of life. It means as well as enrolment in higher education will influence indirectly in reduction of, birth rate, death rate, IMR, and TFR, will increase expectation of life. The regression analysis clearly shows that increase in education level will influence reduction in fertility and mortality indicators and increases health indicator.

To understand the influence of level of education (Higher education) of men and women on health indicator, regression analysis has been used. The results are given in Table 2. Enrolment in higher education of women significantly negatively influences Birth rate (-.985), Death rate (-.958), Infant Mortality Rate (-.978), Total Fertility Rate (-.970) and positively influences Expectation of life .996) reveals that women higher education likely to influence reduction in fertility and increase in longevity.

Table 2
Results of Regression Analysis Showing Influence of Higher Education on Health Indicators by Sex: India

Gender	*Level of Education*	*Health Indicators* Birth Rate	Death Rate	IMR	TFR	EoL
Constant Enrolment in Higher Education						
Women	R^2	.969	.917	.956	.941	.992
	Adjusted R^2	.966	.907	.950	.933	.991
	Beta	-.985	-.958	-.978	-.970	.996
	t	-15.919	-9.417	-13.115	-11.269	31.049
	Sig.	.000	.000	.000	.000	.000
Men	R^2	.935	.944	.955	.908	.969
	Adjusted R^2	.927	.938	.950	.897	.965
	Beta	-.967	-.972	-.977	-.953	.984
	t	-10.710	-11.662	-13.072	-8.899	15.847
	Sig.	.000	.000	.000	.000	.000

Similarly enrolment in higher education of men (Table 2) shows that BR -.967, DR -.972, IMR -.977, TFR -.953, and Expectation of life .984 indicates that higher education among men positively related to health indicators and negatively to fertility indicators.

From the above analysis it was evident that education play a manor role in determining the health .In general presumption that basic and primary education is well enough to improve health outcomes but the findings of this paper shows that secondary and higher education plays quite substantial role in improving the health of masses. Moreover women's education at higher level plays greater role in improving the health of the family as well as women health itself then to the education of a men (Beta of EoL: Women .996 and Men .984, Table 2).

Conclusions

The contribution of education to health improvement is widely recognized. All level of education has a significant and positive role in health improvements however higher levels of education have more to do with health improvements. As has been discussed in the paper that lots of the literature on human development mainly concentrated on the role of literacy and primary education on health improvements, and the role of secondary or higher education was not discussed, assuming that secondary and higher education has no role at all in improving health. But the findings of the paper show that it is secondary and higher education that have larger impact on the health improvements. And it is also true that women's education has strong association with health improvement than education of males. As people with higher education would be more aware of the need for preventive healthcare measures and also would be aware of the availability of general healthcare facilities, leading to the enhanced awareness within households regarding healthcare. Higher level of education can influence the health of the population; other way by providing skilled quality of education to women will have more impact on health conditions of the society leads to human development.

References

Adriana, Lleras-Muney, and Lichtenberg, Frank R. (2002), *The Effect of Education on Medical Technology Adoption: Are the More Educated More Likely to Use New Drugs?* National Bureau of Economic Research Working Paper # 9185, September.

Ethiopia Demographic and Health Survey (2005), *The Impact of Education on Health Outcomes*. Addis Ababa: Ministry of Health Government of Ethiopia.

Kennedy, Steven (2002), *The Relationship between Education and Health in Australia and Canada*. SEDAP Research Paper No. 93.

Kravdal, Oystein (2004), "Child Mortality in India: The Community - Level Effect of Education", *Population Studies* 58(2): 177-192.

Noor, A. (1980), *Education and Basic Needs*. Staff Working Paper No. 450. Washington, D.C.: World Bank.

Sen, A., and Dreze, J. (1995), *India: Economic Development and Social Opportunity*. New York: Oxford University Press.

Sen, A. (1999), *Development as Freedom*. Clarendon: Oxford University Press.

Streeten, Paul (1977), "The Distinctive Features of Basic Needs Approach to Development", *International Development Review* 3: 8–16.

Schultz, Theodore W. (1961), "Investment in Human Capital", *American Economic Review* 51(1): 1–15.

Tilak, J.B.G. (2005), "Post-elementary Education, Poverty and Development in India", International *Journal of Educational Development* 27: 435–445.

UNDP (1990), Human Development Report 1990. New York: Oxford University Press.

World Bank (1980a), *Education Sector Paper,* Washington, D. C.: World Bank.

World Bank (1980b), *Poverty and Human Development,* Washington, D.C.: World Bank.

Annexure - I Data

Table A1
Health Indicators in India

Year	*Birth Rate*	*Death Rate*	*Infant Mortality Rate*	*Total Fertility Rate*	*Expectation of Life at birth (Combined)*
1995	28.3	9.0	74	3.5	61.1
1996	27.5	9.0	72	3.4	61.4
1997	27.2	8.9	71	3.3	61.7
1998	26.5	9.0	72	3.2	61.9
1999	26.1	8.7	70	3.2	62.2
2000	25.8	8.5	68	3.2	62.5
2001	25.4	8.4	66	3.1	62.7
2002	25.0	8.1	63	3.0	63.0
2003	24.8	8.0	60	3.0	63.2
2004	24.1	7.5	58	2.9	63.5

Source: Annual Report of Health Information of India, Ministry of Health & Family Welfare, Government of India

Table A2
Data on Enrolment in Primary, Secondary and Higher Education in India

Year	*Total Enrolment in Primary Education*	*Total Enrolment in Secondary Education*	*Total Enrolment in Higher Education*	*Women Enrolment in Higher Education*
1987-88	119746845	–	–	–
1988-89	121221148	–	–	–
1989-90	123239879	–	–	–
1990-91	131401287	19057399	5043271	1421715
1991-92	136022852	19303198	5265886	1685926
1992-93	148115121	20902815	5534966	1811115
1993-94	144078797	20546677	5817249	1931327
1994-95	149331503	21804395	6113929	2064982
1995-96	150748428	22507501	6574005	2363607
1996-97	151873168	24274490	6842598	2514511
1997-98	–	24890774	7260418	2722062
1998-99	–	25427756	7705520	2932993
1999-2000	–	25826419	8050607	3112090

Source:

1. Selected Educational Statistics, Ministry of Human Resource Development, Government of India,
2. Annual Reports, University Grant Commission.

21

Community Health Management during Natural Disasters

Pradeep Kumar Parida

Introduction

Disasters are rarely expected and can be disruptive to our everyday lives. They can result in property damage, injury, and emotional stress. While we cannot control when or where disasters strike, we can take steps to protect ourselves and our family members. We can learn how to prepare for disasters. The number of people threatened by floods, landslides, volcanic eruptions and other natural hazards has dramatically increased over the last decades. In addition, soil erosion, salinisation, subsidence and other forms of land degradation pose continuous threats to food security and environmental quality. Therefore, natural disaster preparedness, hazard prevention and mitigation have become issues of global importance.

In the last three decades (1970-1990), extreme natural phenomena have caused increasing economic and social losses. For this reason, in 1989, the United Nations General Assembly passed Resolution 44/236, designating the 1990s as the International Decade for Natural Disaster Reduction (IDNDR). This was considered the first universal effort for disaster prevention and mitigation, and it highlighted the idea that human beings have increased responsibility for planning and for regulating what the environment can be exposed to and how it should be used. The United Nations community intensified its efforts to increase and improve information, education, and public awareness around natural disasters. Prevention and early warning systems were strengthened, as were emergency responses, damage restoration, and reconstruction processes. However, in spite of all these efforts and actions, the occurrence and intensity of potentially damaging natural phenomena, such as drought, floods, landslides, tornados, seismic activity, and tropical cyclones, have increased in recent years. These phenomena have caused losses that endanger the development of many communities and have affected, in particular, the poorest sectors of society. This paper examines the disaster situation in India and discusses the health management during disaster situation.

Disaster Situation in India

India has been traditionally vulnerable to natural disasters on account of its unique geo-climatic conditions (Parida, 2002). Floods, droughts, cyclones, earthquakes and landslides have been recurrent phenomena. About 60 percent of the landmass is prone to earthquakes of various intensities; over 40 million hectares is prone to floods; about 8 percent of the total area is prone to cyclones and 68 percent of the area is susceptible to drought (Parida, 2004). In the decade 1990-2000, an average of about 4344 people lost their lives and about 30 million people were affected by disasters every year. The loss in terms of private, community and public assets has been astronomical. Each year disasters also account for loss of thousands of crores in terms of social and community assets. For example to put it specifically, the super cyclone in Orissa in October, 1999 and the Bhuj earthquake in Gujarat in January, 2001 underscored the need to adopt a multi dimensional endeavour involving diverse scientific, engineering, financial and social processes; the need to adopt multi disciplinary and multi-sectoral approach and incorporation of risk reduction in the developmental plans and strategies. One of such endeavours required at present is to enhance the public education programme for acquiring the knowledge and developing appropriate behaviour, attitudes and level of involvement to prevent disasters.

The aim of public education programmes should be to create what is often called a 'culture of safety', where awareness of risk and adoption of risk reducing measures are part of daily life. Obviously, achieving this 'culture of safety' is a long-term process. A programme of activities is needed to reach different target groups, explain and reinforce messages that give people opportunities to think about, question and validate the information they receive. Table 1 reflect the panic of natural disasters in India

Table 1
Damage due to Natural Disasters in India

Year	*People Affected (Lakh)*	*Houses and Buildings Partially/ Totally Damaged*	*Amount of Property Damage /Loss (in Rs crores)*
1985	595.6	2,449,878	40.06
1986	550.0	2,049,277	30.74
1987	483.4	2,919,380	20.57
1988	101.5	242,533	40.63
1989	30.1	782,340	20.41
1990	31.7	1,019,930	10.71
1991	342.7	1,190,109	10.90
1992	190.9	570,969	20.05
1993	262.4	1,529,916	50.80
1994	235.3	1,051,223	10.83
1995	543.5	2,088,355	40.73
1996	549.9	2,376,693	50.43
1997	443.8	1,103,549	n.a.
1998	521.7	1,563,405	.72
1999	501.7	3,104,064	1020.97
2000	594.3	2,736,355	800.00
2001	788.2	846,878	12000.00

Source: NDM Division, Ministry of Home Affairs, 2002.

Disasters and Public Health

According to the International Federation of the Red Cross and Red Crescent Societies, in 2002, international disasters affected 608 million people and killed more than 24,000. Disasters are unusual public health events that overwhelm the coping capacity of the affected community and community population, women and children (Cowen et al., 1973). They are generally classified according to the immediate trigger of the event:

- *Natural disasters,* where the trigger is a natural phenomenon or hazard (biological, geological, or climatic);
- *Technological disasters,* such as chemical spills; or
- *Complex emergencies,* such as civil wars and conflicts.

Health and economic losses from natural disasters disproportionately affect developing countries—which account for more than 90 percent of natural disaster-related deaths—and predominantly affect the poor within those countries. Although the total economic loss in dollars is greater in developed countries, the percentage of losses relative to the gross national product in developing countries far exceeds that of developed nations. Natural disasters are not random. Earthquakes and volcanic eruptions occur along the fault lines between two tectonic plates on land or the ocean floor. And the areas subject to seasonal floods, droughts, or tropical storms (cyclones, hurricanes, or typhoons) are well known, although global warming is redrawing the map of climatic disasters. Local populations, however, may not recognize the risks in these areas. Technological disasters and complex emergencies are less predictable. Few countries are immune to the public health risks from hazardous chemical substances (from insecticides to industrial by-products) or discarded radioactive material. Technological hazards increase rapidly with the largely unregulated industrialization of developing countries and the globalization of the chemical industry, suggesting that chemical emergencies may become a major source of disasters in the 21st century. A population's vulnerability to all types of disasters depends on demographic growth, the pace of urbanization, settlement in unsafe areas, environmental degradation, climate change, and unplanned development. Poverty also increases vulnerability due to lack of access to healthy and safe environments, poor education and risk awareness, and limited coping capacity.

Immediate Health Impact

Short-term losses fall under three categories that have both direct and indirect effects:

1. Illness, disability, and death; 2.Direct losses in infrastructure; and 3. Loss or disruption in health care delivery

The immediate health burden depends on the nature of the hazard. In the aftermath of a major disaster, authorities must meet extraordinary demands with resources that cannot begin to meet even basic health needs and that often have been drained by the immediate emergency response. Disasters related to natural events may affect the transmission of pre-existing infectious disease, but the imminent risk of large outbreaks in the aftermath of natural disasters is often overstated. In the short-term, an increased number of hospital visits due to diarrheal diseases, acute respiratory infections, dermatitis, and other causes should be expected following most disasters. In the medium term, heavy rainfalls may affect the transmission of vector-borne diseases, for example, from residual water that may contribute to an explosive rise in mosquitoes.

Earthquakes can cause a large number of injuries. While most are not life-threatening, the injured do require immediate medical care from health facilities that are often unprepared, damaged, or totally destroyed. Authorities must provide services to a displaced population, rehabilitate health facilities, restore normal services, and strengthen communicable disease surveillance and control. They must also attend to the long-term consequences, such as permanent disabilities, mental health problems, and possibly increases in rates of heart disease and chronic disease.

Tsunamis are catastrophic tidal waves caused by earthquakes on the ocean floor. Waves can travel several hundred kilometres per hour and can be as much as 10 meters high when they reach shore. Damage on shore can be extensive, and usually the number of deaths far exceeds the number of survivors with severe injuries.

Volcanoes cause serious problems, yet are often overlooked because of long periods of inactivity. Eruptions are p receded by a period of volcanic activity, which gives people time for scientific monitoring, warning, and preparation. Some issues, such as ash fall, lethal gases, lava flow, and projectiles, although of public concern, are of minimal health significance. Falling ash affects transportation, communications, water sources, treatment plants, and reservoirs. Volcanic ash and gases can irritate the eye membranes and upper respiratory tract and can exacerbate chronic lung conditions, but usually cause little sickness in the general population. The most important risk is posed by pyroclastic flows (hot gas, ash, and rock travelling with intense speed from the blast) and *lahars*, or gas, ash, rock, and/or mud flows mixed with water, caused by the rapid melting of a volcano's snow cap or by heavy rains on unstable accumulations of ash. Historically, pyroclastic explosions or *lahars* have caused about 90 percent of the casualties from volcanic eruptions. Other concerns are potential contamination of water supplies by minerals from ash; displacement of large populations for an undetermined time; related sanitation problems; and mental health needs.

Climate disasters include seasonal floods, hurricanes, and typhoons. Seasonal floods cause increased incidence of diarrheal diseases, respiratory infections, dermatitis, and snake bites. The risk of compromised water supplies depends on the condition of the community's water supply before the disaster. Saline contamination is a long-term issue following sea surges and tsunamis. Prolonged flooding endangers local agriculture and sometimes means large-scale food assistance will be needed. The primary health concerns are overcrowded living conditions and poor water and sanitation in temporary settlements and other areas where services have deteriorated or are suspended. Sickness and death result from high winds, heavy rainfall, and storm surges caused by tropical storms, such as hurricanes and typhoons. Survivors of such disasters require psychosocial services.

Long-Term Impacts

The health sector bears a significant share of the long-term economic burden from disasters. The value of direct damage and indirect losses together make up the total cost of disasters. Direct damage refers to the material losses that occur as an immediate consequence of disaster: hospital beds lost, equipment and medicines destroyed, health service facilities damaged or affected, and pipes and water plants destroyed. Indirect losses refer to the production of goods and services that are lost as an outcome of the disaster, and to the resulting reduced income. The health burden of disasters includes damage to housing, schools, channels of communication, and industry. Damage to hospitals, health facilities, and water and sewage systems have the biggest impact on health. The long-term health burden includes loss of medical care, interruptions in the control of communicable disease and other public health programs, and loss of laboratory support and diagnostic capabilities of hospitals. A common misperception is that the damage to critical health facilities is promptly repaired, but experience shows that damaged health infrastructure recovers at a slower pace than other service sectors, such as trade, roads, bridges, telecommunications, and housing. Damage to water and sewage systems can also have a great impact on health. In severe flooding, the sudden interruption of these services coincides with the direct effect on the transmission of water-borne or vector-borne diseases. In the case of earthquakes, the number of people adversely affected by water shortage may far exceed those injured or suffering direct material loss. As in the case of health care facilities, the rehabilitation of public water systems is usually slow.

Factors Influencing Health

1. *Overcrowding and Poor Shelter:* Increasing risk of rapid spread of diarrhoeal disease and measles; malaria and risk of hypothermia in infants due to "open to sky" shelter.
2. *Poor Sanitation, Hygiene and Contaminated Water Supply:* Lack of soap and water and clean protected container to carry them.
3. *Breakdown of Health Services:* Increasing the risk that children have missed out on immunization, non availability of treatment of common illnesses, inadequate solid waste disposal increasing the menace of flies and mosquitoes, disturbed and contaminated water supply; and breakdown of drainage system because of cyclone, earthquake and failure of electricity.
4. *Animals:* During such upheavals, even animal populations are displaced and they rush to human habitations carrying with them diseases. Animals even sweep through refugee settlement adding to dirt and unhygienic. Rats and such reptiles are often seen after earthquake.
5. *Generation of Extra Waste:* Remains of the relief rushed to the affected areas generate extra waste, e.g., plastics, bottles, cans, used food packets, papers, clothes etc. Large amount of leftover plastic if embedded in the soil may in due course lead to problems with crop productivity and soil percolation; and may play havoc in natural and artificial drainage of the area.
6. *Disposal of Dead Bodies:* Not properly disposed of bodies being feasted upon by dogs and vultures and such other animals. Traditional burning puts pressure on wood resources and ads to air pollution.
7. *Inadequate Food Supply and Storage:* This increases the risk of malnutrition and susceptibility to infectious illnesses. Food may be contaminated with fungus and bacteria; or may be rotten and fermented.
8. *Change of Environment:* Increases the risk of malaria due to migration to endemic zones and having low immunity.

9. *Vulnerability to Physical Injuries:* Especially in children, elderly persons and pregnant mothers.
10. *Social, Emotional and Psychological Problems:* family separation, displacement, violence or abuse and personal loss of lives and livelihoods.
11. *Lack of Financial Resources at Personal Level:* Loss of living place and working place, physical disability, loss of earning member of family etc. lead to inability to spend on health.

Emotional Health Issues for Victims

Disasters affect people in many ways. In some disaster situations it may mean loss of loved ones, including relatives, friends, neighbours, or family pets. In others, it means loss of home and property, furnishings, and important or cherished belongings. Sometimes it means starting over with a new home or business. The emotional effects life and creates mental illness, and have long term health impact (Rahe, 1979), of loss and disruption may show up immediately or may appear many months later. It is very important to understand that there is a natural grieving process following any loss, and that a disaster of any size will cause unusual and unwanted stress in those attempting to reconstruct their lives.

Disaster Response and Prevention

To alleviate conditions in disaster-stricken areas, environmental health control measures must be undertaken before and in the aftermath of disaster, and whenever possible, during the disaster itself. In determining courses of action at these various stages, a given measure should be judged not only according to its technical feasibility and the availability of resources, but also according to the extent to which the measure is directed at returning environmental conditions to pre-disaster levels.

Factors to consider in making decisions about actions include areas of priority of intervention, the priority of needs for the various environmental health services and the availability of manpower. The major factor that determines the priority of areas for intervention is the presence or absence of disease-related risks in the areas in which disaster victims reside. The highest priority should be accorded to environmental health services that are essential to the protection of the well-being of individuals in high-risk areas. The cooperation of persons in high risk areas should be sought, and they should be actively involved in the provision of services. The minimum levels of necessary services that must be provided are the following:

1. Adequate shelter for the displaced persons
2. Sufficient quantities of accessible drinking water
3. Protection of food supplies against contamination
4. Protection of individuals in affected populations against vector-borne diseases through vector control activities.

Unavailability of appropriate environmental health manpower can be a limiting factor in emergency intervention after a disaster. The use of locally available expert therefore should be given first consideration. Because they are familiar with the pre-disaster and socio-economic conditions in affected areas, and–even more important–because they have experience in working under conditions similar to those of disaster-stricken areas. These individuals are usually best equipped to handle the emergency contingencies caused by natural disaster. In contrast, outside experts often are unfamiliar with both pre-disaster conditions and the particular environmental health standards of a given disaster-stricken area. Their lack of knowledge may in fact hinder the success of relief activities, so caution should be exercised when foreign experts are recruited.

Environmental health problems created by natural disasters should be managed by considering four R i.e., reduction, readiness, response and recovery:

1. *Reduction:* Action to avoid or minimize the adverse health related impacts of events likely to give rise to an emergency.
2. *Readiness:* This includes planning, establishing and maintaining system and undertaking training for an

efficient and effective health sector response to a potential emergency.

3. *Response:* Identifying, mobilizing and deploying health resources immediately prior to or during an emergency, in collaboration with other services to ensure as far as practicable. They are: (a) continuation of essential health services, (b) relief and treatment of people injured or in distress as a result of the emergency and (c) avoidance or reduction of ongoing public or personal health risks to all those affected by the event.
4. *Recovery:* Actions undertaken after an emergency include (a) assessment of the health needs of the affected community, (b) coordinating the health resources made available and (c) managing the rehabilitation and restoration of the affected community's health care services and health status, providing the supportive network by social and psychological services so as to reduce long term and chronic demands on health and social services.

During the disaster preparedness the immediate emergency response is provided under a highly political and emotional climate, and the responsibilities of the national or local health authorities are significant:

- Assessment of the health situation must be rapid, simple, transparent, technically credible, and done in collaboration with nongovernmental actors, donors, and the World Health Organization.
- Effective treatment of mass casualties depends on local preparedness and requires triage of patients to treat those most likely to benefit first.
- Surveillance, prevention, and control of communicable diseases during disasters should be strengthened by quickly and opportunistically resuming and monitoring the routine control programs, rather than resorting to new and expensive measures.

- Prioritizing environmental health—water quality, vector control, excreta disposal, solid waste management, health education, and food safety—is essential, especially in temporary settlements.
- Donations and supplies must be transparently managed to improve the flow of assistance to intended beneficiaries.
- Strong coordination of the humanitarian health efforts maximizes the benefit of the response and ensures it is compatible with the public health development priorities of the affected country.

The need for preparedness cannot be overemphasized. Building local capacity is one of the most cost-effective ways to improve the quality of the national response. Disaster preparedness is primarily a matter of building institutional capacity and human resources, and includes:

- Identifying vulnerability to natural or other hazards;
- Building simple and realistic health scenarios of a possible and probable occurrence;
- Initiating a participatory process among the main actors to develop a basic plan that outlines the responsibilities of each actor in the health sector, identifying possible overlaps or gaps and building a consensus;
- Maintaining close collaboration with these main actors; and
- Sensitizing and training the first health responders and managers to face the special challenges of responding to disasters.

Conclusions

Natural and manmade disasters are occurring with increasing frequency worldwide, but we are lacking in preparedness and post disaster management. The focus has begun to shift from merely providing post disaster assistance to putting in a place a system that will readily swing into action, once disaster strikes. The attitude has to shift from spending money after a disaster to investing in technology that can prevent, control and warn such disaster. While natural calamities are beyond human control, the lives lost for want of proper medical care are a greater disaster.

References

Cowen, E.L. et al. (1973), "Long Term Follow up of early Detected Vulnerable Children", *Journal of Consulting and Clinical Psychology* 41: 438-446.

NDM Division (2002), *Annual Report, 2001.* Ministry of Home Affairs, 2002 New Delhi: Government of India.

Parida, P.K. (2002), "Towards Rebuilding a Post-Disaster Society: A Case Study of Super-Cyclone Affected Coastal Orissa", *The Indian Journal of Social Work* 63(2): 243-262.

Parida, P.K. (2004), "Towards a Sociological Understanding of Flood Disaster in Orissa: A Case Study in Niali Block of Cuttack District", *Man and Development* XXVI (3): 141-154.

Rahe, R.H. (1979), "Life Change Events and Mental Illness: An Overview", *Journal of Human Stress* 5: 2-10.

SECTION – 6

Nutrition and Health

22

Prevalence of Chronic Energy Deficiency and its Consequences on Children's Nutritional Status Among Marginalized Group in India

A.K. Ravishankar, S. Ramachandran, A. Subbiah

Introduction

In recent year, dramatic progress has been made globally in tackling malnutrition, especially in reducing vitamin A deficiency and iodine disorders. However, around 800 million people are chronically malnourished, and more than a billion are sick or disabled because of nutrient deficiencies in the world. Each year, chronic malnutrition is a key factor in the deaths of at least 13 million children under five years of age in the developing world. Maternal nutritional status is important for a host of reasons-for the woman herself, for her capacity to reproduce, and for the development of her children, with implications for the health and reproductive capacity of the next generation's mothers. However, for decades, issues in women's nutrition have centered on nutrition during pregnancy and lactation and much of the concern has thus been for the newborn's health and well-being (Shepard et al., 1996). The nutritional issues of women themselves have rarely been investigated and not many nutritional data are available from non-pregnant women.

In India, more than half of all children under the age of four are malnourished, 30 per cent of newborns are significantly underweight, and sixty per cent of women are anaemic. According to the World Bank Report, in the last 40 years in India the mortality has declined by half and fertility by two-fifths, but malnutrition has only come down by about one-fifth. It is obvious that the further progress in human development in India will be difficult to achieve unless malnutrition is tackled with greater vigor and more rapid improvement in the future than in the past.

In recent decades, India has established a framework of programs with the potential to combat malnutrition, including a Public Distribution System (PDS), an Integrated Child Development Services (ICDS) program, a National Mid-day Meals Program (NMMP), and several employment schemes providing food for work. In India, volumes have been written about the nature and cause of adult and child malnutrition and the means of reducing it. But the role of women's 'chronic energy deficiency' in children's nutritional status has gone largely unnoticed until recently.

In Guatemala, in 1987 (Prentice et al., 1987), the term 'chronic energy deficiency' (CED) was being used as a term to indicate an inadequate household food supply. Since then, attempts to define, measure and assess CED have evolved, using the body mass index (BMI or weight / height^2) of individuals as the index of CED. Therefore, in this study BMI can be used to asses the nutritional status of women. Among children, anthropometry is usually used to track growth or failure to grow (wasting and stunting). Anthropometry is the single most non-invasive method of assessing body composition. It reflects both health and nutrition and predicts performance, health and survival.

India has established a framework of programmes with the potential to combat malnutrition including an ICDS (Integrated Child Development Services) programme, a NMMP (National Mid-day Meals Programme), and a PDS (Public Distribution System) and other some employment schemes providing food for work. Despite these programmes, the India continues to bear a burden of malnutrition - high prevalence of CED and anemia among mothers and more number of severely undernourished children. These situation calls for an exploration of the relationship between CED and children's nutritional status among the marginalized group in India. Hence, an attempt is made here to examine the prevalence of CED and anemia among mothers by using NFHS-3 data.

Objectives

- To study the nutritional status of women in the age group of 15-49 years among marginalized group in India
- To present a nutritional (status) profile of the children less than five years of age in the SC community
- To examines the pattern of food intake practices among ever married Schedule Caste women in India
- To study the degree of 'chronic energy deficiency' and anaemia (severe, mild and moderate) among SC women by selected background characteristics
- To explore the impact of 'chronic energy deficiency' (BMI) of SC women on the nutritional status of their children.

Data and Methods

The data for the present study were drawn from National Family Health Survey-3, a nationally represented large scale sample survey conducted in India during 2005-06 (IIPS and Macro International, 2007). The NFHS III sample covers 99 percent of India's population living in 29 states. Information collected from a nationally representative sample of 109,041 households, 124,385 women age 15-49. A total of 19343 Scheduled Caste women alone were considered for this study. Women who are all currently pregnant and those who have given birth in the month of interview were excluded. In addition, out of 5481 children born to SC women in the four years preceding the survey only 4687 were considered for assessing the nutritional status of children (the height and weight measured children alone).

The use of body mass index (BMI) as a measure of obesity has been widespread and has recently been promoted for assessment of chronic energy deficiency (CED) in adults. The Body Mass Index (BMI) is defined as the weight in kilograms divided by the height in meters squared (kg/m^2). A BMI of less than 18.5 indicates chronic energy deficiency (CED). Women were classified as chronically energy deficient or obese as described by James et al. (1998) and the World Health Organization (1995). Chronic energy deficiency grades I, II, and III correspond to body mass index (BMI) 17.0-18.4, 16.0-16.9, and < 16.0, respectively. Women with BMI 18.5-24.9 were classified as normal. Finally, obesity grades I, and II correspond to BMI 25.0-29.9, and >30.0 respectively. The weight of children and women was measured using a solar-powered digital scale, which gives results with an accuracy of ±100grams. Height/length was measured using an adjustable wooden measuring board that provides accurate measurement to the nearest 0.1 cm.

Three indices of nutritional status were calculated for children: height-for-age, weight-for-height, and weight-for-age. The height-for-age index examines linear growth retardation and is an indicator of chronic under-nutrition. The weight-for height index compares body mass to body length. This index reflects acute under-nutrition. Weight-for-age is a composite measure of both chronic and acute under-nutrition. Under nourished children on the weight-for-age index are referred to as "underweight" on the height-for-age index as "stunted" and on the weight-for-height index as "wasted". The measurements on these three indices are compared with the international reference population as recommended by WHO (Dibley et al., 1987).

Results and Discussion

Women's Nutritional Status in the Study Area

BMIs are most effectively used as indicators to describe the nutritional status of population and as an expression of the magnitude and distribution of under nutrition and over nutrition. Even though there is a progress in the nutritional status of adults, the incidence of CED remains high in India over the past two decades, according to the National Nutrition Monitoring Bureau Survey (2000-01) 37.4 percent of adult males and 39.4 percent of adult females suffered from CED in rural areas of nine sample states. The adult malnutrition is largely a result of poor diets and infection during childhood (Gillespie and McNeill., 1994).

Table 1
Percentage Distribution of Currently-married SC Women in India by their Nutritional Grade (BMI) NFHS-3 Data

Nutritional Grade (BMI)	*Percentage of SC Women*	*Number of SC Women*	*ALL INDIA*
Severe Thinness (less than16.00)	7.3	1356	15.8
Moderate Thinness (16.00 - 16.99)	9.1	1678	
Mild Thinness (17.00 - 18.49)	20.0	3702	19.7
CED (<18.50)	36.3	6736	35.6
Low Normal (18.50-19.99)	18.9	3509	51.8
Well-Nourished (20.00-24.99)	33.0	6126	
I- Degree Obesity (25.00-29.99)	9.4	1747	9.8
II- Degree Obesity (above 30.00)	2.3	418	2.8
Total#	100.0	18536	

Note: # = excludes the women who are all currently pregnant and those who given birth in the month interview

CED: BMI of 18536 ever-married women in the age group15-49 are given in the Table 1. In India, among the 18536 SC women surveyed, more than one-third (36.3%) of women have chronic energy deficiency (CED) which is almost equal to the national average (35.6%). It indicates the high prevalence of nutritional deficiency among the marginalized group. Further, about sixteen percent of the SC women are moderately (9.1%) or severely (7.3%) thin and another one-fifth of the women are mild thinness. At the other end of the spectrum, the women with obesity percentage was lesser (11.7%) than the country's average (12.6%) and the obesity I and II degree were found among 9.4 percent and 2.3 percent of women respectively.

It has been observed only one-third of the women (33%) in the age group15-49 were well-nourished among the marginalized group and more than one-third are seriously under nourished. Finally, the underweight is largely may be the result of poor diets and infection during childhood.

Association between Women's Nutritional Status and Background Factors

Undoubtedly, the socio-cultural and economic characteristics play a significant role in shaping the women's nutritional status. The table 2 furthermore supports this fact that the disparities in background conditions increase women's chances of being malnourished.

CED: Chronic energy deficiency is more serious problem for women in the age group 15-19 (47.3%, Table 2) followed by 20-24 (40.1%). Further, CED is particularly more pronounced for rural women (41.7%) and women who are illiterate (39.8%) and women who are working in agricultural sector (43.6%) and 'not working' (43.3%) categories. More than half of the women in 'poorest' wealth quintile (52.4%) had the nutritional problem (CED).

However, chronic energy deficiency was even more likely among higher educated women (Table 2, 24.3%), women in urban (29.3%), women in the age-group 45-49 (27.8%) and women with richest wealth index (21.7%). The other important findings drawn from this table was that CED grade II (severe thinness) was more widespread among poorest SC women (11.0%), followed by rural and illiterate women (8%) and it was high (9.3%) among women in the young age- group (15-19) and women who are working in the agricultural sectors (9%).

Obesity: According to survey data analysis (Table 2) 11.7 percent of ever married non- pregnant women age 15-49 in Scheduled Caste are overweight and obese. But this percentage is considerably higher for some sub-groups of women, women who have higher education (21.9%), women working in professional jobs (25.7%) and those who fall in the richest category (25.6%). Older age, higher educational

Table 2

Percentage distribution of Currently Married SC Women by their Nutritional Grade (BMI) with their SED Characteristics NFHS-3 Data

Background Characteristics Severe		*Moderate Thinness*	*Mild Thinness*	*Thinness*	*CED*	*Well- Normal*	*Nourished*	*Obesity*
Age**	15-19	9.3	11.2	26.8	47.3	24.2	25.7	2.9
	20-24	7.4	10.1	22.6	40.1	22.8	31.7	5.4
	25-29	6.7	10.1	19.9	36.7	18.4	34.9	10.0
	30-34	6.7	8.0	17.9	32.5	17.7	36.0	13.8
	35-39	6.9	7.3	16.4	30.5	16.2	35.3	18.0
	40-44	6.2	7.0	13.8	27.0	13.9	36.5	22.6
	45-49	6.6	6.5	14.7	27.8	11.7	37.7	22.9
Residence**	Urban	6.1	7.2	16.0	29.3	16.6	36.5	17.7
	Rural	8.2	10.5	23.0	41.7	20.7	30.5	7.1
Religion**	Hindu	7.5	9.1	20.4	37.1	19.1	32.8	11.0
	Muslim	4.7	8.8	17.9	31.4	23.2	33.7	11.7
	Christian	5.5	5.2	14.5	25.2	18.6	36.4	19.8
	Other	6.3	9.5	17.0	32.9	15.7	34.3	17.1
Educational Level**	Illiterate	8.3	9.8	21.7	39.8	19.3	31.6	9.2
	Primary	7.3	8.3	20.3	35.8	19.4	32.9	11.9
	Secondary	6.7	8.9	18.7	34.2	18.8	33.9	13.0
	Higher	4.1	5.8	14.3	24.2	14.8	39.1	21.9
Occupation**	Not working	9.1	11.1	23.4	43.6	22.0	28.6	5.7
	Profe./Others	3.6	4.9	13.3	21.8	20.3	30.1	6.3
	Sales	5.6	7.1	14.5	27.3	18.9	32.9	11.7
	Agri. Empl.	9.1	10.3	23.9	43.3	17.1	38.6	17.0
	Skilled / Unskilled	7.1	9.2	20.0	36.4	13.2	39.2	25.7

Contd.

Background Characteristics	*Severe*	*Moderate Thinness*	*Mild Thinness*	*Thinness*	*CED*	*Well-Normal*	*Nourished*	*Obesity*
Partners' Educational Level**	Illiterate	9.2	10.5	22.7	42.4	22.0	23.5	2.1
	Primary	7.6	8.9	19.2	35.7	21.5	27.1	5.0
	Secondary	5.5	7.7	17.0	30.2	20.3	34.5	8.8
	Higher	2.5	4.6	10.2	17.4	17.4	38.3	15.1
	DK	5.3	8.8	29.2	43.4	14.0	38.7	25.6
Partners Occupation**	Not work	7.3	6.6	18.6	32.5	18.9	33.0	11.7
	Profe./Others	3.0	4.3	11.7	19.0	24.2	25.7	2.9
	Sales	5.3	6.7	13.9	25.9	22.8	31.7	5.4
	Agri. Empl.	9.0	10.5	23.4	42.9	18.4	34.9	10.0
	Skilled / Unskilled	7.0	9.2	19.6	35.8	17.7	36.0	13.8
Wealth Index**	Poorest	11.0	13.0	28.4	52.4	16.2	35.3	18.0
	Poorer	10.4	10.9	25.2	46.5	13.9	36.5	22.6
	Middle	7.5	9.2	19.7	36.4	11.7	37.7	22.9
	Richer	5.0	7.6	16.5	29.1	16.6	36.5	17.7
	Richest	3.8	5.6	12.3	21.7	20.7	30.5	7.1
	Total	7.3	9.1	20.0	36.3	19.1	32.8	11.0

Note: ** = Chi-square test results between SED Characteristics and Nutritional Levels are significant at 1% level.

attainment and richest wealth index are significant risk factor for extreme obesity (grade II). In contrast, the obesity is less common in the early ages of ever-married women and women with poorest wealth index.

On the whole, the Table 2 highlights that there is more than two fold difference in CED between Professional job workers and agricultural laborers women and also registered a four fold difference observed in overweight between these groups. The other interesting observation is that there is more than two fold difference in underweight and more than ten fold differences in overweight observed between poorer and richer wealth index.

Results of Logistic Analysis

The influence of SED variables in determining the prevalence of Chronic Energy Deficiency (CED) are examined by logistic regression. The logistic regression analysis results in the Table-3 show that the odd ratios - Exp(B)s - indicate the effect of each of the predictor variables on the prevalence of CED, controlling for other variables included in the model. Almost in each of the variables the odds decrease with the categories of a variable when compared to the respective variable's first category (except place of residence), indicating a decreasing chance for experiencing CED when improving the background conditions of women.

The wealth index shows the well established link between the variables, when compared the poorest, the prevalence of Chronic Energy Deficiency (CED) on richest women found to be lower (odd ratio .283). Age of the women, women's educational attainment and working status of the women are significantly determining Chronic Energy Deficiency (CED). In respect of current age of women, when compared to reference category (15-19), the probability of having CED at 45-49 age women is low (odd ratio .449) and when compared to not working women, the probability of having CED at professional job women is also low (.621).

Anaemia: Anaemia is characterised by a low level of hemoglobin in the blood. Anaemia usually results from a

Table 3
Odds Ratios from Logistic Regression Examining the Effect of Selected SED Variables on CED Condition of SC Women

					95.0 C.I. for Exp (B)	
SED Variables	*B*	*S.E.*	*Sig.*	*Exp (B)*	*Lower*	*Upper*
Age**						
15-19 (ref.)			.000	1.000		
20-24	-.165	.054	.002	.848	.763	.942
25-29	-.333	.058	.000	.717	.640	.803
30-34	-.570	.061	.000	.566	.502	.638
35-39	-.660	.064	.000	.517	.456	.585
40-44	-.812	.069	.000	.444	.387	.508
45-49	-.801	.075	.000	.449	.387	.520
Residence						
Urban (ref.)				1.000		
Rural	.055	.039	.158	1.057	.979	1.141
Religion						
Hindu (ref.)			.001	1.000		
Muslim	-.276	.122	.024	.759	.597	.964
Christian -.382	.115	.001	.682	.545	.854	
Others	.037	.061	.545	1.038	.921	1.170
Educational Level*						
No Education (ref.)			.006	1.000		
Primary	-.136	.049	.005	.873	.794	.961
Secondary -.132	.045	.003	.877	.803	.957	
Higher	-.188	.095	.047	.828	.688	.998
Occupation**						
Not working (ref.)			.000	1.000		
Agri. Employee	-.242	.061	.000	.785	.696	.886
Sales & Services	-.465	.065	.000	.628	.553	.714
Profe. and Others	-.476	.076	.000	.621	.536	.720
Wealth Index**						
Poorest (ref.)			.000	1.000		
Poorer	-.215	.051	.000	.806	.729	.892
Middle	-.621	.052	.000	.538	.485	.596
Richer	-.911	.059	.000	.402	.358	.451
Richest	-1.262	.071	.000	.283	.246	.325
Constant	.755	.071	.000	2.127		

-2 Log likelihood = 22829.901

nutritional deficiency of iron, foliate, vitamin B12, or some other nutrients. This type of anaemia is commonly referred to as iron-deficiency anaemia. Iron deficiency is the most widespread form of malnutrition in the world, affecting more than two billion people. In India, anaemia affects more than 50 percent of the population. Anaemia may have detrimental effects on the health of women and children and may become an underlying cause of maternal mortality and perinatal mortality. Anaemia results in an increased risk of premature delivery and low birth weight.

Three levels of severity anaemia (Table 4) show that Mild anaemia (10.0-10.9 grams/deciliter for pregnant women, 10.0-11.9 g/dl for non-pregnant women), Moderate anaemia (7.0-9.9 grams/deciliter) and sever anaemia (less than 7.0 g/dl) for pregnant women, 10.0-11.9 g/dl for non-pregnant women). The prevalence of 55 percent of anaemia among the ever married SC women indicates anaemia as a major nutritional problem among these women. Further, more than one-third of the women had mildly anaemic (38.4 percent) and 14.5 percent are moderately anaemic. It is comprehensible that these high levels are attributed to diets that are low in iron content, clear absorption of iron due to inhibitors and increased demand due to the physiological requirements of menstruation, pregnancy and lactation.

Table 4
Percentage Distribution of Ever Married SC Women in India by their Hemoglobin level (G/DL), NFHS-3 data

Anemic Nature	*Number of Women*	*Percentage of Women*		*INDIA*
Severe Anaemic	363	2.0	*Any kind*	1.8
Moderate Anaemic	2653	14.5	*of anemia*	15.4
Mild Anaemic	7003	38.4	54.9	38.9
Non-Anaemic	8009	43.9		46.4

Anaemia is pervasive among SC women in every subgroup shown in the Table 5. More than half of the SC women are anaemic in every subgroup. The incidence of anaemia is highly prominent among women living in poorest wealth index category (63.9%), women with CED (61.2%), women working in agricultural sector (58.8%) and illiterate women (58.2%). On the whole, the incidence of anaemia among the ever married Scheduled Caste women by their background condition also shows the similar pattern as what observed in CED.

Table 5
Percentage Distribution of Currently Married SC Women by their Anaemic Condition with their SED Characteristics

Background Characteristics		*Severe Anaemia*	*Moderate Anaemia*	*Mild Anaemia*	*Anaemic*	*Non-Anaemic*
Age*	15-19	2.1	14.9	38.4	55.4	43.2
	20-24	2.0	16.3	39.2	57.5	41.3
	25-29	1.8	13.0	39.3	54.1	44.6
	30-34	1.7	13.2	38.5	53.4	45.2
	35-39	2.0	14.9	36.3	53.2	46.0
	40-44	2.0	15.8	36.7	54.5	44.4
	45-49	2.5	13.0	40.3	55.8	43.6
Residence**	Urban	2.0	14.2	36.3	52.5	45.3
	Rural	1.9	14.8	40.0	56.7	42.9
Religion**	Hindu	2.0	14.7	39.2	55.9	43.3
	Muslim	1.8	10.7	27.7	40.2	40.5
	Christian	2.1	18.8	33.8	54.7	39.6
	Other	2.1	12.4	32.9	47.4	52.6
Educational Level**	Illiterate	2.2	15.3	39.7	57.2	41.8
	Primary	1.7	15.6	38.9	56.2	42.7
	Secondary	1.9	13.4	37.3	52.6	46.0
	Higher	1.6	13.1	34.0	48.7	49.5
Occupation**	Not working	2.0	14.5	36.4	52.9	45.5
	Agri. Empl	1.9	15.5	41.1	58.5	41.2
	Skilled/Unskilled	2.1	15.0	38.3	55.4	43.5
	Sales	2.4	13.2	38.2	53.8	44.0
	Prof & othe	1.3	12.3	36.2	49.8	48.7
Partners' Educational Level**	Illiterate	2.5	15.9	39.8	58.2	40.5
	Primary	1.7	14.4	42.2	58.3	40.6
	Secondary	1.7	14.2	37.0	52.9	46.1
	Higher	1.4	10.7	37.8	49.9	48.9
	DK	4.5	20.0	40.0	54.5	34.5
Partners' Occupation**	Not work	0.4	18.1	38.1	56.6	43.0
	Prof &oth	1.2	11.9	35.9	49.0	50.2
	Sales	2.2	13.1	38.2	53.5	44.2
	Agri. Empl	1.9	15.4	41.7	59.0	40.5
	Skilled/Unskilled	2.1	15.0	38.4	55.5	43.4
Wealth Index**	Poorest	2.4	16.2	44.5	53.1	36.1
	Poorer	1.9	15.8	40.6	58.3	41.0
	Middle	2.3	14.6	37.9	54.8	44.3
	Richer	2.0	14.3	36.3	52.6	45.7
	Richest	1.4	12.1	34.2	47.7	50.7
BMI**	CED	2.7	17.0	40.6	60.3	38.8
	Normal	2.4	17.3	37.9	57.6	41.1
	Well Nourished	1.5	12.1	37.8	51.4	47.0
	Obesity	0.5	9.0	34.0	43.5	55.6
Total		2.0	14.5	38.4	54.9	43.9

Note: * and ** = Chi-square test results between SED Characteristics and Anaemic levels are Significant at 1% and 5% level, respectively

The importance of nutrition as a foundation for healthy development is often underestimated. Poor nutrition leads to high prevalence of CED and it contributes to further deterioration in their nutritional status. Table 5 clearly shows that women with BMI less than 18.5 have higher incidence of anaemia (60.3%) and this percentage declines with their declining anemic level. Severe and moderate thinness was more pronounced among women who are suffered from severe anaemia. The non-anemic women are found to have high degree of obesity. Hence, it is well clear that the body mass index seems to be highly correlated factor with anaemia.

The logistic regression analysis results indicate (Table 6) that wealth index as the only principle SED variables influencing prevalence of anemia. In respect of wealth index, when compared to reference category (poorest), the probability of non-anemia women among richest wealth index is 1.6 times higher.

Food Intake Practices: Malnutrition reflects an imbalance of both macro and micro-nutrients that may be due to inappropriate intake and/or inefficient biological utilization. Gross imbalance of macro nutrients results in body weight and height that deviate from normal population standards. Latest studies show that in spite of being the world's largest producer of fruits, vegetables and milk and achieving self-sufficiency in cereals, Indians are not eating enough of their own produce to be normally healthy. Table 7 shows about the food practice of Scheduled Caste ever married women in India. The proportion of daily eating practice of green leafy vegetables (60.2%), and pulses or beans (48%) are fairly healthier among the SC women. At the same time, more than one-fourth SC women never eat fish (32.4%), egg (26.6%) and chicken (27.9%) in their life time. The eating of fruits was less common among the SC women about 58 percent of women occasionally eating fruits. About more than one-third of the women did not consume milk or curd, egg and fish even occasionally. In general, the food consumption pattern among the SC women is not adequate

Table 6
Odds Ratios from Logistic Regression Examining the Effect of Selected SED Variables on Anemic Condition of SC Women

SED Variables	B	S.E.	Sig.	Exp(B)	95.0 C.I. for Exp (B) Lower	Upper
Age						
15-19 (Ref)			.001	1.000		
20-24	-.084	.053	.113	.919	.828	1.020
25-29	.087	.057	.125	1.091	.976	1.219
30-34	.136	.059	.022	1.145	1.020	1.286
35-39	.146	.061	.016	1.157	1.027	1.303
40-44	.069	.065	.289	1.071	.943	1.216
45-49	.031	.070	.657	1.032	.899	1.184
Residence						
Urban (ref)				1.000		
Rural	.089	.037	.016	1.093	1.017	1.175
Religion						
Hindu (Ref)			.000	1.000		
Muslim	.257	.123	.037	1.293	1.015	1.646
Christian	-.137	.103	.180	.872	.713	1.066
Others	.276	.056	.000	1.318	1.180	1.471
Educational Level						
No Education (ref)			.580	1.000		
Primary	-.012	.046	.799	.988	.902	1.082
Secondary	.043	.042	.310	1.044	.961	1.134
Higher	.076	.083	.360	1.079	.917	1.270
Occupation						
Not working (Ref)			.403	1.000		
Agricultural	-.055	.060	.357	.946	.841	1.064
Skilled and Unskilled	-.037	.054	.498	.964	.867	1.072
Sales	-.087	.062	.160	.917	.812	1.035
Profe./Others	-.006	.068	.926	.994	.870	1.136
Wealth Index**						
Poorest (Ref)			.000	1.000		
Poorer	.205	.053	.000	1.228	1.108	1.361
Middle	.345	.052	.000	1.412	1.275	1.565
Richer	.428	.057	.000	1.535	1.371	1.717
Richest	.617	.066	.000	1.853	1.628	2.110
Constant	-.660	.069	.000	.517		

-2 Log likelihood = 24511.087.

Table 7
Percentage of Ever Married SC Women by Food Intake Practices

Food Intake Practices	Milk or Curd	Pulses or Beans	Green Leafy Vegetables	Fruits	Fish	Egg	Chicken Meat
Never	13.4	1.3	0.3	3.6	32.4	26.6	27.9
Daily	30.1	48.4	60.2	10.9	6.7	4.3	0.6
Weekly	17.8	39.6	31.3	27.4	25.0	31.6	23.5
Occasionally	38.7	10.8	8.1	58.1	35.8	37.6	48.0

Consumption of a variety of nutritious foods that provide adequate amounts of protein, fat, carbohydrates, vitamins, and minerals is important for women's health. Empirical nutrition studies (Seckler, 1982) show that increase in food energy intake would reduce malnutrition while the other variables are controlled. The relationship between BMI and percent food intake has been examined and the results are given in Table 8.

The Table 8 shows the percentage of ever-married SC women by their Nutritional Grade (BMI) with their Food Intake Practices. It is evident from the table that the proportion of women who never took milk or curd on daily is more likely to have CED than their counterparts. A similar pattern was observed for all other food items. On the other side, the proportion of women who took all food items on daily/weekly is more likely to obesity. The eating pattern of chicken or meat, fruits on weekly clearly establishes the high prevalence of obesity. Therefore, an undoubtedly established fact is a strong association between BMI and food intake practice.

Children's Nutritional Status in the Study Area: Adequate nutrition and health during the first several years of life is fundamental to the attainment of the Millennium Development Goals for child survival and the prevention of malnutrition. Poor nutrition during these critical formative years has both immediate and long-term consequences. A recent authoritative paper on child survival ranked nutrition interventions among the most effective preventive actions for reducing under-five mortality (Jones, 2003). Throughout the world children fail to grow in length and weight in a remarkable similar age-specific pattern, despite vastly different prevalence of low weight-for-age, length-for-age, and weight-for-length between and among regions. Recent estimates show that about 40 per cent of the undernourished children in the world are in India although India accounts for less than 20 percent of the children in the world.

Generally, the prevalence of anaemia is higher during infancy and early childhood than at any other time in the life cycle. The SC representative data from NFHS-III shows

Table 8
Percentage of Ever Married Women by their Nutritional Grade (BMI) with their Food Intake Practices

	*Mother Consumed: Milk or Curd***				
BMI	*Never*	*Daily*	*Weekly*	*Occasionally*	*Total*
Severe Thinness	15.6	25.1	18.7	40.6	1355
Moderate	14.3	24.2	17.8	43.8	1677
Mild	14.4	25.3	18.5	41.8	3702
Nourished	13.4	31.5	16.9	38.1	9634
Obesity	11.4	39.5	19.3	29.8	2165
	*Mother Consumed: Pulses or Beans**				
Severe Thinness	2.1	47.7	40.3	9.8	1355
Moderate	1.7	46.0	41.2	11.2	1677
Mild	1.3	47.4	40.1	11.1	3701
Nourished	1.1	48.2	39.6	11.1	9634
Obesity	1.1	51.1	37.7	10.0	2165
	Mother Consumed: Green leafy Vegetables NS				
Severe Thinness	0.3	59.5	32.5	7.7	1355
Moderate	0.5	58.7	32.6	8.2	1677
Mild	0.3	59.1	32.4	8.2	3700
Nourished	0.3	60.1	31.3	8.3	9634
Obesity	0.3	64.0	28.6	7.0	2164
	*Mother Consumed: Fruits***				
Severe Thinness	3.9	6.2	24.4	65.5	1355
Moderate	4.7	8.5	24.6	62.2	1676
Mild	4.3	7.0	25.4	63.3	3699
Nourished	3.4	11.5	27.7	57.4	9630
Obesity	2.9	19.3	33.1	44.7	2165
	*Mother Consumed: Eggs***				
Severe Thinness	25.6	3.6	32.6	38.2	1354
Moderate	26.7	4.3	29.3	39.7	1677
Mild	26.2	2.9	29.6	41.4	3701
Nourished	27.3	4.2	31.8	36.7	9628
Obesity	26.0	7.7	36.1	30.3	2164
	Mother Consumed: Fish*				
Severe Thinness	29.9	5.1	26.9	38.1	1354
Moderate	31.8	5.2	25.5	37.4	1677
Mild	31.8	5.6	23.6	39.0	3701
Nourished	33.4	7.3	24.7	34.6	9633
Obesity	31.6	9.8	28.1	30.5	2164
Severe Thinness	26.6	0.4	22.2	50.7	1354
Moderate	27.6	0.8	21.9	49.7	1677
Mild	27.9	0.4	19.5	52.2	3701

Contd.

	*Mother Consumed: Chicken or Meat***				
Nourished	28.5	0.6	23.6	47.3	9633
Obesity	26.8	0.7	32.6	39.8	2164
Total	5183 (28.0)	107 (0.6)	4372 (23.6)	8866 (47.9)	18528 (100.0)

Note: * and ** = Chi-square test results between Food Intake Practices and Nutritional Levels are significant at 1% and 5% level, respectively. *NS* = Not Significant.

(Table 9) 70.8 percent of children below 5 years with any kind of anaemia (25.6% had mild, 41.6% had moderate and 3.6% had severe anaemia). The prevalence of anaemia varied from 78 percent in the age group of less than 12 months to 63 percent in the age group of 24-59 months and severe anaemia is highest (5.7%) in the age group 12-23 months. Nevertheless, even though the Indian government performing better child health care programmes, the Scheduled Castes children anemic levels were still high.

Table 9

Percentage Distribution of Children Less Than Five-years of Age Classified by their Anemic Level

Age Groups (in months)	*Children Anemia Level*			
	Severe	*Moderate*	*Mild*	*Non-anemic*
6-11	2.8	49.4	25.6	20.0
12-23	5.7	52.4	22.7	17.5
24-59	2.8	33.5	27.1	35.4
Total	3.6	41.6	25.6	27.6

In terms of nutritional status of children, around forty-seven percent of Scheduled Caste children are underweight and more than two-third of the SC children are stunting (67.4 percent) in India. Further, analysis in the Table 10 shows that underweight and stunting are relatively low for children less than 6 months old and this incidence increases more than four-fold at 12-23 months. Among the marginalized group, only negligible proportion of the children is too thin (wasting). The overall picture discloses the fact that both the acute and chronic under nutrition are a serious concern among the Scheduled Caste children.

Mother's BMI with Incidence of Anaemia: Table 11 highlights the close correlation between mothers's BMI with incidence of anaemia among children. About half of the total severe anemic children are born to the women with BMI less than 18.5 (CED). Further, the table shows that the moderate and mild anaemic children are closely associated with CED. Where as, the severe anaemic nature among children were less common women with obesity (8.3 percent) among the SC community. It is note that the well nourished (and obesity) women have about 46 percent of non-anaemic children.

Environmental and socio-economic factors influence childhood growth in height and weight more than genetic

Table 10
Percentage Distribution of Children Less Than Five-years of Age Classified by their Nutritional Status

	*Wasting***				
Age (in months)	*Severe*	*Moderate*	*Mild*	*Well Nourished*	*Total*
>6 months	3.4	9.1	21.9	65.5	580
6-11	2.6	13.5	29.1	54.7	731
12-23	4.7	19.8	36.4	39.1	1171
24-59	2.1	14.9	43.9	39.1	2205
Total	3.0	15.2	37.0	44.8	4687
	*Stunting***				
>6 months	2.4	8.6	21.4	67.6	580
6-11	9.6	17.5	32.4	40.5	731
12-23	27.4	27.1	23.3	22.2	1171
24-59	18.5	26.5	28.6	26.3	2205
Total	17.4	23.0	27.0	32.6	4687
	*Under Weight***				
>6 months	2.4	7.1	–	90.5	580
6-11	9.7	27.2	–	63.1	731
12-23	21.4	37.6	–	41.0	1171
24-59	16.1	37.7	–	46.2	2205
Total	14.8	32.2	–	53.0	4687

Note: ** = Chi-square test results between Children Nutritional Status and Mother's BMI are significant at 1% and 5% level, respectively.

factors (Habicht et al., 1974). The Table 11 shows linkage between women's BMI and children's anthropometric indices. As expected, women with poorer nutritional status, as indicated by the CED condition, have registered higher risk of severe underweight and severe wasting children (54.9% and 41.3%, respectively). Further, the severe stunting children are also associated with women's BMI. A similar relationship (which witnessed CED with anaemic condition) is also observed in anthropometric indices and, among the well-nourished (and obesity) women who have less significant risk of underweight, stunting and wasting children. So it is clear that the severe underweight children were predominant among low BMI women (around 55%), and a quite significant percentage was also noticed among severe stunting, of around 50 percent.

Table 11
Percentage Distribution of Children's Nutritional Status with the their Mother's Nutritional Grade (BMI)

Children's Nutritional Status		*Mother's Nutritional Grade (BMI)* CED	*Well Normal*	*Nourished*	*Obesity*
Children's Anaemic**	Severe Anaemic	50.3	17.9	23.4	8.3
	Moderate Anaemic	47.2	21.8	26.2	4.8
	Mild Anaemic	40.3	22.0	30.4	7.2
	Non Anaemic	36.1	17.8	36.5	9.6
**Wt/A Standard Deviations	Severe under weight	54.9	20.4	22.2	2.5
	Under weight	47.0	21.5	26.2	5.3
	Well-nourished	33.2	22.2	35.4	9.2
**Ht/A Standard Deviations	Severe Stunting	49.8	20.8	25.1	4.3
	Moderate stunting	46.1	20.0	28.5	5.5
	Mild Stunting	39.0	24.5	30.1	6.4
	Well-nourished	33.9	21.2	35.1	9.8
**Wt/Ht Standard Deviations	Severe wasting	41.3	21.0	34.8	2.9
	Moderate wasting	53.1	21.0	22.9	3.0
	Mild wasting	43.5	22.2	28.1	6.2
	Well-nourished	34.4	21.6	34.8	9.2

Note: ** = Chi-square test results between Children Nutritional Status and Mother's BMI are Significant at 1% and 5% level, respectively

Conclusions

The study's overall goal is to understand the links between women's nutritional status specifically chronic energy deficiency and child's nutrition status among the marginalized group population in India (Scheduled Caste). The prevalence of CED rate was almost equal to (36.6%) to national average (35.6%). Although the incidence of this CED was higher among young age SC women (15-19: 47.3%), rural women (41.7%), uneducated women (39.8%), and women working in agricultural sector (43.3%), women with poorest wealth index (52.4%). A contrast trend was observed in the richest wealth index group (25.6%), women working as professional section (25.7%), and highly educated women (21.9%), that they had high degree of obesity (I degree and II degree). It is therefore concluded that the marginalized women facing the burden of the nutritional disorder.

The food intake patterns confirm that there is an association between BMI and food intake practices. It is also evident that the mother's BMI has a positive association with children's anaemic condition. This risk of having anemic condition among children is more, women with BMI less than 18.5. In addition, the well nourished and obesity women have non-anaemic children. Similarly, the women with poorer nutritional status have infants of severe chronic and acute under nutrition.

In general, under and malnutrition starts in the womb and may extend throughout the life cycle. Malnutrition remains a silent emergency among the marginalised population (SC), though the government of India had made significant progress in the past several decades in improving the health and well-being of its people particularly women and children. The risk of malnutrition is higher among the children whose mothers suffer from chronic energy deficiency. Mother's present nutritional status in turn depends on her childhood nutritional status. Concerted efforts are needed to break the vicious circle (mother-child-mother) of malnutrition among poor. It is emphasized that reduction of child malnutrition would greatly depend on delivery of effective and sustainable interventions to children and their mothers.

At present, too few children and mothers are receiving effective nutrition interventions that could significantly reduce the risk of their malnutrition.

References

Dibley, M.J., N.W. Staehling, P. Neiburg, and F.L. Trowbridge (1987), TInterpretation of Z-Score Anthropometric Indicators Derived from the International Growth Reference", *American Journal of Clinical Nutrition* 46(5): 736-748.

Gillespie, S., and G. McNeill (1994), *Food, Health and Survival in India and Developing Countries*. New York: Oxford University Press.

Habicht J.P., Martorell, R., Yarbrough, C, Malina, R.M., Klein, R.E. (1974), "Height and Weight Standards for Pre-school Children-How Relevant are Ethnic Differences in Growth Potential?", *The Lancet* 304(7871): 47.

International Institute for Population Science (IIPS) and Macro International (2007), *National Family Health Survey (NFHS-3), 2005-06, India*. Mumbai: IIPS.

James, W.P.T., Ferro-Luzzi, A, Waterlow, J.C. (1988), "Definition of Chronic Energy Deficiency in Adults", *European Journal of Clinical Nutrition*.

Jones, G, et al. (2003), "How Many Child Deaths Can We Prevent this Year?", *The Lancet* 362(9377): 65-71.

Prentice, A.M., Cole, T.J., and F.A. Foord (1987), "Increased Birth Weight After Pre-natal Dietary Supplementation of Rural African Women", *American Journal of Clinical Nutrition*.

Seckler, D. (1982), "Small but Health: A Base Hypothesis in the Theory, Management and Policy in Nutrition", In: P. V. Sukhatme, (ed.), *Newer Concepts and Their Implication for Policy*. Pune, Maharshtra: Association for Cultivation of Science.

Shepard, M.J., Bakketeig, L.S., Jacobsen, G, O'Connor, T, Bracken, M.B. (1996), "Maternal Body Mass, Proportional Weight Gain, and Fetal Growth in Parous Women", *Paediatric and Perinatal Epidemiology* 10(2): 207-219.

World Health Organization (1995), *Physical Status: The Use and Interpretation of Anthropometry*. WHO Technical Report Series No. 854. Geneva: WHO.

23

Does Body Mass Index amongst Primiparous Women Affect the Birth Weight of Neonates?

G. Muthulakshmi, R. Swapna, T.R. Gopalan, A.J. Hemamalini

Introduction

Pregnancy is a prime example of physiological synergism in which the mother, fetus and placenta collaborate to sustain and nurture new life. Numerous factors interact to determine the progress and outcome of pregnancy. Although much remains to be learned about the role of nutrition in modifying this process, a mother's food habits and nutritional status before and during pregnancy has been considered an important prognostic indicator of birth outcome (Gottschlich, 2001).

The minimum recommended pre pregnancy weight for an Indian woman is 50 kgs. Low pre-pregnancy weight is a strong determinant of intra uterine growth retardation and premature birth, both of which may result in low birth weight baby. Barker has proposed that prenatal factors that alter or impede fetal growth in utero may lead to long term ramification and may be in part responsible for obesity, diabetes, hypertension, insulin resistance, cardiovascular and heart disease. Intrauterine life is a crucial period which the epidemiological data indicate that a suboptimal intra uterine environment affects future chronic diseases (Matarese and Gottschlich, 1998). The intrauterine environment is assessed crudely by birth weight of infants (Mahan and Escott-Stump, 2003).

Infants with low Birth weight stems primarily from the mother's poor nutrition and health over a long period of time and inadequate maternal weight gain. Low birth weight has been defined by the World Health Organization as weight at birth less than 2500 grams. Generally speaking it is accepted that maternal weight is associated with birth weight (Catalano, 2007) and evidence shows that the incidence of neonates weighing >2500g increases as BMI and gestational weight gain increases (Weiss et al., 2004). Low income and lack of knowledge are also associated with a risk of having low birth weight neonates.

Body Mass Index (BMI) is a measure of body fat based on height and weight. Pre-pregnancy Body Mass Index (BMI) and weight gain during pregnancy reflect nutritional status of pregnant women. Optimal weight gain of the mother during pregnancy is a significant reflection of good nutritional status and contributes to a successful course and outcome. Assignment of an appropriate weight gain is about 11 to 14 kgs and is generally based on the pregnancy body mass index (Williams and Staci, 2008).

Potential causes for a low pre-pregnancy BMI include short stature, low weight for height women as influenced by inadequate nutrient intake, food insecurity, psychological stress, chronic dieting, disturbed eating behaviour, alcohol and drug abuse. It is also an important indicator of nutritional status and reproductive maturity of a pregnant woman and reflects the extent of antenatal care she has received. The causes for low pre-pregnancy BMI status should be identified as early as possible during pregnancy and appropriate nutritional measures to be taken to improve the gestational weight gain and thereby improve the birth weight (Schlenker and Long, 2006).

Several studies have revealed that though the pre pregnancy BMI has been poor, an adequate weight gain during pregnancy according to the recommendations of Institute of Medicine based on individual BMIs; improve the overall outcome of pregnancy with respect to birth weight of the newborn (Suitor, 1991).

Objectives

Keeping above concepts in view an attempt is made to understand the effect of various pre pregnancy Body Mass Index (BMI) categories and corresponding gestational weight gain on newborn birth weight. The Specific objectives are:

- To assess the BMI of the pregnant women from their recorded pre-pregnancy weight
- To study the influence of low pre-pregnancy BMI and gestational weight gain on the birth weight of the newborn

Materials and Methods

A prospective observational study was conducted; where in the pregnant women with appropriate and adequate antenatal check up records were followed up till their delivery and the birth weight of the infants were noted of the pregnant women who are attending Obstetrics and Gynecology Outpatient Department of Sri Ramachandra Medical Centre, Chennai.

All women attending Obstetrics and Gynecology Outpatient Department of Sri Ramachandra Medical Centre, Chennai who are primiparous with in the age group 20-30 years have been identified. Women with Twin gestations, complicated pregnancies and with co-morbid conditions (diabetes mellitus, cardiovascular disease, hypertension) other chronic disorders have been excluded from the study. In all 130 pregnant women with d™ 20 weeks gestation attending antenatal check-ups and having a well maintained medical record were chosen as subjects for the study.

Pregnancy outcome is influenced by the nutritional status of the women which includes maternal age(<16 yrs and >35 yrs), pre pregnancy weight, body mass index, gestational weight gain, and presence of co-morbid conditions like overt diabetes mellitus, gestational diabetes mellitus, cardiovascular disease and pregnancy induced hypertension. Body mass index is influenced by the weight of the patient (Maryam-sadat and Nastaranb, 2004; Ellen et al., 2008). Therefore, the present study excluded subjects who were obese and those with other co morbid conditions to avoid the influence of these factors on the birth weight of the newborn.

Study Parameters and Assessment

The study involved anthropometric assessments such as height, pre-pregnancy weight as recorded in their medical records on the first visit for confirmation, body mass index, gestational weight gain and birth weight of the newborn. The height of the subjects was taken in the ward before or after delivery. A standard height meter fixed firmly on the wall was used to measure the height of the subjects. The pre-pregnancy weight of the subjects was collected as entered in the medical records of the subjects during their first visit to the Obstetric out Patient department for confirmation. Weight before delivery was measured using calibrated weighing scale and measured to the nearest of 0.1 kg. The subject's gestational weight gain was calculated from the difference between the pre pregnancy weight taken and the latest weight taken before delivery.

Body Mass Index (BMI): Based on the pre-pregnancy weight and height, the Body Mass Index was calculated using the following formula (IOM, NAS 1990).

$$BMI = Weight (kg)/ Height (m^2).$$

Table 1
Standard Classification of BMI and Recommended Gestational Weight Gain

Interpretations	*BMI* (Kg/M^2)	*Recommended Weight Gain (Kgs)*
Underweight	<19.8	12.5 - 18
Appropriate weight for height	19.8 -26	11.5 - 15
Overweight	26 - 29	7 - 11.5
Obese	>29	

Birth Weight

Pre-pregnancy BMI and the respective recommended gestational weight gain were categorized based on Institute of Medicine (IOM, NAS, 1990) BMI groups and gestational weight gain guidelines are given in Table 1.

Birth weight of the newborn was recorded from their respective medical records as entered by the attending clinician at the time of birth. Newborn birth weight was grouped into Low birth weight (LBW) (<2,500g) and normal birth weight (2,500-3,999g) (Mahan and Escott-Stump, 2003).

Results

A sample of 130 registered women has been considered for analysis and all of them are in the age range of 20-30 years and 68 percent belongs to 2025 years age group and the remaining was in the age group 26-30 years.

Pre-pregnancy Body Mass Index

Pre-pregnancy BMI is an important factor in predicting pregnancy outcome. It has been observed among 130 sample women 42 percent of women had weight for height in the range of19.8–26 kg/m^2 with mean 21.92 and S.D 1,65. The remaining 58 percent women had a low BMI (<19.8 kg/m^2) with mean 18.36 and SD 1.27. As this study aims at subjects with low BMI and their corresponding gestational weight gain, further analysis was carried out on the 58 percent (76 women) who were found to be with low BMI.

Weight Gain Pattern of Subjects with Low BMI

The gestational weight gain pattern of women with low BMI is presented in table 2. The recommended gestational weight gain range for women with low BMI is between 12-18 kgs. An underweight woman who fails to gain weight adequately during pregnancy is most likely to give birth to a baby with critically low birth weight. From table 2, it was evident 14 percent of low BMI subjects gained a mean weight of about 09.50$\pm$1.12 kg, which is lesser than IOM's weight gain recommendations. However, the weight gained by the remaining subjects was within the recommended range for low body mass index.

Table 2
Weight Gain Pattern Among Low BMI Subjects

Observed Range of Weight Gain (kg)	*N (%) (N=76)*	*BMI (kg/m^2)*	*Weight Gain (kg)Mean ± SD*
Less than 12	11 (14)	16.98 ±1.18	09.50 ±1.12
12.0 - 14.0	39 (52)	18.18 ± 0.93	13.46 ± 0.55
14.1 - 16.0	21 (28)	17.18 ±1.46	15.33 ±0.48
16.1 - 18.0	05 (06)	17.78 ± 2.33	17.60 ± 0.54

Body Mass Index, Gestational Weight Gain and Birth Weight

Infant birth weight is a single most potential indicator of a child's future nutrition and health status. Birth weight is affected to a great extent by the mother's own fetal growth and her diet from birth to pregnancy and thus her body composition at conception. A woman with low pre pregnancy body mass index has a greater tendency to give birth to low birth weight infants, if the recommended range of gestational weight gain is not achieved (Ogunyemi et al., 1998; Ronnenberg et al., 2003). Table 3 presents the gestational weight gain achieved by subjects with lower BMI and the birth weight of their corresponding newborns. The effect of weight gain, by subjects with low BMI, on the birth weight was found to be significant at $p<0.001$ level. Women who started their pregnancy with BMI 19.8-26 and gained weight according to the expected range gave birth to normal weight babies ($P < 0.001$).

Table 3
Body Mass Index, Gestational Weight Gain and Birth Weight

BMI (kg/m^2)	*N=130*	*BMI (kg/m^2) Mean ± SD*	*Weight Gain (kgs) Mean ±SD*	*Birth Weight (kg) Mean ±SD*	*t-value ($p<0.001$)*
Low (<19.8)	76	18.362 ± 1.272	13.68±2.17	2.82±0.26	108.14
Normal (19.8-26)	54	21.919 ± 1.651	11.30±2.34	3.18±0.25	46.33

Gestational Weight Gain Vs Birth Weight

Birth weight of a baby reflects its nutritional environment in the mother's womb and its survival rate once it is born. Infants born with low birth weight have been shown to be more prone to syndrome X, a multiple constellation of diabetes mellitus, hypertension and cardiovascular disease. So it is imperative to improve the birth weight of the infant to improve the health status of the human life on earth. Birth weight of a new born is influenced by various factors, of which maternal nutritional status prior and during pregnancy plays a significant role and her weight gain during gestation has a greater influence on the birth weight (Kramer, 1987). Birth Weight gain among low BMI women with gestational weight gain is given in figure 1. It shows that increase in birth weight with increase in gestational weight gain.

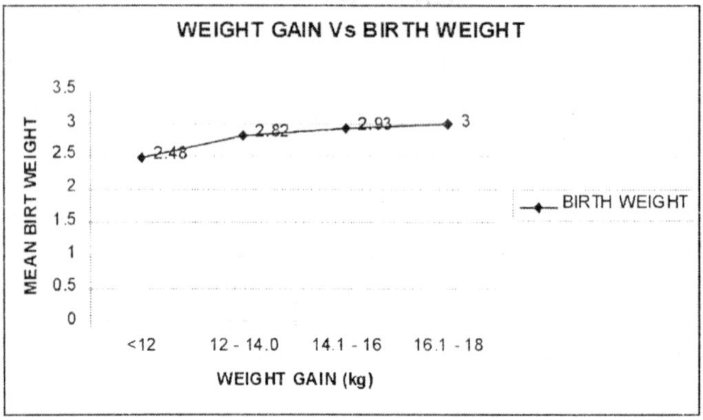

Fig. 1: Gestational Weight Gain in Subjects with Low BMI and Birth Weight of Newborn

To further refine relationship between birth weight and maternal BMI, a further categorisation of the lower BMI was done. Table 4 presents the birth weight of the infants born to subjects with low body mass index. It can be observed from the table, that there were no incidences of low birth weight in general, but among the 11 subjects with a lower pre pregnancy BMI of 16.98 $\pm$1.18 kg/m^2, together with a lower mean weight gain of 09.5 $\pm$1.12 kgs, had delivered babies

Table 4
Gestational Weight Gain in Subjects with Low BMI and Birth Weight of Newborn

BMI (kg/m^2)	*Number (n=76)*	*Range of Weight Gain (kg)*	*Weight Gain (kg) Mean ±SD*	*Birth Weight (kg) Mean ± SD*	*r-value (p<0.001)*
18.18 ± 0.93	39	12-14	13.46 ± 0.55	2.82 ± 0.21	0.1392
17.18 ±1.46	21	14.1 - 16	15.33 ±0.48	2.93 ±0.26	0.3439
17.78 ± 2.33	5	16.1 - 18	17.6 ± 0.54	3.00 ± 0.23	0.6334
16.98 ±1.18	11	< 12	9.5 ±1.12	2.48 ±0.19	0.2078

with low birth weight. The results depicted in table 5 reveals the importance of adequate gestational weight gain to prevent the incidence of low birth weight in case of women starting their pregnancy with a low weight for height, indicated by low body mass index.

It can be observed from the table, that those subjects who have gained greater than and equal to 13 kgs, inspite of having a lower pre pregnancy body mass index, have given birth to infants with normal birth weight compared to their counterparts, who have gained only nine kilograms and given birth to infants with low birth weight. The influence of gestational weight gain of subjects with low body mass index on their respective birth weights of infants delivered was found to be significant at ($p<0.001$) level.

Table 5 presents the mean low BMI observed among the study subjects, their corresponding gestational weight gains and their birth weights of the newborn. For women with pre pregnancy BMI <17 kg/m^2, mean birth weight of newborns was lower for those gaining <12 kg than those gaining > 12.5 kg ($p<0.001$). A significant correlation was found between

Table 5
Pre-pregnancy BMI, Gestational Weight Gain and Birth Weight of Newborn

Parameters (Mean ± SD)	*Birth Weight (kgs) (Mean ± SD)*	*r - value*
Pre pregnancy BMI (kg/m^2) 18.34 ± 1.23	2.81 ± 0.27	0.1906 p<0.001
Maternal Weight gain (kgs) 13.68 ± 2.17		

the gestational weight gain and the birth weight of the newborns, delivered by the subjects with low body mass index.

The observation in this study is similar to those reported by Mitchell and Lerner (1989). Hence it can be represented that even if a woman starts her pregnancy with poor weight for height as indicated by her pre pregnancy body mass index, if she gains adequate and appropriate weight during her gestation, she can give birth to an infant with normal birth weight (Mitchell and Lerner, 1989).

Discussion

Our results confirm earlier reports that birth weight increases as pre-pregnancy BMI increases (Winkvist et al., 2002). Weight gain was significantly associated with birth weight even among low BMI women. Underweight must receive special attention and the need for weight gains of at least 15kg should be stressed (Schlenker and Long, 2006). Despite our small sample size we did identify a reduction in overall adverse outcomes. Our study found 11-13kgs to be appropriate weight gain for women with normal BMI and 13-17kgs for those with low BMI.

Previous studies have shown that pregnancy weight gain within the ranges recommended by IOM is associated with the best outcome for both mothers and infants (Ogunyemi et al., 1998; Merchant et al., 1999). On the contrary, some studies, that retrospectively assessed the sensitivity and specificity of this indictor, concluded that maternal weight gain alone is neither a sensitive nor a specific predictor of poor pregnancy outcomes (Abrams et al., 2000).

Our study suggests that deviation in maternal weight gain can act as a useful marker of newborn weight at birth and, also pre-pregnancy BMI can predict fetal weight especially in women with BMI<19.8 kg/m^2. Ogunyemi et al. (1998) has mentioned that normal BMI and ideal weight gain in pregnancy is associated with decreased perinatal complications and an optimum birth weight. The relation between low pregnancy weight gain and increased risk of preterm birth was previously illustrated by Carmichael and Abrams (1997). Although the biological mechanism underlining this association is unknown, it appears that a rate of pregnancy weight gain below the lower limit of the IOM's recommended range especially in late pregnancy may be related to a higher risk of delivering low birth infants (Abrams et al., 2000). Other studies have found that risk of preterm birth was not associated with maternal BMI (Ronnenberg et al., 2003). In the present study there was no difference between weight gain and birth weight. This may be due to data collection which did not analyse weight fluctuations weekly, and therefore not able to assess any acute inappropriate weight gains, which may have occurred during period of a week.

Pre pregnancy BMI is an independent determinant of birth weight of the child and in this study it was found to be linearly associated with weight gain and birth weight of the child. Unlike many determinants of infant growth, low pre pregnancy BMI is a risk factor that is easily identified. Although it is not known whether efforts to increase low maternal BMI before conception can reduce the risk of adverse pregnancy outcomes, there is evidence that optimized weight gain during pregnancy may help prevent the adverse effects associated with low maternal BMI before pregnancy or in the early months of gestation (Mitchell and Lerner, 1989; Bracero and Byrne, 1998). These findings support the need to balance pre-pregnancy weight and gestational weight gain against the risk of LBW.

Conclusions

Thus in conclusion, efforts should be directed to attain adequate pre-pregnancy weight and gestational weight gain to reduce the likelihood of low birth weight. It is an encouraging fact for women with low BMI that if they achieve an adequate and appropriate weight gain during gestation as per the recommended standards they would be able to deliver a baby with a normal birth weight and thereby decreasing morbidity and mortality and other related complications in future life. Our data support the commonly recommended notion that health care workers and pregnant women should continue to follow patterns of weight gain during pregnancy regardless of pre-pregnancy BMI. Efforts should be directed to attain adequate pre pregnancy weight and maintain recommended weight gain to reduce the likelihood of LBW babies. Nutritional education may be effective on improving weight gain during pregnancy. Special attention should be paid to women with low pre pregnancy BMI and abnormal weight gain as well as illiterate women who are at higher risk for poor weight gain. It is important to identify ways which can minimize risk of adverse maternal and perinatal outcome and so identification of appropriate weight gain for each BMI class allows to counsel better. As abnormal weight gain and BMI were revealed to be associated with severe maternal and neonatal complications that are associated with extra expenses for the society and the family. Maternal nutrition education and consultation to ensure healthy weight gain during gestation seems to be helpful.

References

Abrams, B., Altman, S, and Pickett, K., (2000): *"Pregnancy Weight Gain: Still Controversial", American Journal of Clinical Nutrition* **71:** 1233s-1241s.

Bracero, L. A., and Byrne, D. W., (1998): "Optimal Maternal Weight Gain during Singleton Pregnancy", *Gynecology and Obstetric Investigation* 46: 9-16.

Carmichael, S, and Abrams, B., (1997): *"A Critical Review of the Relationship between Gestational Wight Gain and Pre-term Delivery", Obstetrics and Gynecology* 89: 865-873.

Catalano, P. M., (2007): "Management of Obesity in Pregnancy", *Obstetrics and Gynecology* 109(2, Part I): 419-33.

Ellen, A, Nohr et al., (2008): "Combined Associations of Pre-pregnancy Body Mass Index and Gestational Weight Gain with the Outcome of Pregnancy", *American Journal of Clinical Nutrition* 87(6): 1750-1759.

Gottschlich, Michele, M., (2001): *The Science and Practice of Nutrition Support*. USA: American Society for Parental and Enteral Nutrition, pp. 301-304.

Institute of Medicine, National Academy of Sciences, (1990): *Nutrition during Pregnancy, Part I-Weight Gain and Part II-Nutrient Supplements.* Washington, D.C.: National Academy Press.

Kramer, M. S., (1987): "Determinants of Low Birth Weight: Methodological Assessment and Meta-analysis", *Bulletin of the World Health Organization* 65: 663-737.

Mahan, L. K., and Sylvia Escott-Stump, (2003): *Krause's Food Nutrition and Diet Therapy.* USA: W. B. Saunders Company, pp. 185–189.

Maryam-sadat, Hosseini, and Jameie, Nastaranb, (2004): "Relationship between Pregnancy Outcome and Maternal BMI and Weight Gain", In: *International Congress Series, Volume 1271,* pp. 380-383.

Matarese, L. E., and Gottschlich, M. M., (1998): *Contemporary Nutrition Support Practice: A Clinical Guide.* USA: W. B. Saunders Company, pp. 327-329.

Merchant, S. S., Momin I. A., Sewani A.A., and Zuberi, N.F., (1999): *"Effect of Pre-pregnancy Body Mass Index and Gestational Weight Gain on Birth Weight", Journal of Pakistan Medical Association* 49 (1): 23-25.

Mitchell, M. C., and Lerner, E., (1989): "Weight Gain and Pregnancy Outcome in Underweight and Normal Weight Women", *Journal of American Dietary Association* 89: 634-638.

Ogunyemi, D., Hullett, S., Leeper J., and Risk, A., (1998): *"Pregnancy, Body Mass Index, Weight Gain during Pregnancy, and Perinatal Outcome in a Rural Black Population",* **The** *Journal of Maternal-Fetal Medicine* 7(4): 190-193.

Ronnenberg, A. et al., (2003). *"Low Pre-conception Body Mass Index is associated with Birth Outcome in a Prospective cohort of Chinese Women", Journal of Nutrition* **133**(11): 3449-55.

Schlenker, Eleanor, and Sara Long, (2006): *Williams' Essentials of Nutrition and Diet Therapy.* Amsterdom: Mosby, Elsevier, pp. 262 - 264.

Suitor, Carol, W. (1991): "Perspectives on Nutrition during Pregnancy." Journal of the American Dietetic Association 91:96–98.

Weiss, J. C. et al., (2004): "Obesity, Obstetric Complications and Cesarean Delivery Rate - A Population-based Screening Study", *American Journal of Obstetrics and Gynecology* 190(4): 1091-7.

Williams, Sue Rodwell and Nix, Staci, (2008): *William's Basic Nutrition and Diet Therapy*. Amsterdam: Mosby, Elsevier, pp. 174–181.

Winkvist,.A., Stenlund. H., Hakimi M., Nurdiati, D., and Dibley, M., (2002): "Weight Gain Patterns from Pre-pregnancy until Delivery among Women in Central Java, Indonesia", *American Journal of Clinical Nutrition* 75: 1072-1077.

24

Women and Household Food Safety in India: Inferences from a Nation-wide Study

G.M. Subba Rao, R.V. Sudershan, Kalpagam Polasa

Introduction

It is the basic human right to have access to food that is not only nutritionally adequate but also safe to consume (FAO, 1997). Food safety is therefore a public health priority. In response to the increasing number of food borne illnesses, Governments all over the world are intensifying their efforts to improve food safety (WHO, 2002). The year 2008-09 has been declared as the 'Year of Food Safety and Quality' by the Government of India. Unlike in the west, our food safety concerns are entirely different. In the western countries, people rely heavily on processed foods, which need minimal processing at home before consumption. Whereas, traditionally we are in the habit of procuring raw agricultural produce or semi-processed foods and further process them before making them suitable for cooking/consumption (Achaya, 1994). Hence, safety of foods at household level becomes quintessential in our context (Sudershan et al., 2008; Subba Rao et al., 2007). In the context of growing concerns about a significant proportion of food borne illnesses arising from practices in the home kitchen (Surujlal and Badrie, 2004; Scott, 1996; Bryan, 1998) the role of home food preparers in ensuring food safety becomes all the more important (Medeiros et al., 2004). Throughout the world, women are the ones who most often produce, purchase, handle, prepare and serve food for the family. They are the principal guarantors of food safety and quality of food at household level (FAO, 1997).

Although most food borne diseases are sporadic and often not reported, in India, an estimated 4,00,000 children below five years age die each year due to diarrhoea. Several millions more suffer from multiple episodes of diarrhoea and still others fall ill on account of hepatitis A, enteric fever, etc., caused by poor hygiene and unsafe food/drinking water (UNICEF, 2004). Given this context, the Ministry of Health and Family Welfare, Government of India, with the financial support from the World Bank has carried out a household survey to understand food safety knowledge and practices among the mothers of children below 5 years age in India. The study is unique and perhaps the first of its kind in the Southeast Asian region both by the magnitude and methodology used. The quantitative data was collected from a sample of mother respondents from 20,719 households of five regions spread over 28 states of India. This quantitative data was triangulated with 164 focus group discussions (FGDs) with mother respondents who were not part of quantitative study. The study has given insights in to three main areas viz., Food Safety Awareness, Practices and Enabling Assets, which need immediate attention from the policy makers and food safety educators.

Women Ensuring Food Safety against All Odds

The results of this study reinforce that though women are not always the decision-makers, they are sentinels of health at household level and are responsible for ensuring food safety at household level because it is mostly (>95%) women who cook food in the homes. Most of them have no access to safe cooking fuel; many of them (about 76%) cook using solid fuels like wood, coal and cow dung cakes. Most of the houses are so small that there is no separate designated kitchen leaving them with no other option but to cook in a common place (31%) or verandah (28%). Only 33 percent have access to protected water while ground water is the main source for many (59%). Despite all these limiting factors women ensuring safety of food. Many women (78%) cook food twice a day and more than half of them (53.4%) mange to serve the foods hot. Though refrigerators were owned by a mere 9percent of the households women evolved their own indigenous ways of storing leftover foods, for instance, some women in west and northern regions were in the habit of storing food by keeping the food in cool place or in water or in a porous dish with water on the lid. Some of the women who felt that foodstuffs were more vulnerable to spoilage in summer usually cooked as and when required in less quantity.

Food Safety Awareness and Practices

It is usually assumed that awareness leads to the correct attitudes there by resulting in safe and healthy practices. The Indian experience appears to be proving this wrong. In some instances it was observed that certain food safety measures are traditionally practiced perhaps even without the awareness of scientific rationale behind them. For instance, most families (86%) store the left over cooked food in covered containers (99%) at room temperature (89%) and try to consume it not beyond the next meal (67.8%). Even among the 64.1 percent families who consume non-vegetarian foods (though occasionally), only about half of them store leftover cooked non-vegetarian foods for further consumption. Among them about 51.2 percent store such foods at room temperature. Many of them usually reheat the leftover food before consumption but the importance of thorough heating is hardly known so the practice may not necessarily ensure complete food safety.

Qualitative data also indicated that most of the Indian women seemed to relate washing hands, maintaining personal hygiene and cleanliness of surroundings as the necessary prerequisites of food safety. This is well reflected in the practice of washing hands before undertaking all activities pertaining to food handling. A large proportion of women wash their hands before feeding the child (86%). They (99%) also wash their hands after defecation and cleaning the child's stools. Other activities, which involve exposure to 'dirt' like mopping / dusting the house and handling the cattle are also usually followed by washing of hands (94% and 72%, respectively). Though they knew that washing hands before handling food was a safety measure, more than 75 percent of them wash hands only with water and usage of soap for hand washing was not very common. Even after defecation only 50percent of them use soap. Similarly most of the respondents claimed to wash vegetables (86.8%) and fruits (75.7%) before cutting or peeling. FGDs revealed that some women were in the habit of cleaning them by dipping them in a container of water, while the Dietary Guidelines for Indians (NIN, 1998) suggest that the vegetables should be washed under running water. This clearly indicates that they are aware that washing vegetables and fruits is an essential food safety measure but their practice is faulty because they either do not know the scientific rationale behind washing fruits and vegetables under running water or barely have enough water for drinking. Similarly, in instances where knowledge is not materialising into sound practices, the reasons could be the lack of access to potable water and constraints related to cooking fuel and sanitation.

Food Borne Illnesses

Since there is a possibility of indicating ideal behaviour in the survey and in interviews we made an attempt to cross check by seeking information on the occurrence of food borne diseases. When asked if any of their family members had suffered from symptoms of food borne diseases like vomiting or diarrhoea in the last fortnight (from the date of the study), about 13.2 percent of the respondents replied in affirmative, while about 3 percent reported food borne disease outbreaks in their locality in the last one year. In the focus group discussions most women seemed to have attributed the occurrence of food borne illnesses to consumption of foods outside home and contaminated water.

Action against Food is Adulteration or Contamination

The existing food safety regulation requires the victims of food adulteration to bring the case to the notice of the food inspectors or such grassroots level food safety regulators so that necessary action could be initiated (Chadha, 2004). When asked about the action that they would take in case the food is adulterated or contaminated, as many as 54percent of the women did not know what was to be done. About 29 percent said they 'do not complain'. It was interesting to know from the discussions that some of them pick up a fight with the vendor, but many of them usually return the adulterated foods to the vendor and take something else in exchange.

In FGDs, when the participants were asked about the effectiveness of the Government in curbing adulteration, they felt that the Government machinery was not effective. Many women almost ridiculed the Government fair price shops where they say adulterated stuff is sold.

Knowledge about Food Labels

Although 59.2 percent claim to buy packed foods only 21 percent of them look for the symbols on food labels. As regards the quality symbols on food labels, ISI (Quality Symbol by Bureau of Indian Standards) is known to 77.8 percent of respondents, while AGMARK (Agriculture produce grading and marking) is known to more than half of them only 22 percent know FPO (Fruit Products Order). Over 26 percent always check the list of ingredients on food labels while 43 percent check the same sometimes or rarely and 30.5 percent never check this information on the label. It is encouraging that over 75 percent of them all check the 'best before' date. The findings of the FGDs showed that most of the women were not aware of the measures they should take in case of adulteration. Most of the women never complain anywhere as they seemed to be unaware of what is to be done in such a scenario. In the north though women were aware of quality symbols like ISI and AGMARK, their problem of illiteracy prevented them from actually checking these on food labels. They also did not see the labels as most of the food labels are in English.

Conclusions and Recommendations

Most of the existing food safety measures they practice in their day-today life are innate cultural practices imbibed through generations. Such traditional wisdom is reflected in instinctive cleaning of hands before preparation and handling of food; storing food and drinking water in covered containers; inclination to cook food more number of times per day and serving it hot. Such practices can be strengthened if women are made aware of the scientific rationale behind them. It appears that the 13.2 percent of food borne illnesses reported at the household level are as much attributable to lack of enabling environment as much to the lack of proper food safety awareness.

Although providing enabling environment for food safety is essential it may not be a sufficient condition for ensuring food safety because a review of improved water supplies and sanitation facilities in control of diarrhea diseases among young children has shown that even under the most favorable circumstances the rate of morbidity is reduced only by 27 percent (Esrey, 1985). In this scenario it should be realized that food safety education for women is a powerful and practical means that enables them to make informed choices (Motarjemi and Moaref, 2000). The study also revealed that the *Anganwadi Workers* (Grass-roots level women health functionaries) were the preferred source for food safety education. This women workforce, which has been contributing to the nutritional well-being of mothers, infants and pre-school children, can now be effectively used to empower women with food safety education as well.

Women hold the key to combating to ensuring food safety to all provided they are empowered with enabling environment and supported by sound awareness creation endeavors. Since cooking and dietary practices and cultural activities around that are traditionally viewed as "natural role" for women (Beoku-Betts, 1995), they can play a key role in continuance of these practices for generations. Investing in food safety education for them is an essential and wise investment in 'human capital'.

References

Achaya, K.T. (1994), *Indian food-A Historical Companion*.New Delhi: Oxford University Press, p. 64.

Beoku-Betts, J.A. (1995), "We Got Our Way of Things–Women, Food and Preservation of Cultural Identity among the Gullah", *Gender and Society* 9(5): 535-555.

Bryan, F. (1998), "Risks of Practices, Procedures and Processes that lead to Outbreak of Food-borne Diseases", *Journal of Food Protection* 8: 663-673.

Chadha, D.S. (2004), *The Prevention of Food Adulteration Act and Rules*. New Delhi: Confederation of Indian Industry, pp. 70-72.

Esrey, S.A. (1985), "Interventions for the Control of Diarrhoeal Diseases among Young Children Improving Water Supplies and Excreta Disposal Facilities", *Bulletin of the World Health Organization* 63: 757-772.

Food and Agriculture Organization (FAO) (1997), "FAO and the Right to Food", A Background Paper for an *Expert Seminar on the Right to Food held by the High Commissioner for Human Rights and for the General Discussion on the Normative Content of the Right to Food of the Committee on Economic, Social and Cultural Rights.* Available at: http://www.fao.org/legal/rtf/statemts/paper 97.htm (accessed May 21, 2007).

Medeiros, L.C., Hillers, V.N., Chen, G., Bergmann, V., Kendall, P., and Schroeder, M. (2004), "Design and Development of Food Safety Knowledge and Attitude Scales for Consumer Food Safety Education", *Journal of the American Dietetic Association* 104: 1671-1677

Motarjemi, Y., and Moaref, A. (2000), *Food Borne Disease: A Focus for Health Education*. Geneva: World Health Organization.

National Institute of Nutrition (NIN) (1998), *Dietary Guidelines for Indians - A Manual*. Hyderabad: NIN, India, pp. 52–53.

Scott, E. (1996), "A Review: Food-borne Disease and Other Hygienic Issues in the Home", *Journal of Applied Bacteriology* 80: 5-9.

Subba Rao, G.M., Sudershan, R.V., Pratima Rao, Vishnu Vardhana Rao, M., and Kalpagam Polasa (2007), "Food Safety Knowledge, Attitudes and Practices of Mothers-Findings from Focus Group Studies in South India", *Appetite* 49: 441-449.

Sudershan, R.V., Subba Rao, G.M., Pratima Rao, Vishnu Vardhana Rao M., and Kalpagam Polasa (2008), "Food Safety Related Perceptions and Practices of Mothers-A Case Study in Hyderabad, India", *Food Control* 19: 506-513.

Surujlal, M., and Badrie, M. (2004), "Household Consumer Food Safety in Trinidad, West Indies", *Internet Journal of Food Safety* 3: 8-14.

UNICEF (2004), *Mapping India's Children: UNICEF in Action*. New Delhi: United Nations Children's Emergency Fund, pp. 32-64.

WHO (2002), *WHO Global Strategy for Food Safety: Safer Food for Better Health*. World Health Organization, Geneva.

SECTION – 7

Social Aspects of Health

25

Family Life Education in Schools: An Outlook

N. Dhanabaghyam

Introduction

Adolescent reproductive health received considerable attention at the global level. To promote policy development and program delivery, UNFPA, together with WHO and UNICEF, issued a statement on Action for Adolescent Health there is a growing acceptance of the fact that adolescents need information and education on reproductive health, so that they can protect themselves and make informed decisions regarding their reproductive health. At the same time, it is recognized that parents too have important rights and responsibilities in this regard. Despite such awareness, resistant persist. Some people fear that educating young people about sex and sexuality and providing them with related information and services will lead to a irresponsibility and promiscuity, although studies have shown that reverse is true.

Adolescent is a period of increased risk-taking and therefore susceptibility to behavioural problems. At the time of puberty female adolescents susceptible to more reproductive health problems compared to their male counterparts. They face disproportionate health concerns following puberty; foremost among those are too early pregnancy and frequent child bearing. They are over represented among those obtaining abortion and even more so among those needing medical care for complications of unsafe abortion. The incidence of sexually transmitted disease is also disproportionately high among young people, 1 in 20 adolescents contracts STD each year, and half of all cases of HIV infection take place among people underage twenty-five.

India is the second most populations country in the world, the proportion of young adolescent aged 10-14 is the longest among all young people live in rural areas. Majority of the adolescents still do not have access to information and education on sexuality, reproduction, and sexual and reproductive health rights (Health Promotion and Education in South Asia, 2007). Many adolescents face reproductive health risks. The crude's and social norms, constrain young people's especially young women's access to reproductive health information and services. Creating awareness and providing motivation to create and attitude of healthy sexual practice is going to be a major tool in our battle against AIDS, the point which need to be considered then is so as to which groups should these educational and motivational effort be directed. Now sexual attitudes and practices take a long time to get established in an individual with the seeds being soon during their early adolescence. Sex education or family life education is the best way for change the sexual practices of young people.

Family life education/sex education in its present form aim to impart "necessary" information about human reproduction, contraception and reproductive tract infection/ sexually transmitted infections. Baseline knowledge of the fact of human reproduction is certainly important. However it is essential to understand that such information may have little or no relationship to what young people know and experience as sexuality. In rural Maharastra, general awareness about AIDS was high (91%) but knowledge about correct etiology of AIDS is less (50%) and lack of awareness about RTI/STDs was also noticed. Lancunae in knowledge also existed as regards knowledge about high risk groups, like commercial sex workers, intravenous drug users and commercial blood donors. Durex Global Sex Survey (2005) suggest to 11.7 years as suitable to start sex education and the result also shows that more than one-third believed government should invest in sex education in schools. Studies show that accurate information encourages responsible sexual behaviour, including abstinence among adolescence. Studies conducted in India reveals that knowledge on pre-purbertal changes among girls is very low. Only 38 percent of girls were aware about the growth of auxiliary and pubic hair that accompanied with puberty and menstruation.

Developing countries in all part of the world face serious challenge in addressing adolescent reproductive and sexual health needs. Many adolescents are reluctant to seek help from adults whether with in their families or in professional settings, they therefore do not get information, counseling or services they need. Therefore, in the present study an attempt was made to assess the parents' attitude towards Family Life Education to their children at school.

Objectives

General Objectives

- To assess the attitude of men and women towards teaching of family life education to their children at schools.

Specific Objectives

- To examine the views of men and women about teaching of different components of family life education to boys and girls at schools.
- To assess their opinion about suitable age for introducing of each component of family life education in schools

Data

Data for the present study is drawn from the National Family Health Survey-3 (NFHS-3) conducted in Tamil Nadu during 2005-06 (IIPS and Macro International, 2007). In Tamil Nadu, the survey was conducted in all the 30 districts with a sample population of 6,344 households. Totally, 5,919 woman age 15-49 years and 5,696 men age 15-54 years were interviewed. Opinion about teaching of family life education for their children in schools was gathered through a set of structured questions such as changes in boys' bodies at puberty to boys and girls, changes in girls' bodies at puberty including menstruation to boys and girls, sex and sexual behaviour, contraception, HIV/AIDS and condom use to avoid sexually transmitted diseases. And if yes, the suitable age for teaching the above components were separately asked and analysed.

Results

Attitudes to Teach Family Life Education

In Tamil Nadu, almost all the women (88%) and men (93%) accept to teach family life education to boys at schools. Like that 92 percent of the men and 90 percent of the women had a positive attitude about introduction of family life education to girls at schools. Even though, majority of men and women agreed to teach family life education to girls and boys at schools, they may not have same attitude about teaching of all the components and their views differs in teaching of certain components. Table.1 explains that one-third of the men (33%) said that all the components of family life education should be thought to boys as well as girls in school. Like that 16 percent the women said that all the components of family life education should be thought to boys, but regarding girls the percentage is increase to twenty.

Teaching about HIV/AIDS (87%), changes in boys bodies at puberty (70%) condom use to avoid sexually transmitted diseases (69%) and contraception (63%) were mostly recommended by men for boys. At the same time for girls also they recommend to teach the same components such as HIV/AIDS (86%), contraception (68%), changes in girls' body at puberty including menstruation (72%) and condom use to avoid sexually transmitted diseases (64%). Nearly three-fifths of the men recommend teaching sex and sexual behaviour to boys (59%) and girls (58%) in schools.

Table 1
Attitude towards Teaching Family Life Education in Schools

Components of Family Life Education	*Boys*		*Girls*	
	Yes	*No*	*Yes*	*No*
Men	93.3	6.7	91.9	9.1
Changes in Boys' bodies at Puberty	70.2	29.8	43.1	56.9
Changes in Girls' bodies at Puberty including Menstruation	41.9	58.1	71.7	28.3
Sex and Sexual Behaviour	59.3	40.7	57.7	42.3
Contraception	62.8	37.2	68.0	32.0
HIV/AIDS	86.9	13.1	85.7	14.3
Condom Use to avoid Sexually Transmitted Disease	69.0	31.0	63.8	36.2
All	32.9		33.3	
Women	87.5	12.5	90.4	9.6
Changes in Boys' bodies at Puberty	64.0	36.0	43.0	57.0
Changes in Girls' bodies at Puberty including Menstruation	33.9	66.1	83.2	16.8
Sex and Sexual Behaviour	40.7	59.3	44.1	55.9
Contraception	38.2	61.8	51.2	48.8
HIV/AIDS	76.6	23.4	76.7	23.3
Condom Use to avoid Sexually Transmitted Disease	33.2	66.8	31.2	68.8
All	15.5		20.1	

Women have a different out look on teaching of certain components of family life education compare to men. Like men, women also recommends teaching HIV/AIDS (77%), and changes in boys bodies at puberty (64%) to boys. For girls they recommend to teach changes in girls' bodies at puberty including menstruation (83%) and HIV/AIDS (77%). Compare to men, women shows less interest in teaching of sex and sexual behaviour, contraception and condom use.

Just above half of the women (51%) agreed to teach about contraception to girls at schools compared with 68 percent of men. While considering about the boys the women (38%) differs very much with men (63%). Men show much interest in teaching of sex and sexual behaviour to boys (59%) and girls (58%) compare to women (boys - 41%; girls - 44%). The percentage of men agreed to teach about condom use to avoid STD to boys (69%) and girls (64 percent) is doubled than women who accepts to teach about condom use to boys (33%) and girls (31%). Both men and women show less interest in teaching of changes in boys bodies at puberty to girls (men - 43%; women - 43%) and changes in girls bodies at puberty including menstruation to boys (men - 42% ; women - 34%).

Attitude towards Suitable Age for Giving Different Components of Family Life Education

Respondents' attitude towards suitable age for giving different components of family life education for boys and girls at school are provided in Table 2. Generally, men and women have a holistic approach regarding the age at which the components of family life education to be given. All the men and women agreed the suitable age to give family life education to boys and girls is between 13-16 years.

Mean age suggested by women to start about the education on physical changes in boy bodies at puberty and girls bodies at puberty including menstruation for boys and girls is 13 years and men suggest it as 14 years. According to women suitable age to teach sex and sexuality for boys and girls is 14 years and men suggest one year later (14 years). Men and women uniformly accept to start education on

Table 2
Mean Age to Give Different Components of Family Life Education to Boys and Girls

Components of Family Life Education	*Mean Age (in Years)*	
	Boys	*Girls*
Men		
Changes in Boys' bodies at Puberty	12.5	12.5
Changes in Girls' bodies at Puberty including Menstruation	13.1	12.5
Sex and Sexual Behaviour	14.4	14.1
Contraception	15.3	15.4
HIV/AIDS	14.9	14.9
Condom Use to avoid Sexually Transmitted Disease	15.6	15.7
Women		
Changes in Boys' bodies at Puberty	13.4	13.6
Changes in Girls' bodies at Puberty including Menstruation	14.1	13.6
Sex and Sexual Behaviour	15.0	14.8
Contraception	15.5	15.4
HIV/AIDS	15.0	14.9
Condom Use to avoid Sexually Transmitted Disease	15.6	15.5

contraception and HIV AIDS to boys and girls at the age of 15 years and agreed a mean age of 16 years for giving education on condom use to avoid sexually transmitted diseases.

Results of logistic regression analysis (Table 3 and Table 4) reveal that among all the socio economic and demographic variables, viz., education and standard of living showed significant differences in attitude among men and women towards introduction of family life education to boys and girls at school. Men living in medium and low living standard were less likely interested to introducing family life education to boys at school than men who are in high living standard. Unmarried men were more likely to introduce family life education to boys at school than married men. Men below 20 years were four times more likely interested in teaching family life education in schools than men with 40 and above years. But the results are not significant (Table 3). Women living in high standard and who had high education were more likely interested in teaching of family life education at schools. Women living in slums, who had no living child, with less than five years of marital duration, women married before 18 years, who were living in capital/ large cities are

Table 3
Socio-economic Status of Men and their Attitude towards Family Life Education

Socio-Economic Status	*B*	*S.E.*	*Wald*	*D.f.*	*Sig.*	*Exp (β)*
Residence						
Slum	-0.1477	0.2882	0.2626	1	0.6083	0.8627
Urban	0.1938	0.1896	1.0446	1	0.3067	1.2138
Rural (Ref.)						
Religion						
Hindu	0.0504	0.2636	0.0365	1	0.8485	1.0517
Muslim	-0.1021	0.4089	0.0624	1	0.8028	0.9029
Christian (Ref.)						
Caste						
SC/ST	0.3903	0.4604	0.7186	1	0.3966	1.4774
Backward Caste	0.3321	0.4494	0.5462	1	0.4599	1.3939
Other Caste (Ref.)						
Place of Living						
Large City	-0.2339	0.2429	0.0097	1	0.9215	0.9764
Small City	-0.4556	0.4554	1.0013	1	0.3170	0.6340
Country Side (Ref.)						
Education						
Non-literate	-2.0079	0.4094	24.0567	1	**0.0000**	**0.1343**
Primary School	-1.5969	0.3987	16.0428	1	**0.0001**	**0.2025**
Higher Secondary	-0.7216	0.3894	3.4343	1	0.0639	0.4860
Higher education(Ref.)						
Family Type						
Nuclear	0.0971	0.1342	0.5239	1	0.4692	1.1020
Joint (Ref.)						
Standard of Living						
Low	-0.6644	0.1893	12.3198	1	**0.0004**	**0.5146**
Medium	-0.4964	0.1624	9.3414	1	**0.0022**	**0.6087**
High (Ref.)						
Age (in years)						
< 20	3.6886	15.6873	0.0553	1	0.8141	3.9883
20-24	0.3042	0.3020	1.0145	1	0.3138	1.3556
25-29	0.1230	0.1509	0.6642	1	0.4151	1.1308
30 and above (Ref.)						
Age at Marriage						
< 17	-0.4776	0.2706	3.1155	1	0.0776	0.6203
17-19	-0.3725	0.2437	2.3361	1	0.1264	0.6890
20-21	-0.0406	0.2350	0.0290	1	0.8629	0.9602
21 and above (Ref.)						
Marital Duration						
0-5 years	0.6902	0.3205	4.6384	1	**0.0313**	**1.9942**
> 5 years (Ref.)	-0.0446	0.2053	0.0471	1	0.8281	0.9564
Number of Living children						
0	0.2888	0.2596	1.2380	1	0.2659	0.7492
1	-0.5250	0.2059	6.5033	1	**0.0108**	**0.5916**
2	0.1630	0.1439	1.2837	1	0.2572	1.1771
3 + (Ref.)						

Table 4
Socio-economic Status of Women and their Attitude towards Family Life Education

Socio-Economic	*B*	*S.E.*	*Wald*	*d.f.*	*Sig.*	*Exp (β)*
Residence						
Slum	-0.0619	0.2103	0.0867	1	0.7684	0.9400
Urban	-0.0484	0.1318	0.1351	1	0.7132	0.9527
Rural (Ref.)						
Religion						
Hindu	-0.0804	0.1893	0.1802	1	0.6712	0.9228
Muslim	-0.4326	0.2776	2.4281	1	0.1192	0.6488
Christian (Ref.)						
Caste						
SC/ST	-0.0056	0.4180	0.0002	1	0.9893	0.9944
Backward Caste	-0.0302	0.4104	0.0054	1	0.9413	0.9702
Other Caste (Ref.)						
Place of Living						
Large City	0.1730	0.1682	1.0576	1	0.3038	1.1889
Small City	-0.4722	0.3014	2.4544	1	0.1172	0.6236
Country Side (Ref.)						
Education						
Non-literate	-2.9300	0.4725	38.4523	1	**0.0000**	**0.0534**
Primary School	-2.4187	0.4694	26.5482	1	**0.0000**	**0.0890**
Higher Secondary	-1.8166	0.4633	15.3760	1	**0.0001**	**0.1626**
Higher Education (Ref.)						
Family type						
Nuclear	-0.0799	0.0990	0.6505	1	0.4199	0.9233
Joint (Ref.)						
Standard of Living						
Low	-0.4543	0.1371	10.9860	1	**0.0009**	**0.6349**
Medium	-0.3876	0.1160	11.1659	1	**0.0008**	**0.6787**
High (Ref.)						
Age (in years)						
< 20	0.2615	0.4048	0.4173	1	0.5183	1.2989
20-24	0.2076	0.1893	1.2026	1	0.2728	1.2307
25-29	0.2713	0.1513	3.2155	1	0.0729	1.3117
30 and above (Ref.)						
Age at Marriage						
< 17	0.0889	0.1710	0.2704	1	0.6030	1.0930
17-19	0.0903	0.1502	0.3618	1	0.5475	1.0945
20-21	0.0763	0.1500	0.2590	1	0.6108	1.0793
21 and above (Ref.)						
Marital Duration						
0-5 years	0.0573	0.1428	0.1611	1	**0.0006**	**1.0590**
> 5 years (Ref.)	-0.0343	0.1608	0.0455	1	0.8311	0.9663
Number of Living Children						
0	0.4343	0.1991	4.7567	1	**0.0292**	**1.5438**
1	0.0781	0.1385	0.3183	1	0.5726	1.0813
2	0.1329	0.1032	1.6578	1	0.1979	1.1421
3 + (Ref.)						

more interested to teach family life education in schools than others. Non-literate women and women who had primary education were times less likely to interested in teaching of family life education in schools.

Conclusions

Baseline knowledge about human reproduction, contraception and reproduction tract/sexually transmitted infection in the name of family life education, not in the name of sex education was accepted by majority of the women and men. But, attitude towards teaching of different components of family life education differs wit men and women and for boys and girls. Only one-third of the men and women agreed to teach all the components such as teaching of physical body changes during puberty to boys and girls, contraception (HIV/AIDS), sex and sexual behaviour and condom use to prevent STI/RTI.

Teaching about physical body changes during puberty to boys and girls, HIV/AIDS were invariably accepted by majority of the men and women. Providing knowledge on sex and sexual behaviour contraception and teaching of physical body changes to their opposite sex is not recommended by most of the women and men for both boys and girls. Women and men belong to higher living standard and higher educated are more interested in teaching of family life education in school to boys and girls. Unmarried were more interested in teaching Family Life Education in schools.

References

Durex Global Sex Survey (2005), "Age When First Received Sex Education", In: *Durex Give and Receive 2005 Global Sex Survey 2005*. Accessed from http://www.durex.com/gss

Health Promotion and Education in South Asia (2007).

International Institute for Population Science (IIPS) and Macro International (2007), *National Family Health Survey (NFHS-3), 2005-06, India*. Mumbai: IIPS.

26

Society, Self Image and Risk: A Study of MSM Community in Mumbai

Ashish Kumar Mishra, Arun Kumar Sharma

Introduction

Antiquity and ubiquity of homosexuality is well established. All the sexual minorities (including gay, lesbian and transgender) have been described, acknowledged and even accommodated within all societies (Das, 2005). India is no exception to this. One can invariably find erotic images amongst scenes of epics and legends, which are considered obscene by present day society. Pattnaik (2001) writes that in the Khajuraho Temple one can easily find images of women erotically embracing one another, and men displaying their genitals to each other. One can also find several transgender characters in Indian epics and chronicles, like *Sikhnadini, Mohini, Arjuna (Brihanalla)*, and *Arvan & Krishna*. To him, one may interpret these depictions as repressed homosexual fantasies of a culture. Nag (1996) argues that homosexuality came into existence in India during the Mugal period. According to him some Muslim rulers are reported to have maintained harems of young boys. He also commented and referred to Muslim writings, and particularly to Sufi literature, in which homosexual eroticism was present as a metaphorical expression of the spiritual relationship between God and man.

The recent interest in MSM community, however, arises because of its connection with HIV/AIDS. In 1999, 13 years after the first case of HIV was identified in Madras, Indian government started targeted intervention among high risk groups (HRGs). HRGs were defined as female sex workers (FSW), men having sex with men (MSM), injecting drug users (IDU), truckers, adolescents, youths, migrant laborers, prison inmates, fishermen, street children and people engaged in tourist related jobs. National AIDS Control Policy (NACP)-III focuses particularly on FSWs, MSM and IDUs. Among all the vulnerable groups, MSM is a diverse and hard to reach group. In fact MSM is a general term to encompass wide range of sexual orientations and does not refer merely to homosexuals (Kulkarni et al., 2004). They are most stigmatized and most difficult to identify.

Review of literature shows that as compared to the western countries few studies have been done in India on MSM community. Traditional social norms, beliefs and stigma about same sex behavior and practices make them invisible in society. And due to hidden sexual identity they are supposed to live in isolation and anonymity. This not only makes them vulnerable towards the sexual risk but also elevates them to face many socio-psychological and sexual health consequences. The discrepancy between their sexual orientation and sexual behavior is also responsible for breaking off their social relations including family and marital relations. MSM have to maintain dual identity in life - one social and one sexual - and while maintaining two identities they have to face internal and interpersonal conflicts. Moreover, they are both medically and biologically at higher risk of HIV. Their sexual practices not only make them vulnerable towards HIV infections, but they also carry risk to others. Thus there is a need to study their self-perception, actual behavior, risk and coping strategies. This paper focuses on identities and risk behaviour.

Conceptual Framework

Literature suggests that there is a very little exploration of the social and psychological problems of the MSM. This paper, devoted to study of MSM community, looks at the relationship between social structures, identity and risk behaviour among MSM in Mumbai. It is assumed that both social structure and identity are important determinants of risk behavior; social structure determining behaviour directly as well as indirectly through identity. Thus one cannot ignore the role of social institutions such as marriage and family in understanding MSM behaviour. Both homosexuality and heterosexuality exist in society but due to norms of heterosexuality the issues connected with homosexuality have not been explored adequately.

For MSM, the problem of conflicting identities can be seen at three different levels: society, community and family. All of them influence self-image, actual behavior, risk and coping mechanism. In addition, there are individual level variations that are linked with responses to dissonance between different roles and identities. This paper particularly focuses on how the self-image or self-representation affects risk behaviour with respect to HIV.

Objectives

The main objective of the study is to establish relationship between self image, actualization of self image, risk and coping strategies among MSM in the context of their biographies, and socio-cultural and contextual factors, which are responsible for making them vulnerable to risk of HIV. To the fulfillment of this broader objective the following specific objectives have been set:

- To study the socio-economic and demographic characteristics of MSM in Mumbai;
- To examine if there are pressures on MSM to marry and produce children
- To examine the link between identities and the process of coming out

- To examine the risk behaviour and to examine the relationship between identity and risk behaviour

The Setting

This study was conducted in Mumbai, the capital of Maharashtra, which is one of the most modern Indian cities. In population it is the largest city of India and is known for its mixed, cosmopolitan culture. This city occupies a special niche in India and is considered the commercial capital of India. It has a large centre of industries including 2nd largest film industry in the world, which is popularly known as Bollywood. Over the period, it has been transformed into an entertainment hub, and a leading centre of modernization. Due to a large concentration of industries and a huge population, several other kinds of job opportunities attract thousands of immigrant's everyday from different parts of the country. In most of the cases these migrants are single males from the less developed, poverty stricken states like Uttar Pradesh, Jharkhand and Bihar. Consequently, the immigration has made this city over-urbanised. It is worthwhile to note that nearly 40 percent of the population of Mumbai is living under unhygienic conditions in 570 slums (Bharat and Aggleton, 2002). Poverty being associated with sex trade and risk, no wonder Mumbai alone houses 81 percent of the reported cases of HIV/AIDS infections in Maharashtra. Therefore, it is also known as the AIDS capital of India. It has a largest brothel based industry with more than 15,000 sex workers (Gomarel et al., 2002). Apart from the presence of a large number of FSWs it also has a presence of large number of single male migrants, truck drivers and other high risk groups such as transgender and MSM. Writings of Sharma and others show that Mumbai has had a visible presence of MSM for more than a century. Writers, intellectuals and even freedom fighters were aware of this. Some of them expressed concern about homosexuality among the social workers to Mahatma Gandhi, the father of the nation, who chose not to comment on this (Sharma and Vanita, 2006).

It is notable that the form of sex trade in the city has been changing. Due to closing of dance and disco bars new kinds of establishments are emerging. As a result of closure of dance bars a major shift can be observed from the dance bars based sex work to brothel based or street based sex work. There are several establishments having orchestra where sex work is present but in a disguised manner, creating higher risk of HIV. Interviews with MSM reveal that those clients who visit beer bars are often offered sexual services by MSM at much lower cost than at bars.

MSM activities in Mumbai are rampant at different locations. For those involved in MSM activities it is not difficult to identify other MSM. At several places, one can see them assembled in large groups. Gay bars in posh areas and messages like "Have fun with male" in the compartments of local trains indicate the flourishing MSM activities in the city. In Mumbai there are several formal and informal groups of MSM. There is an informal organization named Gay Bombay for those males who are romantically and sexually attracted towards the other men. This organization has more than 4,000 registered members. The organization usually organizes group meetings and parties for its members at different locations in Mumbai. One may think that in these parties 'sexual activities' are rampant but this is not the case. In fact, the sexual activities in these gay parties are totally banned. They provide a safe space for MSM. Parties are organized for having fun and social intercourse with other MSM. It is worthwhile to mention here that high cost of beer (450 rupees) in these gay bars is enough to suggest that the clientele come from higher socio-economic strata. Gay bars have heightened activity during the weekends. On the other hand, a few low cost gay bars too operate in the posh areas. In these bars sexual activities are not absent. While interviewing the Gay Bombay members it emerged that the higher classes of MSM hesitate to visit these low cost bars because of the fear of social security.

Data and Study Design

This study used both the quantitative and the qualitative methods. For survey among MSM at different sites mixture of probability proportional to size (PPS), and respondent driven sampling method was used. Care was taken to ensure heterogeneity in data. PPS was used for the selection of sites and respondent driven sampling for the selection of respondents. All the data were collected by the first author only who had a prior experience of working among MSM in Mumbai and knew the ways of cruising adopted by them. In addition, help from six community workers and several NGOs were obtained.

Tools of Data Collection

In order to collect the quantitative data from MSM a bilingual structured interview (prepared both in Hindi and English) was used. The structured interview schedule covered issues related to socio-economic and demographic characteristics, identity, risk behavior, coping strategies, awareness of HIV/ AIDS, sexual practices, experiences of STD, and treatment seeking. To gather qualitative data, two separate interviews guides, one for primary key respondents (MSM) and another for other key informants (KIs), were prepared. From the key informants interviews organization related issue were captured. They include: their past experiences about the MSM activities in Mumbai, their opinion on how liberal society is, impact of AIDS on the community, vision and mission of action groups, kind of activities they take up, types of programs run by them, and major sexual health problems faced by MSM. Some information was also collected on their socialization processes, reasons, and the general problems MSM face in society, community and family, how they manage different identities at different levels and at different times, issues related to social stigma, sexual practices and meanings of marriage. Two FGDs were conducted to understand the problems of the MSM community. For this purpose a FGD guideline was prepared.

Results and Discussion

Background Characteristics

Table 1 presents the percentage distribution of the respondents by age, marital status, education, religion, engagement in religious activities, importance of religion, staying pattern and position in the family. The table is self explanatory. It shows that in terms of demographic and socio-economic characteristics MSM are drawn from all sections of society. The age range of the respondents is from 15 to 45 years with a mean of 25.6 years and standard error of .334 (data not given here).

Table 1
Percentage Distribution of Respondents According to Socio-demographic Characteristics

Background Characteristics	*Categories*	*Percent*	*Number*
Age	15-19	11.4	29
	20-24	33.5	85
	25-29	36.6	93
	30 and above	18.5	47
Marital status	Married	29.2	74
	Single	66.5	169
	Others	4.3	11
Education	No education	15.4	39
	Primary	22.8	58
	High school	40.2	102
	Intermediate	9.8	25
	Graduation and above	11.8	30
Religion	Hindu	43.7	111
	Muslim	32.7	83
	Buddhist	10.2	26
	Others*	13.4	34
Religious Activities	Everyday	44.9	114
	At least once in a week	33.5	85
	At least once in a month	13.0	33
	At least once in a year	2.4	6
	Never	6.3	16
Importance of Religion	Very important	60.5	153
	Important	28.9	73
	Not at all important	10.7	27

Contd.

Background Characteristics	*Categories*	*Percent*	*Number*
Staying Pattern	Alone	16.5	42
	With friends/male partner†	23.6	60
	Parents/wife/relatives	59.8	152
Staying with wife	Staying	59.7	43
	Not staying	40.3	29
Eldest son in family	Eldest	42.1	107
	Not eldest	57.9	147
N$		**100.0**	**254**

Note:

* Others include Christian, Jain, Sikh and Parsi

† 11Percent of the respondents are staying as a couple with their male partners.

$ In "importance of religion" there is one missing case, and the total number of those "staying with wife" is 72.

Fluid Identities and Issues Related to Self Identifications

Looking at their subjective perception of self identity, half (50.8%) of the respondents reported that they are effeminate males and identified themselves as *Kothi*, one-fourth (25.2 percent) reported that they are *Bisexual*, 13 percent reported that they are *Panthi* and 10 percent reported that they are *Double Decker*. The qualitative data, however, suggest that these identities are fluid and not fixed. It was found that in the past many *Kothis* have become *Panthis* and some Panthis have become *Kothis*. Among *Kothis* too they have two different types of *Kothis*: *Sari wala Kothi* and *Saathle wala Kothi* (i.e., effeminate MSM who wear the women attire and have make up like women) and the other one is '*Pant Shirt wala Kothi*' (i.e., effeminate MSM who wear men's clothes though during the sexual activity they play role of female partner). Due to societal pressure and social insecurity *Kothis* who wear sari, land up joining *Hijra Gharanas* for their survival. They are easily accommodated in *Hijra Gharanas* as Mumbai has an acceptable position of *Hijras* and these MSM also feel better in their group.

It was observed that *Panthis* face several problems arising due to *Kothi* image of all MSM. During qualitative interviews several MSM expressed worry about how MSM are portrayed in the media and what kind of conceptions general masses have about MSM. On the other hand, *Kothis* have their own woes. As their relationship is not permanent most of the *Kothis* express feelings of insecurity. They think that their partner may go to some other person any day. Many *'Saathle wala Kothis'* have committed suicide for their *Panthis*. Fieldwork shows the emergence of new groups like *Bahrupiya (men who wear clothes of women just for gaining money)* and women who learn clapping for earning money.

Effeminate MSM are likely to join transgender community where they are easily accommodated. After joining *Hijra community,* they have to follow strict rules and regulations of that community. *Hijras* are having different traditions and a hierarchal structure. They have seven different *Gharanas (houses)* and these *Ghranas* are having a clear cut hierarchy in terms of their position within transgender community. One cannot even accept *Paani* (water) from someone belonging to another *Gharana*. As one of the informants reported that *"...if you drink water in the house of any Hijra then you immediately become the member of that Gharana."* The consequences of drinking water can result into ostracisation from the previous *Gharana*. All the *Hijra Gharanas* have a traditional system of *Guru* and *Chela*.

Among *Hijras, Nirvana Hijras* (castrated *Hijras*) have a special niche. Qualitative data reveal that *Nirvana* is a very painful exercise. According to one Key informant, there are two types of *Nirvanas*: *Doctor Nirvana* (performed by a medical doctor), and *Dai Nirvana* (performed by a traditional practitioners). There is a belief in the community that those who go for castration at an early age become more feminine. This was also learnt that not anyone could go for castration. *Guru's* (i.e. leader's) permission is required for the castration. Key informant interviews reveal that due to losing their sexual organ, many *Nirvana Hijras* face problem of depression subsequently and some are known to have committed suicide. Therefore, proper pre-castration and post-castration counseling is necessary for these people.

Issues Related to Disclosure of Sexual Orientation

It is difficult to reveal the stigmatized identity to others. The decision of telling someone about the homosexual orientation can have long lasting impact on the individual. Normally, MSM keep a silence about their status. Whom to reveal and when depends on the evaluation of the social and economic conditions of an individual. A study among a group of sexual minorities shows that gay men are likely to fear that if the members of their parental family suspect or to find out about their sexual preferences then they would withdraw their social and emotional support. Therefore, they feel that hiding identity helps them to maintain interpersonal relationships with their families and friends. The people with a concealed stigmatized identity would carefully choose situations in which they feel comfortable and safe to reveal their identity. This can help them to maintain personal boundaries and provide control over levels of intimacy with others (Kelly and Mckillop, 1996). They can also choose not to reveal their identity if they are concerned about the repercussions, and thus do not have to be constantly on the alert or become the object of prejudice and discrimination.

In society homosexuality is constructed as negative, dangerous and potentially pathological. Social historians have described trans-historical construction of homosexuality as moving from sin to crime to sickness (Weeks, 1986). As a result of heterosexism, revealing stigmatized identity to others may result into breaking off the social relationships. The literature shows that young adolescents do not reveal about their identity even to family members because of fear of economic loss, losing shelter, physical abuse and detachment (Bales, 1985). Researches have also shown that people become uncomfortable when highly personal details are revealed to them too early in the relationships, perhaps because they feel they must also reciprocate with intimate information about them (Collins and Miller, 1994; Cozby, 1973). However, if the stigmatized person waits until a trusting relationship is formed before revealing, the relationship may be hurt because the stigmatized person is seen as not honest or trusting enough to reveal earlier. Jones & Archer (1976) showed that people who are known to hide something, or possessing something that needs to be hidden, are liked less than those who are open and nothing to hide.

A study has shown that MSM have strong desires to come out to their parents but the fear of rejection and negative reactions hold many of them back (D'Augelli et al., 2007). Among MSM effeminate men (*Kothis*) have special problems. *Kothis* can be easily identified by others because of their behaviour and life styles. This study found that only 28.6 percent of them had disclosed their sexual orientation to family members in different ways. Table 2 shows that half of them had told their family members by themselves directly. A substantial proportion (31.9%) of respondents had reported that they had not told parents but they learnt from observations. In some cases friends (11.1%) and relatives (2.8%) had informed the family members about their sexual orientation. The qualitative insights in this study also show that family members would not talk about the matter among themselves even if they are aware of the sexual orientation of their children. Many parents have come to know about son's sexual orientation from his girlish activities but they would keep it a secret; one parent would try to hide it even from the other parent.

Table 2
Mode of Learning about Sexual Orientation of Respondents Among Family Members

Mode of Learning	*Percent*
Self report	50.0
Family members observed	31.9
Through friends	11.1
Through relatives	2.8
Through others	4.2
Total	100.0
N	72

Consequences of Coming Up

Literature shows that those who had concealed their identity from others have relatively better social interaction than those who have revealed their identity (John et al., 1984). Concealment may allow a person to proceed with acquaintance level relationships and activities with fewer burdens than a person with a visible devalued identity. Yet, maintaining a concealed stigmatized identity leads to more cognitive and emotional burdens, while revealing it may interfere with interaction. The studies by Frable et al., (1990) point to the idea that people with concealed, stigmatized identity are quite facile at maintaining positive social interactions despite the additional cognitive burden. Every stigma coping strategy has both costs and benefits. By revealing their identity stigmatized people invite devaluation; by concealing their identity they incur the cost of an extra cognitive burden though they reap the benefit of being considered unmarked in social interaction. Research on the long term health effects of concealing sexual identity for gay men has linked increased concealment with higher rates of cancer and other infectious diseases, and for HIV + men, an accelerated progression of AIDS (Cole et al., 1996).

Members of visible stigmatized groups are able to reach out to others if they so choose. In contrast, people with a concealed stigma have a much more difficult time identifying similarly stigmatized others, and therefore, may miss an avenue of strong social support and comfort. Consequently, people with concealable stigma are expected to show lower self-esteem and more instances of negative affect than those with visible stigma. Thus, as mentioned above, maintaining a concealed identity may make people miss out on optimal medical care and other support.

Effects on Different Aspects of Life

If a group is discriminated against, its members may internalize negative self image. Due to fear of exclusion gay men deny that they were attracted to other males and hide sex relationships with men. Literature shows that gay men have faced humiliation by their parents, brothers and others for not being masculine (Mattison et al., 2005). For hiding they use various survival strategies such as being secretive, pretending, and withdrawing from peer activities although it may be very difficult for gay men to hide their sexual orientation from their close friends. Hiding identity from the friends and acquaintances implies having more sexual encounters with strangers and more risk.

Revealing sexual identity to others may affect the different aspects of human life. Table 3 shows that for some revealing sexual identity had very much affected their sexual life (23.6%), relationship with the male partners (23.6%), social life (45.8%), family life (16.7%), and economic conditions (34.7%). Some of them have also reported that it has affected their emotional and mental state. It may be noted that for nearly a quarter of respondents work life has been (very much or somewhat) affected.

Table 3
Distribution of Respondents Who Reported Change in Different Aspects of Life

	Extant of Change in Life after Disclosing Status			
	Very much	*Some what*	*Not at all*	*Total*
Aspects of Life	*Percent*	*Percent*	*Percent*	*Percent*
Sexual life in general	23.6	18.1	58.3	100.0
Extramarital relationship	2.8	8.3	88.9	100.0
Relationship with the male partner	23.6	8.3	68.1	100.0
The way I perceive myself	8.3	5.6	86.1	100.0
Work life	12.5	12.5	75.0	100.0
Family life	16.7	8.3	75.0	100.0
Social life	45.8	13.9	40.3	100.0
Economic condition	34.7	16.7	48.6	100.0
Emotional state	12.5	12.5	75.0	100.0
Mental state	13.9	18.1	68.1	100.0

MSM face difficulties at their work place. *Kothis* particularly face discrimination at the work place because of their looks and appearances. Sometimes the exploitation turns into providing sexual satisfaction to others.

In the study a question was asked to those respondents who have revealed their identity to someone about how they rate their current relationships with the other people. Table 4 shows that a very few have reported having good relationship with their wives (22.2%). Yet, it is satisfactory to note that a substantial proportion of the respondents have reported having good relationships with their family members (59.7%), relatives (54.2%), friends (84.7%), colleagues (86.1%) and neighbors (70.8%) though.

Table 4
Distribution of Respondents According to Rating of Relationship with Different Members

	Rating				
Relationship	*Good*	*Bad*	*No Relations*	*NA*	*Total*
Wife	22.2	9.7	4.2	63.9	100.0
Family members	59.7	25	9.7	5.6	100.0
Relatives	54.2	30.6	11.1	4.2	100.0
Friends	84.7	6.9	5.6	2.8	100.0
Colleagues	86.1	4.2	1.4	8.3	100.0
Neighbours	70.8	12.5	9.7	6.9	100.0

Issues Related to Family and Marriage

Among MSM issues related to family formation and marriage of great significance. Young and unmarried MSM are apprehensive about the consequences of getting married and exposing their sexual orientation to family and society. The social responsibilities, however, create enormous pressure on them to marry. Forced marriages of MSM create unimaginable odd situations for both the parties. Their family exists in society. Family also has a strong expectation from them to prove their masculinity by procreating children. MSM get married to women not because of their desire for marriage with a woman but due to mounting societal pressure through which they are compelled to get married and for fulfilling the societal needs they have to produce a child. Since MSM have no attraction towards women, marriage creates a very uncomfortable situation in front of them. Wife's knowledge about husband's homosexual status can lead to divorce between husband and wife. In extreme cases, conflict between husband and wife, when the wife came to know about sexual orientation of the husband, has led to suicide. Some MSM are hiring boys for providing sexual satisfaction to their wives. In such situations, it is very difficult to say who the victim is and who the victimizer is. This is a matter of serious concern to planners as this affects the dignity of wife also. This also affects the power structure of family especially with regard to husband-wife relationship. In-depth interview with one MSM shows that MSM are also most concerned about the marital relationships. He also suggests that allowing gay marriage might solve several problems of marriage and family like property inheritance and adoption of children.

The acceptance of MSM by their family members depends on their needs. These needs could be in the form of money, emotional or physical. If some needs of family members are satisfied from MSM then the family members may ignore their sexual orientation. The family members react more when there is a gap in fulfillment of their wishes. Therefore, adjustment problems are more associated with the family demands or expectations. MSM respondents think that they cannot live their life as per their own desire as homosexuality will never be accepted in society. Due to social needs they sacrifice their desires and try to fulfill the family expectations by following the norms of society.

In Indian situation most families hold to tradition. Their value system is often reinforced by the religious belief system. In the current system one has to follow heterosexual life styles and family members are expected to marry and continue the traditional system even when heterosexual marriage creates unnecessary pressures on them. They leave very little space for men and women to enjoy their choice and compel married MSM to remain married. Moreover, they have also known that at the later stages of life unmarried MSM face problems of loneliness. Single persons face difficulty in maintaining social relationships. Sometimes, they are cut off from their social circle.

Factors in Sexual Self Image

The above discussion shows how societal norms and perceptions affect the family life of MSM. David Greenberg (1988) argues in his book *Construction of Homosexuality* that in general, homosexuality is considered as evil, sick or undesirable and the corresponding efforts to punish, cure, or prevent it make homosexuality deviant. Consequently, in society a homosexual is labeled as deviant, mentally ill, and an incomplete man. This makes a MSM develop self-image of deviant. In psychology the self-image has been defined as the "total subjective perception of oneself, including an image of one's body and impressions of one's personality, capabilities, and so on" (Coon, 1994). One's self-image is one's mental picture of one's physical appearance, and the integration of one's experiences, desires, and feelings. Mead looks at self as an ongoing social process with two distinct phases: the *'I'* who is described as spontaneous response of the individual to social situation, and *'Me'* a socially structured, conscious self-image. For Mead, the *'I'* is a source of novelty and creativity, vital for the affirmation of individuality, while me refers to the set of organized social attitudes within one. For this study the *self-image is defined as the positive and negative perceptions about oneself because of one's sexual orientation.* This is not to deny that variety of individual, family and societal factors play crucial role in shaping one's perceptions about oneself. Those who are having positive self-image are more likely to tolerate discrimination, condemnation, and misperception by others. The negative self-images could result into high substance use, low safe sexual practices, unsatisfactory relationships, feeling of underachievement, feeling of guilt and shame, fear of rejection, depression, feeling of being inferior and suicidal feelings (Alexander, 1997).

Analysis shows that those who reported lesser number of partners are more likely to maintain heterosexual identity in society. Those who are having higher number of male partners are more likely to maintain homosexual behavior in public places. Further, those who received exchange during the last sexual encounter, higher proportion of them maintain heterosexual image in public. Risk related actions also show significant variations between the categories of homosexual and heterosexual; it shows that a higher proportion of those who do not practice any risk reduction action are maintaining heterosexual identity. HIV testing is also related to image in public. It shows that those who have reported to go for testing are more likely to have homosexual identity. *Kothis* are more likely to maintain homosexual identity in public as compared to their *Panthis* and *Bisexuals*. There is a caveat here. It is difficult to say whether the social and risk characteristics are causes or consequences of public image. They are both.

Initiation of Sex, Subjective Identities, and Risk

Table 5 shows the results of analysis of multiple partner sex and its relationship with their subjective identities, initiation of sex and characteristics related to current sexual practices. It shows significant variation in the practice of multi-partner sex for all the characteristics. *Kothis seem to have* more number of partners (10.6) in last 30 days as compared to *Panthis* (6 partners) and *Bisexuals* (5.3 partners). The others, however, have the maximum number of partners (18 partners). Analysis of relationship of multiple partner sex with age of feeling of being homosexual shows that the relationship is inverted U-shaped. Those who felt that they are homosexual between 9-14 years of age have more number of partners than those who felt so earlier or later. Age of involvement in MSM activities seems to be negatively associated with multiple partner sex. Those who involved in sex with male at older ages have lower number of partners than those who had sex earlier. All other relationships are along expected lines. Multiple partner sex is associated with having first sex in one's own social circle, recent sex, unknown marital status, casual sex and exchange of cash and kind in last sex.

Table 5
Average Number of Male Partners in Last 30 Days by Self Identity, Age of Initiation of Sex and Current Sexual Practices

Background Characteristics	*Mean*	*N*	*SD*	*F*	*Sig.*
Self Identity					
Kothi	10.6	129	11.3	6.11	0.001
Panthi	6.0	33	12.8		
Bisexual	5.3	64	7.6		
Others	18.4	28	32.4		
Total	9.5	254	15.1		
Age of Feeling of Being Homosexual					
0-9	12.3	26	13.6	5.1	0.007
9-14	13.2	82	17.0		
15 and above	7.0	146	13.7		
Total	9.5	254	15.1		
Age of Involvement in Sex with Male					
0-9	26.3	3	37.9	4.69	0.010
10-14	14.2	42	13.8		
15 and above	8.3	209	14.7		
Total	9.5	254	15.1		
First Sexual Relationship with Male Partner					
Social Circle	8.8	224	13.6	10.01	0.002
Anonymous 19.9	20	26.5			
Total	9.7	244	15.3		
Number of Days Having Last Sex					
Less than 7days	12.4	160	1.8	8.57	0.000
7 to 15 days 4.6	62	3.9			
More than 15 days	4.5	32	7.2		
Total	9.5	254	15.1		
Marital Status of Last Partner					
Known marital status	6.3	171	7.3	27.07	0.000
Unknown marital status	16.2	83	22.9		
Total	9.5	254	15.1		
Type of Relationship with Male Partners					
Stable	3.8	76	6.1	13.86	0.000
Stable with multiple partners	6.6	54	5.4		
Casual	14.3	124	19.6		
Total	9.5	254	15.1		
Received Cash/Kind during Last Sex					
Yes	14.0	109	17.4	17.8	0.000
No	6.2	145	12.1		
Total	9.5	254	15.1		

Conclusions

This study shows how the social structure dominated by heterosexual discourse leads to various health risks among the MSM. In day-to-day interaction MSM adopt dual images in public and private life. Due to these dual images and conflicts between them, they face negative emotions such as guilt and anger. Information about sexual identity of a homosexual son kills the honor of the family. Its knowledge results in a great shock. In some cases it may lead to severe psychological problems and heart attack. In this milieu, heterosexual norms create a conflict between sexual and social identities and whether a person should come out or not. In both the cases it leads to tremendous psychological stress on the mind of the person. If he comes out he faces discrimination, stigma and prejudices. If he does not come out he suffers from the feeling of being a liar, a criminal. What a person does eventually depends on family environment, experiences and social circumstances. Many members of the MSM community are forced to marry to maintain family honor and this not only victimizes the person but this also ruins the life of his wife and in the process many people are adversely affected. In the context of conflict between sexual and social identity and abnormal self-image the members of sexual minorities develop subsequently, they tend to lose agency and are found engaging in risk behavior affecting their health as well health of many others who come in their contact - wife, partners, etc. This calls for appropriate action on the part of government and civil society actors.

References

Alexander, L. (1997), "Self-injury and Its Function in a Non-Clinical Population: Preliminary Findings". Paper Presented at the *Meeting of International Society for the Traumatic Stress*, Montreal, Canada.

Das, Amara, (2005), *Tritiya-Prakriti: People of Third Sex*. USA: Galva-108 Inc.

Bales, J. (1985), "Gay Adolescents Pain Compounded", *APA Monitor* 16(12).

Bharat, S., and P.J. Aggleton (2002), "Community Responses to HIV/AIDS in Mumbai City", In: Smiran Panda, Anindya Chatteerjee and Abu S Abdul-Quader, (eds.), *Living with the AIDS Virus: The Epidemic and Response in India.* New Delhi: Sage.

Cole, Steve W., Margaret E. Kemeny, S.E. Taylor, and B.R. Visscher (1996), "Elevated Physical Health Risk among Gay Men Who Conceal Their Homosexual Identity", *Health Psychology* 15(4): 243-251.

Collins, N.L., and L.C. Miller (1994), "Self Disclosure and Liking: A Meta-analytic Review", *Psychological Bulletin* 116(3): 457-475.

Coon, D. (1994), *Essentials of Psychology*, St. Paul, Minneapolis: West Publishing Co.

Cozby, Paul. C. (1973), "Self Disclosure: A Literature Review", *Psychological Bulletin* 79(2): 73-91.

D'Augelli, A.R., H.J. Rendina, K.O. Sinclair, and A.H. Grossman (2007), "Lesbian and Gay Youth's Aspirations for Marriage and Raising Children", *Journal of LGBT Issues in Counselling* 1(4): 77-96.

Greenberg, David F. (1988), *The Construction of Homosexuality* Chicago and London: University of Chicago Press.

Frable, D.E., S.T. Blackstone, and C. Scherbaum (1990), "Marginal and Mindful: Deviants in Social Interactions", *Journal of Personality and Social Psychology* 59(1): 140-149.

Gomarel, M, A. Bmne, and J. Thanekar (2002), "Adopting Strategic Approach for Reaching out to Inaccessible Population viz., Sex Workers in the Brothel-based Industry with Comprehensive Package of Services in Mumbai, India". Paper presented at the *X1V International Conference*, Barcelona.

John, P.D., Michael G., and Shively (1984), *Bisexual and Homosexual Identities: Critical Theoretical Issues*. Philadelphia: Haworth Press.

Jones, E.E., and R.L. Archer (1976), "Are there Special Effects of Personality Self-Disclosure?" *Journal of Experimental Social Psychclogy* 12(2): 180-193.

Kelly, A.E., and K.J. Mckillop (1996), "Consequence of Revealing Personal Secrets", *Psychological Bulletin* 120(3): 450-465.

Kulkarni, Vinay, Sanjeevani Kulkarni, and Spaeth R. Kenneth (2004), "Men having Sex with Men: A Study of Urban Western

Maharashtra", In: Ravi Verma, (ed.) *Sexuality in the Time of AIDS: Contemporary Perspectives from Communities in India.* New Delhi: Sage.

Nag, Moni (1996), *Sexual Behaviour and AIDS in India.* New Delhi: Vikas Publishing House.

Pattnaik, Devdutt (2001), *The Man Who Was a Woman and Other Queer Tales from Hindu Lore.* Philadelphia: Haworth Press

Sharma, Pandey Bechan, and Ruth Vanita (2006), *Chocolate: And Other Writings on Male-Male Desire.* New York: Oxford University Press.

Weeks, J. (1986), *Sexuality.* London: Routledge.

27

The Green- Eyed Monster: Understanding the Meaning of Jealousy in Romantic Relationship

Anindita Chowdhury

Introduction

The ensuing introduction entails definitions, theories and variables that are associated with understanding and explaining jealousy in romantic relationship, followed by researches that are relevant for the present study. The rationale for carrying out this study has been mentioned at the end of the introduction.

The Nature of Jealousy in Romantic Relationship

Jealousy is an intrinsically relational phenomenon (Guerrero et al., 1993). Jealousy is defined as 'a complex of thoughts, emotions and actions that follows loss or threat to self-esteem and/or the existence or quality of the romantic relationship' (White, 1980). Romantic jealousy is a set of thoughts, emotions and responses following a perceived threat to a romantic relationship by a rival (Guerrero and Andersen, 1998a). Jealousy occurs when a person desires to protect a relationship with someone perceived as already possessed, in contrast to envy, which involves the desire for something or someone not currently possessed (Guerrero and Andersen, 1998a). Several emotions comprise the jealousy complex, including anger, fear, and sadness (Guerrero and Andersen, 1998b; Sharpsteen and Kirkpatrick, 1997). Jealousy is associated with loss of affection, rejection, suspiciousness, insecurity and anxiety (Peretti and Pudowski, 1997). External manifestations of jealousy include crying, retaliating, leaving, using surveillance or even becoming violent (Guerrero and Andersen, 1998b; Pines, 1998). These responses can be both direct and indirect (Guerrero et al., 1995). In sum, jealousy is an involuntary emotion that typically follows some sort of real or perceived relationship threat. The potentially destructive nature of this threat is well established (Afifi and Reichert, 1996; Peretti and Pudowski, 1997). Indeed, jealousy is the most commonly attributed cause of relational violence. However, research also suggests that jealousy is sometimes associated with positive relational outcomes (Buss, 2000; Pines, 1998; White, 1980). For example, some partners believe that jealousy is a reflection of how much a partner values and loves them (Staske, 1999). One study found close to three-quarters of respondents reported attempting to make their partner jealous at some times or another (Sheets et al., 1997).

More pertinent to the present study are the studies concerning jealousy and its effects on relationship status. Research findings on the association between relationship satisfaction and jealousy, relationship status or length of relationship have been somewhat conflicting. Many studies report that jealousy increases at the point where a developing relationship becomes serious or exclusive (Braiker-Stambul 1975). A study conducted by Mathes (1986), indicate a positive relation between jealousy and romantic love, suggesting that jealousy preserves and promotes love. Review of literature shows that couples that are seriously dating or living together experience and express more jealousy than individuals who are casually dating, married or are opposite-sex friends (Aune and Comstock, 1991; Guerrero et al., 1993).

Relationship intensity also affects jealous experiences. For example, jealousy tends to be more prevalent among individuals in love (Mathes and Severa, 1981), who are more emotionally dependent (Guerrero and Andersen, 1998a), and whose partners have invested less time, money, and emotion (White, 1981). These diverse findings are consistent with an evolutionary conception in which jealousy serves functions such as mate guarding, expressing commitment, or attempting to elicit such signs from one's partner (Guerrero et al., 2004).

Relatively little research has directly examined whether, why or how people might make others jealous. The type of the relationship (married vs. unmarried) is believed to have a close relationship to jealousy Guerrero et al. (1993) found that unmarried individuals display more intense emotional and cognitive reactions to jealousy than their married counterparts. Buunk (1981) showed that unmarried women showed more jealousy symptoms than married women.

Studies Focused on Conceptualization of Jealousy:

Gehl and Watson, (2003) derived a conceptualization of jealousy using the data driven method of factor analysis that was not entirely novel. Buunk, (1997) based upon prior conceptualization proposed three different types of jealousy: reactive, preventive and anxious. Radecki et al, 1990, studied the effects of adult attachment and Depression of Quality of Relationships and romantic jealousy found higher levels of dispositional jealousy correlate with depression. A study conducted by Knobloch, 2001 on relationship development and attachment in the experience of jealousy found relational uncertainty and intimacy linked to cognitive and emotional jealousy respectively. A number of scales have also been formulated to measure jealousy. Boekhout et al., 2003 developed the Relationship Issues Scale (RIS) to explore infidelity. Pfeiffer et al, 1989conducted studies to investigate the psychometric properties of Multidimensional Jealousy scale (MJS), which provides separate assessment of cognitive, emotional and behavioral jealousy.

Objectives

The objective of this research was to understand the dynamics of this construct in romantic relationship by:

- Coming to a conceptualization of the term from the perspective of the participant
- Identifying the context (s) that gives rise to it.
- The impact it has on oneself and the partner
- The impact it has on the relationship.

Underlying assumptions on which the objective was based were:

- Jealousy is a negative physiological, emotional and mental state, experienced at least at some point in the relationship by all individuals (Pines and Aronson, 1983).
- Jealousy is universal in nature; its ramification is found extensively in romantic and intimate relationship.
- From the review of literature it was well evident that it is not a simple concept but a combination of emotions and reactions.
- The role of culture in understanding this construct seemed of paramount importance since it falls within the purview of relationship which is determined by culture and societal norms.

In the present study, the exploration was narrowed down only in terms of romantic relationship and did not explore the connotation and dynamicity of this concept in marital relationship. Romantic relationship in this study was viewed as a complex ratio of passion intimacy along with commitment. Review of literature shows that jealousy and its various correlates had been studied quantitatively, from a western perspective. Role of culture is a very important factor since the concept of jealousy is found to be associated and determined by cultural factors. Rationale for the preset study is based on the paucity of research of jealousy from an individual perspective following qualitative approach, keeping the Indian perspective and sensitivity in mind.

Method

Sample: The current study was based on 8 Unmarried postgraduate students of Delhi University. (4 male, 4 female) who were either currently involved in a romantic relationship, or were in a romantic relationship. Purposive sampling technique was used in this study. The Choice of unmarried sample was based on the findings of the research carried out by Guerrero et al 1993. The participants belonged to the age range of 21- 25 years.

Method used in the study: In the present study qualitative method of enquiry was adopted, since it enabled deeper engagement vis -a -vis the subject which was the focal point of the study. In the process of meaning making, the author's role as a co-creator facilitated the process of dialogue. Moreover the acceptability of the researcher's own subjectivity and frame of reference was not a source of contamination, which would compromise the objectivity of the research. Another significant reason of choosing qualitative method was the desire to obtain rich data, based on the faith of kaleidoscope of human experience.

Last but not the least was the fact that available literature on this subject was completely quantitative in nature, from the assumption that the method of study determines the result and the findings, the novelty of the process of the data and themes that would emerge from the narratives were the chief areas of interest.

Nature of Data: Data was in the form of narratives, which were verbatim in nature. The use of a tape recorder allowed the privilege of storing the intensity of each participant's experience, that they revealed in the interview, in uncontaminated form. The flow of the interview was left upon the comfort level of the participant. Semi- structured interview was conducted to collect the Data.

Data Analysis: Grounded Theory

Procedure: Each participant was interviewed twice and in certain cases thrice.

There was no fixed time limit kept for the interview, in a way it was left open to the flow of the conversation. The enquiry was framed as "If you were writing an autobiography about your romantic relationship what are some of the significant chapters that you would include or write about? What are some of the issues that you would mention? What are the landmarks that define and make your relationship different from others? What are some of the problem areas and silver linings in your relationship?"

This seemed un-provocative and at the same time gave a lot of control to the participant. They felt easier to relate to it. They started right from the way how the relationship started. This memory was one of the happiest for all of them, and it put them in a good mood. It gave them a frame, to come up with the issues as an when they happened in the relationship. In the process they mentioned the way jealousy affected their relationship. Strangely enough very few mentioned the term jealousy; they spoke of it experientially rather than conceptually.

Transcribing: This took place simultaneously with the data collection. After each transcription the basic analyzing of the data was taken up. Going through the transcription at least thrice, the process of coding was initiated notes were jotted at the right side of the lines or paragraph, they became the open codes. Further readings refined them.

Next similar concepts that each paragraph contained were clubbed; they became themes or axial codes. The themes were the underlying similarity in the concepts and categories, which were further specifications of the concepts. The participants were re-interviewed in case of any clarification/ addition/ elaboration for certain instance. More focused interviews were conducted after open coding.

After finishing the coding and data analysis using the grounded theory approach, the next participant was approached and the same procedure of data collection and simultaneous analysis was followed. The next stage after analysis of the data was that of discussion, where the common themes were amassed to understand the processes and come to a broader understanding of the dynamics. Due to lack of rich data and other factors only the last 5 interviews were used for data interpretation and discussion.

Interpretation of Results

A brief case study of the 5 participants whose narrative had been analyzed have been presented in the following section, followed by a discussion chart of one participant (Chart-I) whose various themes have been amassed to come to various variables operating on the relationship.

Case Study 1: Raj has been in the relationship with Anu for 7 years, and he feels that the magic is still there. The relationship started from high school. It was not love at first sight but a gradual affection, which metamorphoses in love catalyzed by the chemistry they share. The relationship went through its tests successfully. The fact that it was able to transcend the problematic dimension of long distance 5 years after its commencement made it more special. Long distance was not stated as a problem, but the issue regarding the "other" was an area, which had challenged the relationship time and again and had almost terminated it. The rival who had qualities, which he envied, and the capacity to replace him was a constant threat in the relationship. His own circumstantial inadequacy made him feel threatened.

Case Study 2: Pakhi, 23 has been in the relationship for 9 years, two years of which was before Vivek got married, while the rest 7 ensued after his marriage. In a way jealousy marked both the start of a serious relationship and the reason for termination. In this dynamics of jealousy operated in an ego destructive fashion. Issues regarding the concept of fidelity as understood from gender perspective evolved. Conceptualization of trust, mistrust and coping strategies used in relationship for mate retention came to the forefront through the narratives.

Case Study 3: Smita, aged 22, was in the relationship for two years with Sohan, which started from friendship and later turned into a romantic attachment. Issues of possessiveness, and partner exclusivity were the major factor for falling out. Her style of attachment and over indulgence seemed to make her undesirable in the eyes of the partner. Her main difficulty in the relationship was over sharing Sohan even with his friends, she wanted him exclusively to herself and considered every one coming between them in any way a threat to herself and the relationship. Link between attachment style and romantic relationship was one of the important dimension was explored in the discussion.

Case Study 4: Sonya aged 23 narrated her relationship with Rohit, which was just over two years. It was long distance relationship right after three months of commencement. The progression being from class mates –city mates-long distance lovers- to cross continent lover. Main issues in the relationship were regarding ex boyfriends and her ongoing friendship with them. Rohit found it overbearing owing to his introvert nature and the fact that she was his first lady friend. According to her, he felt his territory violated whenever there were instances of her past cropping up in the relationship even in the form of platonic friendship.

Case Study 5: Ana, 22 years was in the relationship with Karan for over one and a half years. She is the one who had taken the first step. Being the silent kind he was not very sure if she would reciprocate his feelings, so he had stayed put. In a way she harbors this feeling of not having been won over like she had desired in her heart. Her feelings are a clash between what she wants and what she has. Her insecurities about the relationship and love are often put to litmus test of jealousy, which she skillfully manipulates to constantly reassure herself on both grounds.

Discussion

The process surrounding the construct of jealousy have been elaborated in terms of conceptualization of the construct, tracing the factors that arouse it, the effect of it on the person experiencing as well as on the partner and finally the effect of it on the relationship.

Individual conceptualization of jealousy was obtained from the instances that aroused it either in oneself or on the partner. Its effect on the relationship was dependent on the behavior of the couple in response to each other, and the situation. The study had been conducted keeping in mind the Indian

Chart I: Conceptualization of Jealousy - Raj

Conceptualisation of Jealousy	*Reason Attributed for Jealousy*	*Effect on Self*	*Effect on Partner*	*Effect on Relationship*
The fear of losing the loved one to some else	Comparison with other more successful relationship	Pretense of normality and nonchalance	Unawareness of the true feelings of the partner	Relationship initiation
Being the second fiddleThe information regarding existence of desirable men in the life of the loved one other than oneself.	Comparison with rival and information about his resources	Striving to keep the partner all to self	Comparison with other romantic relationships	Bitterness and souring
Intrusion of a potential rival in the private space extracting quality time from partner.	Speaking of the opposite sex in flattering terms	Non participation in conversations	Crying	Reduced desirability of partner and relationship
Inability to keeping partner exclusively to one self	Partner considering the rival as perfect match	Hatred and aggressive feelings directed towards the rival	Re-evaluating the desirability of the partner and the relationship	Seeking alternatives
Too friendly overtures of other men directed at my partner		Entertaining Doubts of partner and relationship uncertainty	Renewed faith and security in the relationship	Re-establishment of love and need for partner
		Desire to get back at the partner	Giving more power and control to the partner	Tilting balance of power
		Losing faith in relationship	Reassurance of love and need for the partner	Strengthening and preservation of relationship
		Feeling animosity towards the partner	Choosing partner over desirable alternatives	
		Partner and the relationship losing its desirability		
		Attempts to salvage male ego		
		Substance abuse		
		Forcing the partner to take a decision		
		Demanding more control of the partner		
		Re- evaluating partners desirability in the light of new evidence		
		Giving the partner the benefit of the doubt		

Context, which had not been taken up by any previous research. As a researcher the object was to conceptualize jealousy from the narratives, in the process of which, the understanding developed that the subjective meaning jealousy, has for an individual determines not just his behavior in the relationship but also that of his partners and thereby the fate of the relationship. Thus subjective conceptualization of jealousy can be considered the overarching frame, which explains all the other dynamics of jealousy in the relationship.

The processes formulated in this study are resonant with the theoretical model of Investment given by Rusbult (1980; 1983), Interdependence theory (Thibaut and Kelley, 1959; and Ellis' model (1998) of partner-specific investment (PSI), which is grounded in evolutionary theory. In the process of meaning making eight interviews had been taken but only five were used for the purpose of interpretation. The reason behind this was that the mode of interview was reorganized and improved based on the learning's and shortcomings of the previous interviews. Out of the three interviews that were not used in the process of analysis, two were un- recorded transcripts. The participants had refused to allow recording and didn't go into the intricacy of their romantic relationship as a result the data obtained was not rich enough for analytic purpose.

Another feature of this study was the use of exploratory mode of enquiry while addressing individuals. The qualitative method of enquiry gives the freedom and due space for using ones own subjectivity to enter into the phenomenological world of individuals. It helped in tapping the range of emotions and understanding the significance and implication of the meaning of the construct in the life and personal space of the individual. After the process of individual data analysis, the understanding of interdependency of conceptualization and the context was well established. That is context determines the experience of jealousy in an individual while the other face of the coin was that the conceptualization of the jealousy, which has personal meaning for the individual determines the context under which it is aroused.

Based on the understanding an effort has been made to diagrammatically bring out the meaning of jealousy and thereby its dynamics in a romantic relationship (See Fig. 1). Depending upon the behavior adopted by the couple in either situation, the course of the relationship was determined, which was eithers enhanced or terminated. Thus behavior of the partner in response to ones felt jealousy or induced jealousy determines the effect on the relationship. The direction taken for the resolution of the context in which jealousy operates determines the fate of the relationship.

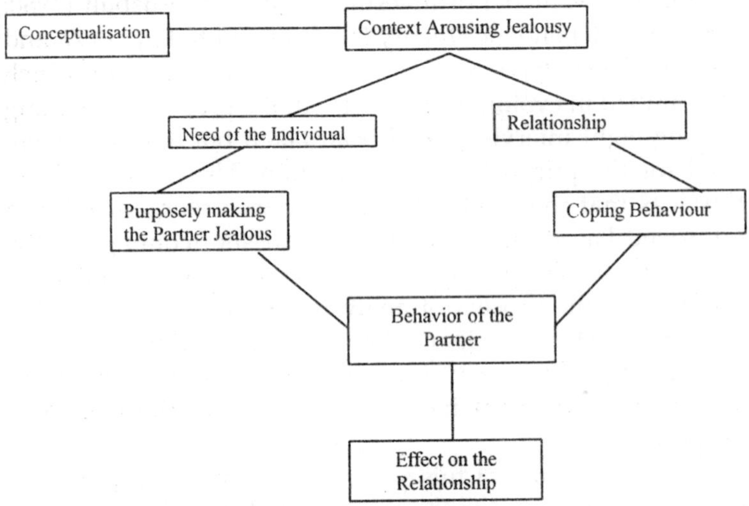

Fig. 1: The Dynamics of Jealousy

In accordance to the framework the common themes around the conceptualization of jealousy were:

- Evidence of love, and desirability of oneself and the relationship in the eyes of the partner.
- Fear of loss of partner or the relationship.
- Threat to the relationship from a potential rival, which involves the desirability of the alternative relationship as against the current.
- Possessiveness and need to make the partner exclusively ones own.

From the instances taken out of the narratives, the conceptualization of jealousy crystallized around the factor of love, dependency, insecurity and inequity in terms of investment into the relationship, be it tangible or symbolic. This is in accordance with the findings of Guerrero and Anderson (1998b). All of these conceptualizations corroborate the fact that jealousy tends to be prevalent among individuals in love who are more emotionally dependent and whose partner have invested less in time money and emotion, which makes the individual insecure and uncertain about the commitment of the partner. With regards to the narrative everybody other than Raj, considers that their partner have not invested as much as them in the relationship. This sets apart the conceptualization obtained from Raj's narrative from those of the others. For him the experience of jealousy is greater when the relationship is threatened by a potential rival who has resources, which the partner finds desirable. The next conceptualization of jealousy as formulated from the narrative of Ana, and Pakhi, was that of desirability of oneself and the relationship in the eyes of the partner, or the need to evidence love through manifestation of possessiveness. The feeling of jealousy in such relationships made the relationship desirable and the partner committed. The effect of jealousy, in such instances, was associated with positive relational outcome, since it enhanced the relationship making the individual feel more secure (Buss, 2000; Pines, 1998; White, 1980). Individual's operating with this conceptualization, deliberately tried to make the partner feel threatened in the relationship just to test their love and commitment. This implies that jealousy for these individuals served a personal need with an underlying motive for certain strategic outcome (Fleischmann et al., 2005).

In all the narratives the feeling of jealousy was associated with possessiveness or partner exclusivity, which was found to increase at the point when a developing relationship becomes serious and exclusive. Another conceptualization of jealousy that came about was that of the feeling of jealousy, which aroused an emotional need to getting back, what was once possessed. "*...the fact that he was married and that somebody who was all mine all this while was now somebody else's triggered off all the emotions like how can I let something that is mine go away, so it was more of an emotion of getting back getting it back.*" This feeling of possessiveness and retention of the partner goes to the extent where she justifies even his cheating on her. Pakhi operated on the evolutionary understanding of human sexual behavior. According to which, women consider emotional commitment with rival as a sign of infidelity. The study conducted by Meyer's et al. (2000), assumed that women infer emotional infidelity from the partner's spending time and exploring common interest with the third party. So to prevent the development of any form of emotional attachment with the rival, who was the wife in this case, Pakhi, bound him to the terms of the contract, which was psychological in nature. Operating on the belief that he was still emotionally faithful she chose not to terminate her relationship with him even after the birth of his son. But Rohit (her boy-friend) didn't want show her the same forgiveness when she had sexual relationship with another man. He wanted to end the relationship. The study conducted by Harris et al. (1996) showed similar pattern of sexual difference in response to jealousy. According to this study women thinking that man can have sex without love would think in terms that having sex does not imply that he has fallen out of love with her. The same scenario when encountered in Sonya's relationship created difficulty for Rohit to cope with. Thinking along the lines that a woman has sex only when in love, he had reasons to believe that since his partner had had sex with another man, she must have been in love with that man. Extrapolating on that he felt that the old love would be re- evoked if she kept in touch with her past. So for him, the issue of her past relationships seemed like a constant threat to the relationship's fate. These finding are consistent with an evolutionary conception in which jealousy serves the functions of mate guarding, expressing commitment or attempting to elicit such signs from one's partner.

Having framed the conceptualization of jealousy, grounded in individual narrative, there were certain points of departure that set each of the relationships apart. That is, it (jealousy) enhanced certain relationships while led to break up in others. This can be understood when analysed from the perspective of theoretical models. The reason accounted for jealousy in a relationship was based on certain factors, which can be divided in to individual and relationship variables.

Individual based variables were those which aroused the feeling of jealousy in partner purposely and sometimes without reflection. The jealousy, in these instances was conceptualized as demands that would fulfill certain needs of the individual. So more often than not it took the form of goal directed behavior aimed at fulfilling that need.

- The need of the individual may be to get attention,
- To sustain attention,
- To bolster self esteem,
- To reinstate the feeling of indispensability, and
- To reinstate exclusive rights on partner or to establish new rules in the relationship to broaden the area of control over partner.

Relationship Variables: This was dependent upon the degree of presence or absence of security in the relationship and the stage of the relationship i.e. in terms of being a developing, serious or exclusive relationship. Therefore in this case the following instances resulted in making an individual feel jealous.

- Uncertainty in terms of future with the partner.
- Lack of commitment, or allowed license of trust given by the partner.
- Presence of an alternative, which led to conflicts about the desirability of the current relationship.
- To get back at the partner for some past infliction of a similar kind.
- To score a point during an argument.
- Feeling the relationship slackening.

- As a way out of the relationship due to reasons that makes the previously desirable relationship currently less desirable.

Behavior of either partner depends on the reason accounted for the feeling of jealousy in the relationship. The individual who functions on the basis of the individual based variable uses behavior strategies, which are goal directed, based on the success rate of past experience and accurate intuition of the partner's response. Some such behavior, found were:

- Developing more dominating behavior.
- Demanding more control.
- Use comparison actively.
- Make the partner feel threatened to make them realize his or her importance.
- Inform presence of attractive alternatives beyond the relationship.
- Use various techniques that make the partner reiterate their love, based on past effectiveness.

The individual feeling jealousy due to relationship variable develops a form of behavior, which is coping in nature. It has the following features:

- Trying to incorporate the positive or the desired feature of the rival unto self to sustain the attention of the love interest.
- Inflicting pain on self, like self mutilation, which is used as a form of blackmail
- Using suicidal threats.
- Threats to terminate relationship.
- Withholding affection or becoming distant and reducing various forms of expected intimacy.
- Setting boundaries like asking partner not to talk, or spend time with rival.
- Reduce the chances of emotional attachment with the rival.

- Constant vigilance.
- Communication of indifference.
- Seeking out relationship alternatives.
- Getting back at the partner.

Depending upon the frame from which the individual is operating i.e. individual need or relationship issues the recipient partner resorts to crying; giving more control to the partner; agreeing to any terms and condition laid down by the partner to win him / her back; making choices, albeit forced upon them; which are in keeping with the demands of the partner; being more attentive; changing lifestyle to reduce the issues i.e. forsaking a certain lifestyle which were non acceptant to the partner; or reanalyzing the desirability of the relationship.

The last factor of analysing the desirability of the relationship determines the fate of the relationship; it is psychological and completely dependent upon the individual's own perception and needs. Its content cannot be specified with accuracy.

According, to Interdependence Theory (Kelley, 1979; Thibaut and Kelley, 1959) individuals evaluate their partners and relationships based on the perceived consistency between a priori standards or expectations and perceptions of the current partner and relationship. This is done by using the two standards: the comparison level (CL) and the comparison level for alternatives (CLalt). The former determines the attractiveness of and satisfaction in the current relationship while the latter refers to what the individual will obtain if they indulge in the alternative relationship available to him / her.

The relationship of Sohan and Smita didn't work out because Sohan perceived his CLalt higher than his current relationship hence he became indifferent. The current relationship had lost its attractiveness for him, owing to the constant fights and excessive possessiveness that Smita exhibited.

In the case of Pakhi, the relationship had developed from the mutual investment in which both of them had made tangible as well as symbolic investment. The switch in orientation that the relationship underwent following his marriage had made it more desirable. Since Pakhi had not been interested in any form of long term commitment before his marriage the relationship functioned on an exchange basis wherein rewards was based on the principle of equity. This became communal: a relationship in which people reward their partner out of direct concern and to show caring; when the future of the relationship was considered. But when Vivek in the later stage refused to reciprocate it was seen as a violation of commitment and caring. But the reason she continued with the relationship can be understood from the point of view of the Interdependence and Social Exchange theories of relationship commitment. This theory posits that's when relationships end, it is possible to recover items left at a partner's apartment, or divide marital assets, but it is not possible to retrieve the time spent doing things with, or for, partners. These types of "un-bankable" relationship investments play a pivotal role in determining relationship commitment (Rusbult and Buunk, 1993). Specifically, the more people invest in their relationships, the more likely they are to stay in those relationships. This was the reason Pakhi didn't terminate the relationship, in spite of wanting to move out of it at various points of time. The evidence of Vivek cheating on her also didn't change her mind.

Vivek, on the other hand considered his alternative relationship more attractive since if he let go of Pakhi then he would stand the advantage of forming emotional bonding with his wife and child, whereas if he continued with Pakhi he would lose on both fronts. Pakhi's physical involvement with a man other than him was something that he had difficulty dealing with. This adversely affected both his dependency on her and his commitment to her, and made him re-consider his alternative relationship which became more promising in comparison.

In case of Raj and Anu, the relationship being that of a committed one, individual monitoring of possible alternatives to their current relationship influenced interaction with current partner (Thibaut and Kelly, 1959; Buss, 2000), he believed that his partner would be difficult to replace, this made him resort to constructive coping strategies. Incase of Sonya, she depended completely on Rohit, she considers her relationship extremely attractive given the fact that he understands every small nuances of her mood like no one else. As specified by the Interdependence Theory (Thibaut and Kelley, 1959; Kelley, 1979), dependence reflects the degree to which outcomes obtained in one's current relationship surpasses one's CLalt, for her this relationship was the first of its kind, in which she completely felt secure and trusting unlike her previous other relationships. As a result she felt more satisfied with her relationship and engaged in behaviors that promote greater long-term relationship well-being (Drigotas and Rusbult, 1992). She gave up her freedom to a great extent. She even gave him the control to set boundaries which would govern her social life. With him she resolved issues in a manner that it would be in his favor because she perceives him to have valuable personal attributes, which surpassed her best available alternatives. For Ana, the litmus test of jealousy was enough to reassure herself about her importance and indispensability to the partner, which was an added boost to her making the relationship and the partner extremely desirable.

Limitations of the Present Study

- The study uses only unmarried couple thus the dynamics only relate to one aspect of intimate relationship.
- This study could not delve into the childhood relationship and attachment pattern of the participant.
- The narratives are just one side of the story; the dynamics of jealousy can be better understood if both the participant and his /her partner can be interviewed.

Conclusions

Individual data analysis and compilation revealed that individual conceptualization of jealousy was based on the factor which evokes it, that is whether it is self evoked or situational based, this determines the behavior of the individual experiencing it as well as his or her partner. The behavior can be goal directed when jealousy is tried to be purposely induced unto the partner tc fulfill an ulterior motive, or it can coping behavior which is adopted to deal with the jealousy aroused by the situation. Depending upon the behavior adopted by the couple in either situation, the course of the relationship was determined, which was either enhanced or terminated. Thus behavior of the partner in response to ones felt jealousy or induced jealousy determines the effect on the relationship. The direction taken for the resolution of the context in which jealousy operates determines the fate of the relationship.

References

Afifi, W. A., and Reichert, T., (1996): "Understanding the Role of Uncertainty in Jealousy Experience and Expression", *Communication Reports* 9: 93-104.

Aune, K. S., and Comstock, J., (1991): "Experience and Expression of Jealousy: Comparison between Friends and Romantics", *Psychological Reports* 69(1): 315-319.

Boekhout, Brock A., Susan S. Hendrick, and Clyde Hendrick, (2003): "Exploring Infidelity: Developing the Relationship Issues Scale", *Journal of Loss and Trauma* 8 (4): 283-306.

Braiker-Stambul, H. B., (1975). "*Stages of courtship: The development of premarital relationships*". Unpublished doctoral dissertation, University of California at Los Angeles, Cited in White, G. L., and Mullen, P. E. (1989)

Buss, D. M., (2000): The Dangerous Passion. New York: Free Press.

Buunk, B., (1981): "Jealousy in Sexually Open Marriage and Alternative Lifestyles", *Family Relations* 4: 357-372.

Buunk, Bram P., (1997). "Personality, Birth Order and Attachment Styles as Related to Various Types of Jealousy", *Personality and Individual Differences* 23(6): 997-1006.

Drigotas, S.M., and Rusbult, C.E., (1992): *"Should I stay or should I go?: A dependence model of breakups", Journal of Personality and Social Psychology* 62(1): 62-87.

Ellis, B.J., (1998). "The Partner Specific Investment: An Evolutionary Approach to Individual Difference in Investment", Journal of Personality 66(3): 383-442.

Fleischmann, Amy A., Spitzberg, Brian. H, Andersen, P.A., and Roesch, Scott C., (2005): "Tickling the Monster: Jealousy Induction in Relationships", *Journal of Social and Personal Relationships* 22(1): 49-73.

Gehl, B.K., and Watson, D., (2003). "Defining the Structure of Jealousy through Factor Analysis", Poster Presented at the *Society of Personality and Social Psychology Annual Meeting.*

Guerrero, L.K., and Andersen, P.A., (1998a): "Jealousy Experience and Expression in Romantic Relationships", In: P. A. Andersen and L.K. Guerrero, (eds.), *Handbook of Communication and Emotion: Research, Theory, Applications, and Contexts.* San Diego, CA: Academic Press, pp. 155-188.

Guerrero, L. K., and Andersen, P. A., (1998b):"The Dark Side of Jealousy and Envy: Desire, Delusion, Desperation, and Destructive Communication", In: B. H. Spitzberg and W. R. Cupach, (eds.), *The Dark Side of Close Relationships.* Mahwah, NJ: Erlbaum, pp. 33-70.

Guerrero, L.K., Andersen, P.A., Jorgensen, P.F., Spitzberg, B.H., and Eloy, S.V., (1995): "Coping with the Green-eyed Monster: Conceptualising and Measuring Communicative Responses to Romantic Jealousy", *Western Journal of Communication* 59: 270-304.

Guerrero, L.K., Eloy, S.V., Jorgensen, P.F., and Andersen, P.A., (1993): "Hers or His? Sex Differences in the Experience and Communication of Jealousy in Close Relationships" In: P. Kalbfleisch, (ed.), *Interpersonal Communication in Evolving Interpersonal Relationships.* Hillsdale, NJ: Erlbaum, 109-131.

Guerrero, L.K., Spitzberg, B.H., and Yoshimura, S.M., (2004): *Sexual and Emotional Jealousy,* London: Sage Publications.

Harris, C.R., and Christenfeld, N., (1996):*"Gender, Jealousy, and Reason", Psychological Science 7*: 364-366.

Kelley, H. H., (1979). *Personal Relationships: Their Structures and Processes.* Hillsdale, NJ: Erlbaum.

Knobloch, L.K., Solomon, D.H., and Cruz, M.G. (2001): "The Role of Relationship Development and Attachment in the Experience of Romantic Jealousy", *Personal Relationships* 8(2): 205–224.

Mathes, E.W., (1986): "Jealousy and Romantic Love: A Longitudinal Study", *Psychological Reports* 58(3): 885-886.

Mathes, E.W., and Severa, N. (1981): "Jealousy, Romantic Love, and Liking: Theoretical Considerations and Preliminary Scale Development", *Psychological Reports* 49(5): 23-31.

Meyers, L.S., and Nannini, D. K., (2000): "Jealousy in sexual and emotional infidelity: An Alternative to the Evolutionary Explanation", *Journal of Sex Research*

Peretti, P. O., and Pudowski, B. C., (1997):"Influence of jealousy on male and female college daters", *Social Behavior and Personality* 25(2): 155–160.

Pfeiffer, S. M., and Wong, P. T. P., (1989): "Multidimensional Jealousy", *Journal of Social and Personal Relationships* 6(2): 181–196.

Pines, A., and Aronson, E., (1983): "Antecedents, Correlates, and Consequences of Sexual Jealousy", *Journal of Personality* 51(1): 108–136.

Pines, Ayala M., (1998): *Romantic Jealousy: Causes, Symptoms, Cures.* New York. Routledge.

Radecki-Bush, Joseph P., (1990): "Quality of Relationships and Romantic Jealousy: Effects of Adult Attachment and Depression". Paper presented at the *Annual Convention of the American Psychological Association.* 99th, San Francisco, CA, August 16-20, 1991).

Rusbult, Caryl E, and Buunk, P., (1993): "Commitment Processes in Close Relationships: An Interdependence Analysis", *Journal of Social and Personal Relationships* 10(2): 175-204.

Rusbult, C.E., (1980): "Investment Model and Sexual Risk Behavior of Gay Men in Steady Relationships", *Journal of Applied Social Psychology* 36(1): 22-40.

Sharpsteen, D.J., and Kirkpatrick, L.A., (1997):"Romantic jealousy and adult romantic attachment", *Journal of Personality and Social Psychology* 72(3): 672-640.

Sheets, V.L., Fredendall, L.L., and Claypool, H.M., (1997): "Jealousy Evocation, Partner Reassurance, and Relationship Stability: An Exploration of the Potential Benefits of Jealousy", *Evolution and Human Behavior* 18: 387-402.

Staske, S.A., (1999): "Creating Relational Ties in Talk: The Collaborative Construction of Relational Jealousy", *Symbolic Interaction* 22: 213–246.

Thibaut, J.W., and Kelley, H.H., (1959): *Social Psychology of Groups.* New York: Wiley.

White, G.L., (1980). "Inducing Jealousy: A Power Perspective", *Personality and Social Psychology Bulletin* 6(2): 222-227.

White G.L., (1981): "Relative Involvement, Inadequacy, and Jealousy: A Test of a Causal Model", *Alternative Lifestyles* 4: 291-309.

28

Socio-Political Historiography and Corruption on Health Aspects in India: From Colonial Era to Globalised Era

Sangram Kumar Rout

Introduction

When the countries of South Asia freed themselves from the grip of colonial rule to reshape their destinies, they adopted two pronged strategies towards development. One component was the use of structural reforms at the social level. These included land reforms, protective legislation for the vulnerable religious and caste groups, provision of education for all and building of infrastructures to provide basic services such as public health (including medical care), transport, electricity, housing and drinking water. The other component was the promotion and use of technology to increase the outputs in all areas of primary, secondary and tertiary production. These two legs of development strategy were used in different combination by various countries depending upon their specific context and political formation. With this, the article is divided into two sections. But as a whole, it deals with the interrelationship between politics, economics and development of health systems of the Third World countries, an issue (health service) that has been marginalised in much of contemporary social analysis and policy making. It reflects the concern over the deliberate neglect of historical forces in policy debates and analyses the macro linkages in the Third World and other domains. The predominance of the neo classical economic paradigm in health policy and the politics of aid in the region are explored. But, the whole paper emphasized the need for an autonomous and people-centered development in the health sector.

The first section traces the evolution of health services in India within the political historiography from the colonial era. Before World War II, most Third World countries had what can be called a colonial pattern of health services systems. Colonial powers had brought with them the western system of medicine. The launching of the health services in these countries was subservient to the overall imperial policy of the colonial powers. Unlike the industrial European countries, the colonial countries were plunged directly from a pre-industrial health culture to a complex, alien pattern of colonial based health culture.

As the people rapidly became pauperized, they were unable to maintain the health services that they had developed earlier as a component of their overall way of like. This vacuum was filled by faith healers, sorcerers, magicians and other quick medical practitioners, who exploited the suffering of people for their own gains. In addition, unlike in European countries, colonial rulers were not overly concerned about public opinion because the population was subjugated by the sheer brute force of the colonial government. Many serious flows in the health services system of affluent countries have been identified by so many scholars. They have also made a critical analysis of health services systems in these countries in terms of their political economy. It is, however, significant that despite all the flaws and influence of certain political forces in these countries, health services have evolved as an organic component of a given social structure. Perhaps, the most distinctive feature of the growth of health services in Third world countries is that these services have been profoundly influenced by affluent countries. In this process, such influence has severely inhibited the growth of health services in Third world countries as organic components of their respective social structure.

In these Third world countries, Health services and introduction of western medicine set in motion very complex interaction within each country. The introduction of western medicine also causes complex interaction between it, on the one hand and the pre-existing health culture of the population, on the other. The far-reaching political, social, cultural and economic consequences of colonialism and imperialism, which have been associated with the introduction of western medicine in most Third World countries from another major category of factors that also influenced the process of interactions leading to the formation of health services in these countries in the colonial and post colonial eras. Health services were shaped on the western model. The medical establishment not only generates new health needs, it also determines how these needs are to be met. Due to increasing the commercialization and professionalization of health services in affluent countries, which were actively promoting the dependence of people on health professionals, the elite-oriented services in third world countries also acquired these elements. In this process, they swallowed more and more scare resources. The excessive preoccupation of the leadership at political, bureaucratic and technocratic levels with urban health services system led to the neglect of rural health services.

The Indian Scenario (Health Services)

In the field of health, the new rulers promised to take active steps to make benefits available to the masses, particularly, to the weaker sections. In fact, they continued to follow the old colonial tradition and the urban health services systems continued to receive much greater attention in the development of both the curative and the preventive aspects in contrast to the rural health services system. The generation of internal tension in the ruling classes and because of some awakening among the masses, political leadership in the Third

World is now realizing that it is no longer possible to perpetuate the present social order without making some 'concessions' to the masses. Imposition of a state emergency in India in June, 1977 showed that a major crisis had developed within the prevailing social and political system. The area of health services has been singled out for making concessions on the presumption that, unlike such sensitive areas as land reforms, minimum wages and democratization, it will not pose much of a threat to the social system. In India, for example, the leaders who took over political power in March, 1977 by taking advantage of the deep-seated resentment and revulsion of the people to the family planning excesses in previous months, redeemed their election pledges and initiated a new programme based on village level community health workers, entrusting "people's health in people's hands". This is a remarkable development, though it is obvious that the existing social structure and prevailing 'culture' of the elite-oriented professionalized health system of the country are grossly incompatible with such a philosophy.

The political leadership and health administrators in third world countries sought an aura of social legitimacy for their lopsided health services development by getting ill-defined or often not very relevant social, cultural and psychological issues raised by social scientists and health educators. Social scientists dutifully raised such value-loaded issues as "modernization" as against traditionalism and urban culture as against rural folk culture. These could be used to justify the urban and privileged class orientation of health services in these countries on grounds that backward, superstition-ridden, uneducated villagers first have to be educated by a corps of "well-trained" health educators from the cities on the virtues of 'modern' health services. Health services are only one of the many factors that influence the health status of a population, it is also influenced, sometimes even more significantly, by such social and economic factors as nutrition, water supply, waste disposal, housing, education, income and its distribution, employment, communication and transport and the social structure. Second, just as other factors influence health status, so the health services of a community are usually a function of its political system.

In a political system where there is a commitment to extend the process of democratization and involve the entire population in decision making, the circumstances for formulating an alternative health services are basically different. In the first place, there is considerable enthusiasm among people to actively participate in the shaping of their health services system and in running it. Second, the very process of democratization ensures that those working at technological levels are impelled to evolve an alternative technological framework more meaningful to the entire population, particularly to the weaker sections. No doubt, more often than not, this commitment to democratization is used as a mere façade to perpetuate old unjust social relations. It is also very likely that under such political conditions formulation of an alternative system, however scientific and relevant, becomes at best an academic exercise. None the less, even an academic exercise can become a useful instrument for bringing pressure to bear for sided political change by offering concrete, well-thought out alternatives. It can in any case, serve as a blueprint for action when political changes take place.

The second section of this article is to place political issues (corruption) concerning health and health sector in India. First and foremost, analysis of health services must be located in the socio-cultural, ecological, economic and political settings of the countries.

Political Issues of Concern in India

India remains the World Bank's largest single borrower. Its lending to our country had touched $2.9 billion in financial year 2005. For the second time in less than two years, the World Bank has alleged rampant corruption, involving bribery to fraud, fake NGOs to tampered documents, to its five health sector projects it funded, including control of aids, tuberculosis and malaria. A Detailed Implementation Review (DIR), launched by the World Bank in 2006 and supported by the Government of India, has found "significant indicators of fraud and corruption" that include "collusive behavior, bid-rigging, bribery and manipulative bid practices. World Bank Investigation in 2005 into a Reproductive and Child Health Project had found similar instances of corruption, including alleged kick backs to government officials. Following those findings, the Bank withheld funds worth nearly $2 billion meant for pending proposals in the health sector. The important cases highlighted in the report as follows;

Food and Drug Capacity Building Project, $54 Million (2003-2008)

Project was meant to upgrade food testing labs and technicians. The report alleges questionable procurement practices in contracts representing 88% of value of equipment procured; shifting of bidding deadlines and favoritism; widespread deficiencies in delivery and installation of equipment in all 15 labs; more than half of 282 equipments uninstalled or delivered.

Orissa Health Systems Development Projects, $82.1 Million (1998-2006)

This was only the state level project that sought to improve health in Orissa which has the highest infant morality rate in the country. Project, meant to renovate healthcare facilities, supplying additional medical equipment, was marred by fraud. As high as 93 percent of the 55 project hospitals had problems like uninitiated or incomplete work, leaking roofs, crumbling ceilings and molding walls and non-functional sewage system; and yet all were given completion certificates. The report cites 17 types of equipment that violated project technical specification including autoclaves that could explore and neonatal equipment that lacked adequate electrical grounding, exposing babies and medical staff to electrical shocks.

Second National AIDS Control Project, $193.7 Million (1999-2006)

Project aimed to reduce the spread of HIV infection in India and strengthen country's capacity to respond to HIV/AIDS.

The review found that selection and oversight of NGOs chosen for workshops and targeted interventions was corrupt. Procurement officials demanded and received bribes in exchange for awarding contracts. Many NGOs were not qualified to carry out HIV prevention activities and some did not even exist. They furnished false certificates to show their eligibility. Fraud was detected in 82% of the 217 locally procured contracts.

Malaria Control Project, $114 Million (1997-2005)

Project sought to assist National Malaria Eradication programme by introducing effective mechanisms to control malaria. Review found bid-rigging, bribery and collusion in procurement of medicines, bed-nets and pharmaceuticals. Same firms debarred by the bank for collusive behavior in the earlier review were found indulging in similar practices here.

The irregularities exposed in World Bank aided health projects in India are only a tip of the ice-berg. The bigger scams got exposed, when somebody gets a chance to dig deep. The standard response is that an inquiry has been ordered and strict action will be taken and then afterwards all are forgotten. Regrettably, neither the public nor the politicians feel outraged at the high level of corruption in the Government or the agencies or NGOs funded by the Govt. The culture of cut from any grant given or aid given is the unsaid, but very eloquent culture in most government offices. From the other side, the Public Sector Undertakings (PSUs) are often made to sing and dance to their ministers 'tunes is well known. But for the first time ever, Chief Vigilance Commissioner in November 2003 complained to the Prime Minister that six cabinet ministers, handling key infrastructure ministries, were allegedly harassing PSUs chiefs for "personal favors". In some cases, they were even asking for pay offs. All these complaints were made to the CVC by the PSUs chiefs themselves. Ministerial or parliamentarian corruption, from where everything flows downward is not known. We had the case of eleven MPs being expelled from the parliament and losing their seats for demanding cash for asking questions in the parliament. Corruption, which is a serious issue deserving investigation, trial and prompts conviction, has become institutionalized. In fact, it is no more an issue for any politician or a political party in any election.

A survey reports that one-sixth of public think that citizens/users of government services themselves are responsible for corruption. They believe that there is no active and sustained civil society movement. The efforts are more sporadic, localized and short-lived and have never acquired a character of a large movement. One-third of citizens think that corruption is "an obvious fact" where both giver and taker are familiar with modalities. The citizens' charter promising certain performance standard on the basis of "where to go, How to proceed," is a recent initiative. But the charter, as it is made out is neither directly relevant nor are citizens aware of such a thing.

What is to be Done?

The prime movers for action to improve the situation must come from within the countries concerned. Regional and International cooperation in health service development must be based on a solid foundation of endogenous public health. If there will be some agenda for action for India, then in my words, adoption of a simplistic approach to such a complex system is must. The most urgent and important measure will be to create political conditions which will impel the political leadership to initiate steps to undo the enormous damage that has been inflicted on the system. To respond to such political demands, the leadership will have to create conditions for some of the most competent people of the country to come together, in some or all the key institutions, to form "critical masses" to rejuvenate the training, research and education activities of these institutions should be groomed to fill key positions in the top administration of the health services, both at the union and state levels. The current vertical programmes should be integrated with the general health services with a view to their ultimate transfer to the state health services.

Similarly, the Family Planning Department should be merged with Department of health at the union and state levels. The question of increased budgetary allocations is being deliberately left to the last because funding should be increased only after it is ensured that the system has become efficient enough to make effective use of funds that are already available.

Of the recommendations that will require extended time frames, top priority is to be assigned to the people. The response of the people to epidemiologically assessed health problems should be used to choose people-oriented technologies, which in turn will determine the organizational structures and management strategies. Another very crucial element of the prescription for improvement will be to ensure that the programmes taken up for implementation are cost-effective. Programmes for manpower development will have to conform to the requirements of the cost-effective, optimized systems. An associated priority area will be the development of a more appropriate healthy service cadre structure. Enforcement of ethical standards through the Medical Council of India and policy issues in the promotion of indigenous systems of medicine are other areas of concern.

Conclusions

Despite India's claiming to become a new destination for global investors, 38 percent of over 5,400 companies' representatives surveyed by the global consultancy firm Price Water House Coopers said they were asked to pay bribes to get licenses and orders. It is a way of life for some Government Officials in power. Bribe has to be given to obtain free government services. The employees of any government department that has more powers earn more money in terms of bribes. Despite the discussion about Indian culture, philosophy and time-tested spiritual values how can the individuals so stinking with corruption as a nation? Poverty in India is wedded to corruption, whether it is education or health or roads or public distribution sector. Due to epidemic corruption, funds meant for development end up in the pockets of custodians of public trust. This system has to go. But how does it go? It can go only if there is a prompt justice and prompt punishment. If people know that wrong doing will meet retribution immediately, they will think twice before indulging in any crime.

Bibliography

Banerji, D. (1975), "Social and Cultural Foundation of Health Services Systems of India", *Inquiry* 12.

Banerji, D. (1978), "Façade of the Rural health care scheme of India as an opportunity", *Yojana* 22.

Banerji, D. (1978), "Political Issues in Health, Population and Nutrition", *Social Scientist* 7.

Banerji, D., (1982): *Poverty, Class and Health Culture in India*. New Delhi: Prachi Prakashan.

Banerji, D. (1984), "The Political Economy of Western Medicine in Third World Countries", In: John Mckinslay, (ed.), *Issues in the Political Economy of Health Care*. London: Tavistock Publication.

Banerji, D. (1988), *"New Public Health"*, *Journal of Sociological Studies* 7.

Baru, R. (1997), *Private Health Care in India: Social Characteristics and Trends*. New Delhi: Sage Publication.

Bose, A. (1978), *Assessment of the New Rural Health Scheme and Suggestions for Improvement*. New Delhi: Institute of Economic Growth.

Government of India (2000), *Economic Survey, 1999-2000*. New Delhi: Economic Division, Ministry of Finance.

Government of India (1980), *Annual Report, 1977-78*. New Delhi: Ministry of Health and Family Welfare.

Patnaik, P. (1994), "Notes on the Political Economy of Structural Adjustment", *Social Scientist* 22.

Prasad, N. Purendra (2007), "Medicine, Power and Social Legitimacy: A Socio-historical Appraisal of Health Systems in Contemporary India", *Economic and Political Weekly* Aug 25.

Singh, Joginder (2008), "Corruption in Health Sector", *South Asian Politics* 7(1):

Index

T

U